PATHOLOGY
RECALL

PATHOLOGY RECALL

EDITOR

ANIKAR CHHABRA, MD
Resident in Orthopaedic Surgery
University of Virginia
Charlottesville, Virginia

RECALL SERIES EDITOR
AND SENIOR EDITOR

LORNE H. BLACKBOURNE, MD
General Surgeon
Fayetteville, North Carolina

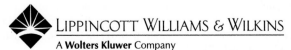
LIPPINCOTT WILLIAMS & WILKINS
A **Wolters Kluwer** Company
Philadelphia · Baltimore · New York · London
Buenos Aires · Hong Kong · Sydney · Tokyo

Development Editors: Emilie Linkins, Virginia Barishek, Martha Cushman
Managing Editor: Marette Magargle-Smith

Copyright © 2002 Lippincott Williams & Wilkins

351 West Camden Street
Baltimore, Maryland 21201-2436 USA

530 Walnut Street
Philadelphia, Pennsylvania 19106 USA

Printed in the United States of America

Library of Congress Cataloging-in-Publication Data

Pathology recall / senior editor, Lorne H. Blackbourne ; editor, Anikar Chhabra.
    p. ; cm. — (Recall series)
    Includes index.
    ISBN 0-7817-3406-1
    1. Pathology—Examinations, questions, etc. I. Blackbourne, Lorne H.
II. Chhabra, Anikar. III. Series.
    [DNLM: 1. Pathology—Examination Questions. QZ 18.2 P2973 2001]
RB31 .P335 2001
616.07'076—dc21

                         2001038244

We'd like to hear from you! If you have comments or suggestions regarding this
Lippincott Williams & Wilkins title, please contact us at the appropriate customer service number listed below, or send correspondence to **book_com-
ments@lww.com.** If possible, please remember to include your mailing ad-
dress, phone number, and a reference to the book title and author in your
message. To purchase additional copies of this book call our customer service
department at **(800) 638-3030** or fax orders to **(301) 824-7390.** International
customers should call **(301) 714-2324.**

                                  02 03 04 05
                         2 3 4 5 6 7 8 9 10

Advisor and Associate Editor

Brian D. Blackbourne, MD
Forensic Pathologist
San Diego, California

Contributors

James E. Boyer
Gordon M. Bussard, MD
Robert G. Canady
Sandhya Chhabra, MD
C. April Collett, MD
Peter A. deSchweinitz, MD
Hiwot B. Desta, MD
Christopher Gasink, MD
Shawn A. Gregory, MD
Sameena Hassan, MD
Holland McBryde Mason, MD
Brooke E. McMinn, MD
Clinton R. Nichols, MD
J. Stewart O'Keefe, MD
Tara Nayak Palmore, MD
Peter F. Robinson, MD
Sita M. Sundaresan
Harrison F. Warner, MD
Wendy M. Wilson, MD

Preface

Pathology Recall is written in the Recall Series format for "rapid-fire" acquisition and review of pathology facts. The Recall format uses two columns with the questions on the left and the answers on the right. The bookmark is used to cover the answers while you answer the question in your head. This process should be repeated until you have mastered the material.

Pathology Recall can be used to test your knowledge before a major exam or before the USMLE Step 1 examination. We hope that you will find it a great tool to maximize your study time.

The Authors and Editors have dedicated their work to the late Dr. Gaffney of the Department of Pathology at the University of Virginia. It is our hope that his enthusiasm for teaching medical students and residents will be reflected in our work.

Anikar Chhabra, M.D.
Resident in Orthopaedic Surgery
University of Virginia
Charlottesville, Virginia

Lorne H. Blackbourne, M.D.
General Surgeon
Fayetteville, North Carolina

P.S. Please let us know if you have any correction, memory aids, or suggestions for making this book better. Contact ELINKINS@LWW.com

This book is dedicated to the memory of **Michael James Gaffey, M.D.,** Associate Professor of Pathology at the University of Virginia. Dr. Gaffey was born July 18, 1955. Dr. Gaffey received his Doctorate of Medicine, magna cum laude, from the University of Maryland in 1983. There he was a member of Alpha Omega Alpha and the recipient of the Milton L. Sacks Memorial Award in Medicine and Hematology.

Dr. Gaffey was a resident in Internal Medicine and then Pathology at the University of Virginia Health Sciences Center, Charlottesville, Virginia. Following a Fellowship in Surgical Pathology at the City of Hope National Medical Center, he returned to the University of Virginia School of Medicine as Director of Transplantation Pathology. Dr. Gaffey was an active academic surgical pathologist serving numerous professional organizations including the American Society of Clinical Pathologists and the United States and Canadian Academy of Pathology. He authored or coauthored several book chapters and numerous journal articles.

Dr. Gaffey enjoyed a full and intensely active life with his wife and two children. He brought his infectious competitive spirit to bicycling, scuba diving and motorcycling. He died in a motorcycle accident on December 20, 1997. Dr. Gaffey is best remembered as an enthusiastic teacher of medical students and housestaff. This book is an expression of Mike's "get to the essence, just the facts, Jack" approach to learning medicine.

Donald J. Innes, Jr., M.D.
Professor of Pathology
University of Virginia
Charlottesville, Virginia

To my father, an outstanding teacher and motivator: thanks for guiding me into the field of medicine. I would never have gotten this far without your support.

To my mother: you have taught me the value of persistence, and to never be satisfied until the end result is perfect.

To Bobby, my brother, the most caring doctor I have ever met: I can only hope I am half as good an orthopaedist as you are.

To Avni, my sister: your zest for life is inspiring; you have taught me to live life to the fullest every day.

Thanks for your support on this project. I could never have done it without any of you.

Anikar Chhabra, M.D.

Table of Contents

SECTION III. PATHOLOGY ATLAS

Abbreviations

ASD	atrial septal defect
ATP	adenosine triphosphate
AV	atrioventricular
CA	carcinoma
CCl$_4$	carbon tetrachloride
CGD	chronic granulomatous disease
CHD	congenital heart disease
Cl	chloride
CO	carbon monoxide
COX	cyclooxygenase
Cr	creatinine
CrCl	creatinine clearance
CREST	calcinosis, Raynaud phenomenon, esophageal involvement, sclerodactyly, and telangiectasis
CSA	cell-surface antigen
CT	computed tomography
C3a, C5a, C3b	members of the complement cascade
DNA	deoxyribonucleic acid
ECG	electrocardiogram, electrocardiography, electrocardiographic

ECM	extracellular matrix
EM	electron microscopy
ESR	erythrocyte sedimentation rate
Fc	Fragment of complement
FNA	fine needle aspiration
GI	gastrointestinal
G6PD	glucose-6-phosphate dehydrogenase
H	hydrogen
HCl	hydrochloric acid
HDL	high-density lipoprotein
HETE	hydroxy-eicosatetraenoic (acid)
HIV	human immunodeficiency virus
HMW	high molecular weight
HOCl	hypochlorous acid
HPETE	hydroperoxyeicosatetraenoic acic
hpf	high-powered field (microscope)
5 HT	5-hydroxytryptophan (serotonin)
Ig	immunoglobulin
IHC	immunohistochemistry
IHD	ischemic heart disease
IL	interleukin
ISH	in situ hybridization
ISH-PCR	in situ hybridation-polymerase chain reaction
LADCA	left anterior descending coronary artery

LCCA	left circumflex coronary artery
LDH	lactate dehydrogenase
LFTs	liver function tests
LOX	lipoxygenase
LTB$_4$, LTC$_4$, LTD$_4$, LTE$_4$	types of leukotrienes
MBP	major basic proteins
MHA-TP	microhemagluttination-*Treponema pallidum*
MI	myocardial infarction
MPO	myeloperoxidase
NADPH	reduced nicotinamide adenine dinucleotide phosphate
O	oxygen
OH	hydrocorticosteroid
PAF	platelet activating factor
PCB	polychlorinated biphenyl
PDA	patent ductus arteriosus
PGI$_2$	prostacyclin
PKD	polycystic kidney disease
PKU	phenylketonuria
PMNs	polymorphonuclear neutrophils
PT	prothrombin time
PTT	partial thromboplastin time
RBC	red blood cell
RCA	right coronary artery
RDS	respiratory distress syndrome

RNA	ribonucleic acid
RPR	rapid plasma reagin (test)
SIADH	syndrome of inappropriate secretion of anti-diuretic hormone
SLE	systemic lupus erythematosus
TB	tuberculosis
TNF-α	tumor necrosis factor α
TxA$_2$	thromboxane A
UV	ultraviolet
VDRL	Venereal Disease Research Laboratory (test for syphilis)
VSD	ventral septal defect

Section I

General Pathology
and Diagnostic
Techniques

1

Pathology Diagnostic Techniques

INTRODUCTION

Pathologic tissues sent to the laboratory in what 2 forms?

1. Gross specimens
2. Cytologic specimens

When possible, how should specimens be transported?

Fresh tissues in saline should be rapidly transported.

Name the 5 common techniques used to analyze tissues.

1. Cytology
2. Immunohistochemistry
3. Flow cytometry for DNA analysis
4. Electron microscopy
5. Hybridization procedures for DNA analysis

TECHNIQUES USED TO ANALYZE TISSUES

CYTOLOGY

What is cytology?

The use of various cells scraped from the lining of orifices or obtained by fine needle aspiration (FNA) to study disease processes.

What imaging techniques are often used for needle guided biopsies?

CT, US

How invasive is cytology?

Minimally invasive. Cells can be taken from any secretions, brushings of lesions. If FNA is required, an extremely thin needle may be used.

Is cytology helpful in diagnosing cancer?

Yes, it is necessary to visualize changes in neoplastic cells.

Name 3 common uses of FNA.	Obtaining diagnostic tissue samples of 1. Breast masses 2. Hepatic nodules 3. Lung lesions

IMMUNOHISTOCHEMISTRY (IHC)

What is IHC?	The use of antibodies to tissue markers (antigens) for diagnostic purposes.
What types of antibodies can be used?	1. Polyclonal antibodies 2. Monoclonal antibodies
What are two methods for detection of these antibody-antigen interactions?	1. Fluorescent probe (immunofluorescence) 2. An enzymatic system such as peroxidase (immunoperoxidase)
How are these tissues stored?	1. Frozen tissue 2. Paraffin-embedded tissue

IMMUNOFLUORESCENCE

This technique is commonly used with what 3 tissues?	1. Skin 2. Kidney 3. Lung
What dye is most frequently used?	Fluorescein isothiocyanate
What uses does immunofluorescence have (5)?	1. Detection of autoantibodies 2. Localization of tissue antigens 3. Identification of microorganisms in tissues 4. Identification of immune complexes deposits 5. Identify complement proteins

IMMUNOPEROXIDASE

Describe the action of immunoperoxidase.	It catalyzes a substrate, making a product at the site of the antigen.
How is it activated?	A secondary antibody, which is conjugated to peroxidase, attaches to the primary antibody-antigen complex.
What other enzyme is often used to catalyze a substrate?	Alkaline phosphatase

What are some common uses for alkaline phosphatase (8)?

1. Identifying the cells of origin, oncofetal antigens, tissue specific markers, or loss of an antigen in neoplasms
2. Detecting hormones or hormone receptors
3. Localizing enzymes
4. Differentiating types of lymphomas
5. Detecting amounts of a type of cell
6. Finding autoantibodies
7. Identifying viral antigens
8. Identifying microorganisms

What are the advantages of alkaline phosphatase over immunofluorescence?

1. Higher sensitivity
2. The preparations are permanent
3. Paraffin-embedded tissues are better for visualizing cell details.
4. Lesser amounts of antibody are used because of higher dilution rates.

FLOW CYTOMETRY

What is flow cytometry?

Analysis of cell populations by treating cells with specific antibodies and passed through a laser. The light is then analyzed to give properties of the cells.

What is this technique used for?

To determine the DNA ploidy of neoplastic tissues.

Why is this important?

The ploidy of a tumor often predicts the nature of a tumor.

Reactive and benign lesions are always what ploidy?

Diploid. However, not all diploids neoplasms are benign.

What is the usual ploidy of neoplastic and malignant lesions?

Aneuploid.

What types of tissue can be used?

1. Fresh tissue
2. Formalin-fixed tissue

What is the first step after a sample has been obtained?

Cell nuclei are extracted from a tissue sample.

What is done with these nuclei?

They are stained and analyzed in a flow cytometer.

What is the next step?

The amount of emitted light of a specified wavelength determines the amount of DNA per cell.

What can be constructed from this data to determine the number of cells in each phase of the cell cycle and the ploidy of the cells?

A DNA histogram

ELECTRON MICROSCOPY (EM)

Why is this technique important?

It allows the study of tissues at the ultrastructural level.

What is it used for?

1. Evaluation of rare infections
2. Diagnosis of immune complex disease
3. Diagnosis of neoplasms by showing alterations in cellular structure

What are several disadvantages of EM?

1. Expense
2. Special tissue preparations are necessary
3. Tests often require several days
4. Sampling error is high because it only looks at a minute portion of the sample

HYBRIDIZATION PROCEDURES

What can these procedures do?

Isolate and identify DNA fragments

What are these procedures used for?

1. Identification of microbes using DNA probes
2. Gene studies of inherited conditions, such as sickle cell anemia
3. Determination of compatibility of gene alleles for transplant tissue typing
4. Identification of lymphoproliferative disorders by using gene arrangements for B and T cell disorders

Name the common types of hybridization procedures?

1. Southern blot tests
2. DNA gene rearrangement assays
3. In situ hybridization
4. In situ hybridization—polymerase chain reaction

Southern blot tests

How are DNA fragments from tissue abstracts separated?

Electrophoresis

What does a probe consist of?

1. A known DNA or RNA sequence
2. A labeled radioisotope

What does a probe combine with?

The complementary sequences on the blot

How are the unknown nucleic acid sequences identified?

Autoradiography

DNA gene rearrangement assays

What are these assays used for?

For detection of lymphomas and leukemias

How do they do this?

In a technique similar to in situ hybridization, in which probes are hybridized to fresh tissues, lymphomas and leukemias show gene arrangements while nonmalignant disorders will show a germline (nonrearranged) immunoglobulin or t-receptor genes.

In situ hybridization (ISH)

Why is this technique important?

It allows examination of a tissue section, as opposed to a tissue extract. The exact location of the probe in the tissue can be found.

What is often detected? Why?

Viral infections, because multiple copies of DNA per cell are present.

What is often difficult to detect because multiple copies are not always present?

Oncogenes of tumors

Because of this, what can be done?

In situ hybridization—polymerase chain reaction

In situ hybridization—polymerase chain reaction (ISH—PCR)

How is this different from ISH?	Small pieces of DNA or RNA which cannot be detected by ISH can be amplified using specific probes, allowing detection

POWER REVIEW

Name the 5 common techniques used to analyze tissues.	1. Cytology 2. Immunohistochemistry 3. Flow cytometry for DNA analysis 4. Hybridization procedures for DNA analysis 5. Electron microscopy
Define 1. **Cytology** 2. **Immunohistochemistry** 3. **Flow cytometry for DNA analysis** 4. **Hybridization procedures for DNA analysis** 5. **Electron microscopy**	1. The use of various cells from orifices or by fine needle aspiration to study disease processes 2. The use of antibodies to tissue markers (antigens) for diagnostic purposes 3. Diagnostic technique using wavelengths to determine the DNA ploidy of neoplastic tissues 4. Diagnostic technique used to isolate and identify DNA fragments 5. The study of tissues at the ultrastructural level
Name the common types of hybridization procedures?	1. Southern blot tests 2. DNA gene rearrangement assays 3. ISH 4. ISH-PCR
Why is ISH important?	It allows examination of a tissue section, as opposed to a tissue extract.
How is this ISH-PCR different from ISH?	Small pieces of DNA or RNA can be amplified using specific probes, allowing detection.
Name 3 common uses of FNA.	To obtain diagnostic tissue samples of 1. Breast masses 2. Hepatic nodules 3. Lung lesions

Immunofluorescence is commonly used with what 3 tissues?

1. Skin
2. Kidney
3. Lung

What is immunoperoxidase IHC?

An enzyme catalyzes a substrate, making a product at the site of the antigen.

If possible, how should biopsy specimens be sent to pathology?

Fresh in saline

What technique is best used to differentiate

Prostate CA from gastric CA?

IHC

Lymphoma from carcinoma?

IHC or electron microscopy

Adenocarcinoma from mesothelioma?

IHC or electron microscopy

2   Inflammation

ACUTE INFLAMMATION

What is inflammation?

A protective vascular response to injured tissue

What are the 4 cardinal signs of inflammation?

1. Rubor (redness)
2. Calor (heat)
3. Tumor (swelling)
4. Dolor (pain)

What is the sequence of vascular events in acute inflammation?

1. Transient reflex vasoconstriction
2. Vasodilation secondary to PGI_2 and nitric oxide-mediated smooth muscle relaxation leads to increased blood flow (rubor, calor)
3. Increased capillary permeability leads to exudation of fluid into interstitium, which leads to edema (tumor)
4. Stasis of blood flow secondary locally to increased viscosity

What are the 7 cellular (leukocyte) responses in acute inflammation?

1. Margination = rolling along endothelium
2. Pavementing = lining endothelium
3. Adhesion = sticking to endothelium via cellular adhesion molecules (e.g. selectins)
4. Emigration = diapedesis (extravasation) between endothelial cells into interstitium
5. Chemotaxis = migration along chemical gradient of cytokines, leukotrienes, bacterial products, complement products
6. Phagocytosis = ingestion of cells, bacteria, debris by PMNs and macrophages, often facilitated by opsonization
7. Intracellular killing/degradation of microbes or debris

What is opsonization?	Coating of particles by opsonins, molecules that bind receptors on phagocytes. Promotes engulfment of a particle by immobilizing it on the surface of the phagocyte.
Name 2 important opsonins.	1. IgG 2. C3b
What cells are present in acute inflammation?	Early on, PMNs. After 24–48 hours, they are replaced by macrophages and lymphocytes.
In what type of infection do lymphocytes predominate?	Viral infection
In what type of infection do eosinophils predominate?	Parasitic infections (Eosinophils also predominate in allergic reactions.)

CHEMICAL MEDIATORS OF ACUTE INFLAMMATION

What are the anaphylatoxins	C3a and C5a
Why are they called that?	They mediate release of histamine via basophil and mast cell degranulation.
Name 2 important vaso-active amines.	Serotonin and histamine
Why are they "vasoactive"?	They stimulate contraction of endothelial cells which leads to increased capillary permeability (leakage between endothelial cells)
What cells release histamine?	Basophils, mast cells, platelets
What triggers histamine release in each?	Basophils and mast cells: binding of IgE, anaphylatoxins, IL-1, heat or cold Platelets: aggregation
What cells release 5-HT?	Serotonin (5-hydroxytryptophan) is released from platelets during aggregation.
What does platelet activating factor (PAF) do?	PAF, released from granulocytes, macrophages, basophils, and endothelial

cells, triggers platelet aggregation, vasoconstriction, bronchospasm, and arachidonic acid pathways.

Where is arachidonic acid found?

Attached to cell membrane phospholipids

How is it released?

Released by phospholipase A_2

Name the 2 key pathways of arachidonic acid metabolism.

Cyclooxygenase (COX) and lipoxygenase (LOX)

What are the products of the COX pathway?

Prostaglandins and thromboxanes

What does PGI_2 do?

PGI_2, also known as prostacyclin, vasodilates and inhibits platelet aggregation.

What does TxA_2 do?

Vasoconstricts and stimulates platelet aggregation

What is an important intermediate product of LOX pathway?

HPETE (hydroperoxyeicosatetraenoic acid).

What are the products of the LOX pathway and their actions?

Leukotrienes and HETE. LTB_4 and HETE are chemotactic agents. LTC_4, LTD_4, LTE_4 vasoconstrict, bronchoconstrict, and stimulate capillary permeability.

What are cytokines?

Proteins, produced by macrophages, that mediate the systemic inflammatory and immune responses. IL-1 and TNF-α are examples of two common cytokines.

What systemic inflammatory effects do cytokines have?

Fever, leukocytosis, and synthesis and release of acute phase proteins

What are the acute phase proteins?

C-reactive protein, complement, fibrinogen, prothrombin, ceruloplasmin, α-1-antitrypsin, α-2-macroglobulin

Which cytokine stimulates their synthesis?

IL-6 from inflammatory fibroblasts, macrophages, and endothelial cells mediates their synthesis by the liver.

What is the pathway of kinin synthesis?

Factor XII converts prekallikrein to kallikrein. Kallikrein cleaves HMW kininogen to bradykinin.

What are other functions of Factor XII?

It is also involved in clotting cascade and fibrinolytic system

What is the eponym for Factor XII?

Hageman factor

What does bradykinin do?

Stimulates vasodilation, capillary permeability, and pain

What does C3b do?

It is an opsonin; it triggers phagocytosis by binding to specific cell-surface receptors.

What does C3a do?

It is an anaphylatoxin and is responsible for basophil and mast cell degranulation and release of histamine

What does C5a do?

It is an anaphylatoxin and a chemotactic agent; it activates the cascades that lead to the LOX pathway

What does C5b-9 do?

It is the membrane attack complex (MAC), which lyses bacteria

What cytokine induces eosinophilia?

IL-5

What are the potential outcomes of acute inflammation?

1. Resolution
2. Abscess formation—when area of inflammation is walled off from circulation
3. Nonhealing opening—ulcer or fistula
4. Scar
5. Chronic inflammation

CHRONIC INFLAMMATION

What always precedes chronic inflammation?

Nothing necessarily precedes it. It can be preceded by recurrent or unresolved acute inflammation or it can be a primary response itself.

When is chronic inflammation a primary response?

Viral infection, malignancy, autoimmune disorders, and parasitic or fungal infections

What cell types are characteristic of chronic inflammation?	Lymphocytes, plasma cells, macrophages, proliferating endothelial cells, and fibroblasts
What is the role of macrophages in chronic inflammation?	Macrophages are long-lived; they proliferate in the inflammatory site, phagocytize debris, activate lymphocytes via cytokines, and stimulate plasma cell production.
What is a granuloma?	A circumscribed collection of epithelioid macrophages, usually surrounded by a rim of lymphocytes, often with multinucleated giant cells

How does granulomatous inflammation arise?

1. Organisms (bacteria) or foreign objects appear that PMNs cannot digest.
2. These are ingested by macrophages, which likewise cannot degrade them, but sequester them permanently.
3. Macrophages present antigen to CD4+ T-cells.
4. T cells produce lymphokines (γ-interferon and IL-4) that keep macrophages there and transform them into epithelioid and giant cells.

Name 6 infections associated with granulomatous inflammation.	Tuberculosis, leprosy, histoplasmosis, blastomycosis, cat-scratch disease, syphilis
Name 2 noninfectious causes of granulomata.	Foreign bodies and sarcoidosis
What type of granuloma is seen in sarcoidosis?	Non-caseating granulomata
What is the indigestible agent responsible for sarcoidosis?	Unknown
What is the key characteristic of a mycobacterial granuloma?	Caseous necrosis
What is a feature of syphilitic granulomata?	Gummatous necrosis

What are Langhans cells?

Multinucleated giant cells with nuclei in a horseshoe, characteristic of tuberculous granuloma

How do foreign body giant cells differ?

They have scattered nuclei.

MECHANISMS AND DISORDERS OF INTRACELLULAR KILLING

What are the 2 kinds of intracellular degradation and killing?

Oxygen-dependent and oxygen-independent. Oxygen-dependent killing is more effective and can be myeloperoxidase (MPO)-dependent or MPO-independent.

What mediates oxygen-independent killing?

Proteins and enzymes, such as lysozyme, lactoferrin, major basic protein (MBP), defensins, and lysosomal hydrolases

Describe the steps in MPO-dependent killing.

Oxidative burst→superoxide anion→H_2O_2→hypochlorous acid, which oxidizes proteins and disrupts membranes:
$2O_2 + NADPH →2O_2^- \cdot + NADP^+ + H^+$ (NADPH oxidase)
$2O_2^- \cdot + 2H^+→ H_2O_2 + O_2$ (superoxide dismutase)
$Cl^- + H_2O_2 →HOCl$ (MPO in presence of halide)

What mediates MPO-independent killing?

Superoxide anion $O_2^- \cdot$ produced by oxidative burst and hydroxyl radical OH $\cdot$ from H_2O_2

Why do patients with MPO deficiency have nearly normal infection rates?

Absence of lysosomal MPO is compensated by increased H_2O_2 levels and MPO-independent killing. (autosomal recessive)

What is the defect in chronic granulomatous disease (CGD) of childhood?

PMNs are missing a portion of NADPH oxidase, which is needed to generate H_2O_2. Without H_2O_2, PMNs can ingest but not kill, thus resulting in chronic granulomata. CGD of childhood is X-linked and autosomal recessive.

Why can CGD patients fight catalase-negative but not catalase-positive microbes?

Catalase converts H_2O_2 into O_2 and H_2O. Catalase-positive bacteria degrade their own H_2O_2 so neutrophil MPO cannot use it to make bactericidal HOCl. Catalase-negative bugs provide the neutrophil with H_2O_2 it needs for normal killing.

What is Chédiak-Higashi syndrome?

An autosomal recessive disorder with abnormal lysosomes and defective microtubule function. WBCs have giant cytoplasmic granules and impaired chemotaxis and degranulation. Repeated fungal and bacterial infections, neutropenia, albinism, and neuropathies occur.

POWER REVIEW

What are the 4 cardinal signs of inflammation?

Rubor, calor, tumor, dolor

What is the correct sequence of leukocyte responses in acute inflammation?

Margination→pavementing→adhesion→ emigration→chemotaxis→phagocytosis

What are the two key opsonins?

IgG and C3b

What type of cells predominate in viral infection?

Lymphocytes

In parasitic infection?

Eosinophils

Which cells release histamine?

Mast cells, basophils, platelets

What are the endogenous pyrogens?

IL-1 and TNF-α

What are the anaphylatoxins?

C3a, C5a

What are the slow reacting substances of anaphylaxis (SRS-A)?

LTC_4, LTD_4, LTE_4

What pathway produces the SRS-A?

LOX

What pathway does aspirin inhibit?

COX

What is HPETE?	An intermediate of the LOX pathway
What cell types show up during acute inflammation?	Initially, PMNs. After 1–2 days, macrophages and lymphs take over.
What are C-reactive protein and fibrinogen?	Acute phase proteins
Where are acute phase proteins synthesized?	In the liver
What factor is key to the clotting cascade, fibrinolytic system, and bradykinin synthesis?	Factor XII (Hageman factor)
What are the steps in bradykinin synthesis?	Factor XII converts prekallikrein to kallikrein. Kallikrein then cleaves HMW kininogen to bradykinin.
What is C5a?	Anaphylatoxin, activator of LOX, and chemotactic agent
What is C5b-9?	The membrane attack complex (MAC), which lyses bacteria
What bactericidal agent does MPO produce?	HOCl (hypochlorous acid)
Of oxygen-dependent and oxygen-independent killing, which is more effective?	Oxygen-dependent killing
What cells predominate in chronic inflammation?	Lymphocytes, macrophages, plasma cells, fibroblasts, and endothelial cells
What cells are found in a granuloma?	Epithelioid macrophages, multinucleated giant cells, and lymphocytes
What type of necrosis is found in a TB granuloma?	Caseous necrosis
What type of giant cell is found in a TB granuloma?	Langhans cell
What type of giant cell is found in a granuloma surrounding a particle of silica?	Foreign body giant cell

What idiopathic disorder is characterized by non-caseating granulomata?	Sarcoidosis
In what disorder can patients fight catalase-negative but not catalase-positive bacteria?	CGD of childhood
What is the defect?	Dysfunction of NADPH oxidase
In what disorder do leuko-cytes have large bizarre granules?	Chédiak-Higashi syndrome
How is CGD of childhood transmitted?	X-linked

3

Cellular Injury And Death

MECHANISMS OF CELL INJURY

Name 3 important causes of cell injury.

1. Ischemia
2. Free radicals
3. Chemical toxicity

What causes cellular hypoxia/anoxia?

Arterial obstruction, decreased oxygenation of blood (lung disease), decreased oxygen-carrying capacity (anemia, CO poisoning), inadequate tissue perfusion (heart failure, hypotension)

What is the cause of ischemic cell injury?

Increased intracellucar calcium. The progression can be detailed as follows:
1. Hypoxia→decreased oxidative phosphorylation→decreased ATP→decreased membrane integrity and pump failure→loss of ion gradients→Ca influx.
2. Decreased oxidative phosphorylation→anaerobic metabolism→lactic acid production. This further results in chromatin, organelle, and membrane damage which leads to calcium release from mitochondria and Ca influx.

Why are free radicals dangerous to cells?

A free radical has an unpaired electron in its outer orbit, which makes it unstable and highly reactive. The free radical initiates protein crosslinking, lipid peroxidation, and amino acid oxidation in propagated chain reactions. This damages cell and organelle membranes.

What are sources of free radicals?

1. Normal metabolism
2. Chemical toxicity

3. Reperfusion injury
4. Ionizing radiation
5. O_2 therapy
6. Immune response/inflammation (PMN oxidative burst)

Name 2 important free radicals.

1. Superoxide $O_2 \cdot {}^-$
2. Hydroxyl radical OH^-

Name 4 antioxidants and describe their mechanism of action.

Glutathione, vitamin E, transferrin, and ceruloplasmin. They inhibit lipid peroxidation.

Name 3 free-radical scavengers and describe their mechanism of action.

Superoxide dismutase, catalase, and mannitol. They bind and inactivate free radicals.

How does CCl_4 cause hepatocyte injury and death?

CCl_4 is processed by P450 system and releases $CCl_2 \cdot$. This leads to peroxidation of intracellular membrane lipid and loss of membrane function. Ribosome disaggregation leads to decreased protein synthesis, which further leads to cell swelling and Ca buildup, which result in cell death.

RESPONSES TO CELLULAR INJURY

Name 4 adaptive responses to stress.

Hyperplasia, hypertrophy, atrophy, metaplasia

Are adaptive responses to stress reversible?

Yes

What is hyperplasia?

Enlargement of a tissue secondary to an increase in the number of cells

Give examples of 2 types of hyperplasia.

Endometrium in the menstrual cycle (caused by physiologic stimuli), and hand callouses (caused by mechanical stress)

What is hypertrophy?

Increase in cell size and functional capacity

Give examples of 2 types of hypertrophy.

Skeletal muscle and myocardium (increased functional demand), and lactating breast (trophic hormones).

What is atrophy?

Decrease in cell size and function

Give examples of 4 types of atrophy.

Muscle (denervation), vaginal mucosa (decreased trophic hormones), kidneys (ischemia),and brain (aging)

What is metaplasia?

Replacement of one differentiated cell type by another in response to chronic irritation and inflammation

Give examples of 2 types of metaplasia.

Bronchial mucosa replaced by squamous epithelium (smoking) and cervical columnar epithelium replaced by squamous epithelium (cervicitis).

What is dysplasia?

Dysregulation of cell proliferation and development of atypical features secondary to irritation and inflammation, often in metaplastic tissue

Give 2 examples of tissue where dysplasia can occur.

Cervical epithelium (chronic cervicitis), and bronchial epithelium (smokers)

Are dysplastic lesions worrisome?

Yes. When severe, dysplastic lesions are considered premalignant.

What are 4 signs of early hypoxic injury?

1. Hydropic change: pale, distended cytoplasm secondary to increased H_2O content (failure of plasma membrane barrier)
2. Swelling of endoplasmic reticulum
3. Swelling of mitochondria (dissipated energy gradient)
4. Ribosomal disaggregation (leads to failed protein synthesis).

What are signs of late, but still reversible, hypoxic injury?

1. Cell blebs: bubbles in cell membrane
2. Myelin figures: swirled blobs of denuded membrane

What is the point at which the progression of ischemic cell injury becomes irreversible?

Massive calcium influx leading to mitochondrial and membrane damage

How long does it take ischemic injury to become irreversible in the heart, liver, brain, and skeletal muscle?

Myocardial cells and hepatocytes: 1–2 hours
Neurons: 3–5 minutes (especially hippocampus and Purkinje cells)
Skeletal muscle: variable (2–8 hours)

CELLULAR ACCUMULATIONS

What causes materials to accumulate abnormally in cells?

1. Failure of the mechanism involved in removal or metabolism of normal substance
2. Inability to remove or metabolize abnormal substance

What causes fatty change in the liver?

Imbalance of production, utilization, and mobilization of fats:
1. ↑ entry of fatty acids into cells
2. ↑ synthesis of fatty acids
3. ↓ use of fatty acids
4. ↓ mobilization of fatty acids [↓ apoprotein synthesis (e.g., in CCl_4 toxicity or malnutrition)]

What are the terms for abnormal cellular accumulation of the following?

Bilirubin

Kernicterus

Iron

Hemosiderosis (macrophages), hemochromatosis (parenchymal cells), jaundice (tissues)

Melanin

Suntan

Lead

Plumbism

Silver

Argyria

Water

Hydropic change

What is the "wear-and-tear" pigment?

Lipofuscin. The breakdown product of lipids which accumulate in atrophic cells of elderly people as "brown atrophy."

Name 2 types of abnormal calcification.

1. Metastatic calcification—hypercalcemia resulting in deposition of calcium in living tissue.
2. Dystrophic calcification—deposition of calcium in damaged tissue.

NECROSIS

What is necrosis?

Death and degradation of cells from severe environmental insult

What is apoptosis?

Programmed, energy-dependent cell death

Give 2 examples of apoptosis.

Embryogenesis (excess tissue is killed off during apoptosis); shedding of endometrium during menstrual cycle.

What is heterolysis?

Digestion of necrotic cells by enzymes from leukocytes or bacteria

What is autolysis?

Degradation of cells by their own lysosomal enzymes

How is autolysis different from necrosis?

Autolysis follows cell death; autolysis and heterolysis help to dissolve necrotic tissue.

What cytoplasmic change occurs in necrosis?

Increased eosinophilia (and decreased basophilia) secondary to loss of RNA and denaturation of proteins by ↓ pH.

What nuclear changes take place in necrosis?

1. Pyknosis: condensation of chromatin (ball sitting in nucleus)
2. Karyorrhexis: fragmentation of nucleus
3. Karyolysis: fading of chromatin secondary to dissolution by proteolytic enzymes
4. Nuclear loss

What are 6 types of necrosis?

Coagulation, caseous, liquefaction, gangrenous, fibrinoid, and fat

What does early coagulation necrosis look like?

Tissue architecture is preserved, cytoplasm is eosinophilic

Where and when does coagulation necrosis occur?

Heart, lung, kidney, or spleen, usually after infarction.

How does liquefaction necrosis differ from coagulation necrosis?

Loss of architecture occurs in liquefaction necrosis: tissue is softened and liquefied by autolysis ± heterolysis.

What is a typical site of liquefaction necrosis?

CNS (autolysis), suppurative infection (heterolysis)

What is caseous necrosis?

A combination of coagulation and liquefaction necrosis. Caseous (cheeselike) refers to resemblance to cottage cheese.

What causes caseous necrosis?

Granulomatous inflammation caused by mycobacteria

What are the 2 types of gangrene?

1. "Wet gangrene" (liquefaction necrosis)
2. "Dry gangrene" (coagulation necrosis)

What are typical sites of gangrene?

Bowel wall and lower limbs (secondary to acute ischemia)

What is fibrinoid necrosis?

Deposition of fibrinous material in damaged arterial walls

What causes fat necrosis?

Hydrolysis of fat by lipases liberates fatty acids, which form Ca salts (saponification)

Under what circumstances does fat necrosis occur?

1. Hemorrhagic pancreatitis—liberated enzymes digest pancreatic fat
2. Trauma to fatty tissue (e.g., breast)

POWER REVIEW

Name 2 free radicals.

Superoxide O_2^- and hydroxyl radical OH

Name 3 free-radical scavengers.

Superoxide dismutase, catalase, mannitol

Name 4 antioxidants.

Glutathione, vitamin E, transferrin, ceruloplasmin

How long can hepatocytes and myocardial cells survive ischemia?

1–2 hours

What is hydropic change?

Abnormal accumulation of water in cells

What is lipofuscin?

Breakdown product of lipids. It builds up in atrophic cells of elderly people.

What are the nuclear changes in necrosis?

1. Pyknosis (chromatin clumps)
2. Karyorrhexis (nucleus fragments)
3. Karyolysis (chromatin dissolves and fades)
4. Nuclear loss

What happens to cytoplasm in necrotic cells?

Increased eosinophilia

What is Barrett esophagus an example of?

Metaplasia: squamous epithelium leads to gastric glandular mucosa secondary to acid reflux.

What is the harbinger of irreversible cell injury?

Massive intracellular buildup of calcium

How does autolysis accelerate cell death?

It doesn't. Autolysis takes place when a dead cell's enzymes digest it.

What kind of necrosis takes place in an abscess?

Liquefaction necrosis

What is pus?

Product of liquefaction necrosis: dead cell debris, PMNs, monocytes, lysosomal enzymes in an exudative, purulent soup

What type of necrosis is seen in tuberculous granulomata?

Caseous necrosis

What type of necrosis might cause a hard breast mass after an auto accident?

Fat necrosis saponification

What adaptive cellular change takes place in the heart of a chronically hypertensive man?

Hypertrophy

In which type of necrosis is tissue architecture preserved?

Coagulation necrosis

What type of cell death prevents us from having webbed fingers and toes?

Apoptosis

What type of adaptive response do foot cells have to uncomfortable shoes?

Hyperplasia (corns)

4

Repair and Healing

What are the 2 possible outcomes of healing and repair?

1. Regeneration of parenchyma
2. Organization of parenchyma

Can all cell types regenerate?

No, only certain cell types have potential for proliferation.

What are labile cells?

Actively dividing cells capable of regeneration

Give 2 examples.

Mucosal cells, hematopoietic cells

What are stable cells?

Cells that rarely divide under normal conditions but remain capable of division and regeneration when activated

Give 4 examples.

Hepatocytes, renal tubular epithelium, endothelial cells, endocrine cells

What are permanent cells?

Terminally differentiated cells that are incapable of division and regeneration

Give 3 examples.

Myocardial cells, neurons, lens cells

During healing, what is organization?

Replacement of damaged tissue by scar tissue

What cell types are responsible for organization?

Fibroblasts and capillaries grow into infarcted or inflamed tissue or thrombus and then proliferate to form a scar.

What is granulation tissue?

New, highly vascular connective tissue formed by the ingrowth of endothelial cells and fibroblasts into a tissue defect. It is the reddish-pink layer that bleeds when you pick off a scab.

What is the relationship between granuloma and granulation tissue?

None! Don't confuse these!

What is wound contraction?	Reduction in the surface area of a wound by myofibroblasts
What is healing by first, or primary, intention?	Healing of a clean surgical incision with edges in apposition and minimal damage to tissues

Describe the progression of healing by first intention at the following time intervals

0–24 hours?	Polymorphonuclear neutrophil (PMN) migration, fibrin deposition
24–48 hours?	Epithelial cell migration and proliferation
3 days?	Wound contraction begins, proliferating fibroblasts deposit type III collagen, capillaries proliferate
5 days?	Granulation tissue is established
2 weeks?	Fibroblasts deposit type I collagen
1 month to 1 year?	Scar remodeling
What is the term for formation of new capillaries?	Angiogenesis
What is scar remodeling?	Simultaneous deposition, breakdown, cross-linking of collagen
Why do scars often look paler than normal tissue?	They are devascularized as they are remodeled.
What percent of original tensile strength can be achieved by a scar?	70%–80%
What is healing by secondary intention?	Repair of a large tissue defect with separated edges (e.g., gouge wound)
Name 4 ways in which healing by secondary intention differs from healing by primary intention?	1. There is a greater degree of inflammation. 2. There is a large amount of granulation tissue to fill the defect. 3. Wound contraction is slower. 4. A large scar results.

What is a keloid scar and who gets it?	Abnormal, excessive scar extending beyond the wound. It is more common in African Americans, and often recurs after excision. May be caused by a block in the healing process.

GROWTH FACTORS INVOLVED IN HEALING

What are the effects of fibroblast growth factor (FGF)?	Increased synthesis of the extracellular matrix (ECM) by fibroblasts, endothelial cells, and macrophages Increased proliferation of fibroblasts, endothelial cells, and smooth muscle cells
What effect does epidermal growth factor (EGF) have?	Increased proliferation of epithelial cells and fibroblasts
What effects does transforming growth factor (TGF-) have?	1. Increases proliferation of epithelial cells and fibroblasts. 2. Regulates the repair process by inhibiting growth of many cell types. 3. Increases fibroblast division and collagen deposition.
Where does platelet derived growth factor (PDGF) come from and what does it do?	It is released by platelets, monocytes, and endothelial cells. It enables a competent response of fibroblasts and smooth muscle cells to other growth factors ("competence factor").
What are the effects of macrophage-derived growth factor (MDGF) and where does it come from?	Increased proliferation of fibroblasts, endothelial cells, and smooth muscle cells. Secretion of MDGF is stimulated by fibronectin and bacterial products.

EXTRACELLULAR MATRIX (ECM)

What is the ECM?	A complex of macromolecules surrounding epithelia and connective tissue
What is the function of the ECM?	It plays a critical role in structural support, cell-cell interactions, and wound healing.
Name the 5 components of ECM and give the main example for each.	1. Collagen (extracellular protein) 2. Elastic fibers (elastin) 3. Structural glycoproteins (fibronectin)

4. Basement membrane
5. Proteoglycans (mucopolysaccharides)

What does basement membrane consist of?

Laminin and type IV collagen

What are the functions of proteoglycans?

Maintain tissue turgor and filter materials in and out of the ECM

What is fibronectin?

An ECM glycoprotein that links other ECM constituents to each other and to cells via integrins. Also promotes angiogenesis and migration of fibroblasts and endothelial cells.

What are integrins?

Glycoprotein cell-surface receptors that bind and interact with ECM components for cell-cell and cell-matrix adhesion and communication.

COLLAGEN

What are the 4 important types of collagen and their locations?

Type I—Tendon, skin, bone, mature scar
Type II—Cartilage
Type III—Early wound healing, blood vessels, GI tract, uterus
Type IV—Basement membranes only
(Types V and VI are also widely distributed.)

What are the steps of collagen synthesis?

1. Pre-procollagen forms on endoplasmic reticulum-bound ribosomes and cleaves to procollagen chains.
2. Three procollagen chains form a procollagen molecule in ER.
3. Intracellular processing occurs, including hydroxylation of proline and lysine and helix formation.
4. Secretion into ECM occurs.
5. Extracellular processing occurs, including cleavage of N- and C-terminal peptides.
6. Collagen fibers are formed by aggregation and lysine oxidation cross-linking.

What part of collagen synthesis is vitamin C-dependent?

Chain hydroxylation of proline residues. Vitamin C deficiency results in scurvy, characterized by poor wound healing.

What part of collagen synthesis is copper-dependent?	Lysyl oxidase, responsible for extracellular cross-linking to strengthen collagen fibers

FACTORS THAT AFFECT WOUND HEALING

What local factors influence wound healing and how?	1. Nature of wound (size, location, sharp versus blunt) 2. Vascular supply (poor supply prevents healing) 3. Infection (slows or prevents healing) 4. Movement (persistent trauma slows healing) 5. Ionizing radiation (damages vessels, inhibits cell proliferation) 6. Ultraviolet (UV) light (speeds healing!)
What systemic factors affect wound healing?	1. Nutritional status (deficiency of vitamin C and zinc impairs healing) 2. Diabetes mellitus(type I or II; impairs healing) 3. Infection (impairs healing) 4. Steroids (impair healing)
Does age affect wound healing?	Not by itself; however, the elderly are more likely to have one of the above factors that retard wound healing.

POWER REVIEW

What cell types cannot regenerate?	Permanent cells: neurons, lens cells, myocardial cells
What cell types are in a constant state of renewal?	Labile cells: GI mucosa, bone marrow cells
What is organization?	Replacement of damaged tissue by a scar
What cell types are responsible for organization?	Endothelial cells and fibroblasts
What is granulation tissue?	New connective tissue formed by growth of capillaries and fibroblasts into damaged tissue

What cells mediate wound contraction?	Myofibroblasts
When does deposition of type III collagen begin in wound healing?	Day 3
When does deposition of type I collagen begin?	2 weeks
Does injured tissue have its full tensile strength restored 5 years after healing?	No. Scarred tissue can have only 70%-80% of its original tensile strength.
What type of healing takes place in a clean surgical incision?	Healing by primary, or first, intention
What is more rapid, healing by primary (first) or secondary intention?	Primary (first)
What growth factor has inhibitory effects on cell proliferation?	TGF-η. Also promotes fibroblast division and collagen deposition.
What growth factor stimulates synthesis of ECM?	FGF
What are the components of ECM?	1. Collagen 2. Elastic fibers (elastin) 3. Structural glycoproteins (fibronectin) 4. Basement membrane (made of laminin and type IV collagen) 5. Proteoglycans
What does fibronectin bind?	All other ECM components, in addition to cell surface integrins
Where are the proline residues of collagen hydroxylated?	In the ER
What disease results from defective proline hydroxylation?	Scurvy, caused by vitamin C deficiency

Where does lysine oxidation cross-linking take place?

In the ECM

What are the 4 important types of collagen?

Type I-Tendon, skin, bone, mature scar
Type II-Cartilage
Type III-Early wound healing, blood vessels, GI tract, uterus
Type IV-Basement membranes only

How do steroids speed wound healing?

They don't! Steroids, malnutrition, infection, and diabetes all impair wound healing.

Does movement accelerate wound healing?

No, it slows it because it causes repeated trauma to wound edges.

How does ionizing radiation impair wound healing?

It damages capillaries and inhibits cellular proliferation.

5   Neoplasia

DEFINITIONS

Neoplasia	Uncontrolled, autonomous proliferation of cells
Cancer	Term that refers to any malignant neoplasm
Tumor	Any swelling or mass (not limited to neoplastic processes)
Benign	Having no potential for invasion or metastasis
Malignant	Having the potential for invasion and metastasis
Invasion	Infiltration of neoplastic cells into adjacent tissue
Metastasis	Spread of neoplastic cells to non-contiguous sites
Carcinoma	Malignancy of epithelial or glandular origin (e.g., skin, gastrointestinal system, breast, pancreas)
Carcinoma in situ	Lesion where the neoplastic cells are confined to the epithelium without invasion across the basement membrane
Sarcoma	Malignancy of mesenchymal origin (e.g., bone, muscle, fat)
Leukemia	Malignancy of blood cell lines (WBCs, RBCs, platelets)
Lymphoma	Malignancy of lymphoid tissues

Grade	Pathologic classification of a tumor based on histology and cytology of a sample of cells, examining specifically for the degree of differentiation. Scale ranges from grade I through IV, where I = well-differentiated and IV = highly anaplastic
Stage	Clinical classification of a patient's disease based on the size of the primary tumor and extent of invasion or metastasis. Scale ranges from stage I through IV where I = local disease, and IV = metastatic
Hypertrophy	An increase in the size of individual cells
Hyperplasia	An increase in the number of cells
Differentiation	Maturation of cells toward their "adult" cell type
Metaplasia	Reversible change of one differentiated cell type to another (e.g., ciliated respiratory epithelium changes to squamous epithelium in the respiratory tract of smokers)
Dysplasia	Reversible change in the development of a cell line marked by disorderly architecture; variability in nuclear size, shape, and staining; and abnormal mitoses. Dysplasia is a precursor lesion of neoplasia.
Anaplasia	Complete lack of differentiation
Pleomorphism	Variability in the size, shape, and staining of cells or nuclei
Transformation	Conversion of normal cells to neoplastic cells
Carcinogen	A substance that either directly or indirectly leads to the transformation of cells
Tumor suppressor gene	A gene encoding a protein product involved in the control of the cell cycle (considered recessive since two mutations are needed for carcinogenesis)

Oncogene	A gene that encodes a protein involved in cell signaling pathways or control of the cell cycle (considered dominant since one mutant allele will lead to uncontrolled cell growth and division)
Papillary	Frondlike in appearance
Medullary	Soft, cellular
Scirrhous	Hard, fibrous
Colloid	Glutinous or mucoid

NOMENCLATURE

How are neoplasms named?	By combining a prefix and a suffix: Prefix denoting the **cell type** (e.g., fat, muscle) or **architectural pattern** (e.g., glandular, squamous) Suffix denoting the **malignancy** of the neoplasm
Identify the 3 suffixes used for neoplasms and give the meaning of each.	1. -oma: benign neoplasm 2. -carcinoma: malignant neoplasm of epithelial or glandular origin 3. -sarcoma: malignant neoplasm of mesenchymal origin
Give the prefix for the following cell types or patterns.	
fat	lipo-
smooth muscle	leiomyo-
striated muscle	rhabdomyo-
bone	osteo-
cartilage	chondro-
glandular	adeno-
bile duct	cholangio-
Name a benign neoplasm of smooth muscle.	Leiomyoma

Name a malignant tumor of smooth muscle origin.	Leiomyosarcoma
Name a benign neoplasm of cartilage.	Chondroma
Name a malignant neoplasm of the glandular epithelium of the stomach.	Gastric adenocarcinoma

There are several notable exceptions to the neoplastic nomenclature rules as follows. Please define each.

Melanoma	Skin carcinoma derived from melanocytes
Lymphoma	Malignancy of lymphoid tissue
Hodgkin disease	A type of lymphoma
Leukemia	Malignancy of blood cell lines
Wilms tumor	Malignant tumor of the kidney
Seminoma	Malignancy of the testes
Hepatoma	Malignant liver tumor

BENIGN VS. MALIGNANT

What are 4 characteristics of benign processes?

1. Have no potential for invasion or metastasis
2. Are usually well-differentiated (cells closely resemble tissue of origin)
3. Grow by compression (not invasion) of surrounding tissues
4. Are usually well circumscribed

What are 3 characteristics of malignant processes?

1. Have the potential for invasion and metastasis
2. Are usually poorly differentiated
3. Grow by invasion

What are the cytologic clues that a sample is malignant?

Malignant cells exhibit anaplasia marked by cellular atypia, pleomorphism, increase in the nucleus:cell size ratio, abnormal mitoses, prominent nucleoli, hyperchromatism (dark staining of the nucleus), and irregular clumping of chromatin.

What is the SVC syndrome? External compression or direct invasion of the superior vena cava (SVC) by a tumor.

How is it caused? It is usually caused by primary lung carcinoma, but can also be caused by non-Hodgkin lymphoma, or metastatic disease.

What are the symptoms? Symptoms include fullness or swelling of the head, dyspnea, cough, or chest pain.

Name the 3 major routes of metastasis.
1. Hematogenous
2. Lymphatic
3. Direct extension through serous cavities

What are the steps involved in hematogenous and lymphatic metastasis?
1. Carcinoma in situ
2. Penetration through the basement membrane by binding to elements of the extracellular matrix (laminin, fibronectin, collagen) with cell surface proteins (integrins) and lysis of the basement membrane via release of proteases
3. Invasion into adjacent tissue—may involve cell motility by extension of pseudopodia
4. Invasion into vessels—usually thin-walled capillaries, venules, or lymphatics
5. Embolization of clusters of malignant cells and deposition downstream in a capillary bed or lymph node
6. Attachment and invasion of the vessel endothelium
7. Growth and survival of the lesion through angiogenesis or neovascularization [angiogenic growth factors (i.e., platelet-derived growth factor, transforming growth factor) are released by malignant cells]

What are the 2 most common sites of hematogenous metastasis and why?

Liver and lung; tumor cells invade the venous system, embolize, and tend to lodge in the first capillary network they encounter. Therefore, tumors that invade into the portal system (gastrointestinal system, pancreas) will embolize to the liver, while tumors invading into the systemic circulation (sarcomas, melanoma, breast) will embolize to the lung

Which tumors characteristically metastasize to bone?

Breast and prostate

What presenting complaints might indicate a metastasis to a vertebral body?

Pain, pathologic fracture, or spinal cord compression

Which primary tumors most commonly metastasize to the brain?

Lung and breast

What is carcinomatous meningitis?

Diffuse seeding of the leptomeninges by metastatic disease (most often from breast, lung, or lymphoma). The classical presentation is multifocal neurologic deficits.

What is the prognosis for a patient with carcinomatous meningitis?

Poor prognosis; the median survival is 4–6 months.

What is the pattern of metastasis through the lymphatic system?

Cells invade lymphatic channels and tend to grow in local lymph nodes, but also may present with metastasis to distant nodes ("skip" metastasis).

What is Virchow node?

Metastasis to a left supraclavicular node indicative of gastrointestinal malignancy

What is Sister Mary Joseph's node?

Metastasis to a periumbilical node indicative of intra-abdominal malignancy

What is the most common route of metastasis of carcinomas?

Lymphatic

What is the most common route of metastasis of sarcomas?	Hematogenous
What type of tumor is particularly prone to metastasis through the serous peritoneal cavity?	Ovarian cancer; it often presents with ascites and widespread intra-abdominal metastasis as a result of shedding of tumor cells and implantation at distant sites within the peritoneum.

CARCINOGENESIS

What is a proto-oncogene?	A normal gene that is involved in signal transduction and/or the regulation of growth and differentiation.
What is the genetic change responsible for Burkitt lymphoma?	An 8:14 translocation. The c-*myc* proto-oncogene of chromosome 8 is translocated to chromosome 14 where its production is enhanced. This leads to overproduction of c-*myc* and dys-regulation of the cell cycle.
How is the Philadelphia chromosome involved in carcinogenesis?	The 9:22 translocation (the Philadelphia chromosome) is seen in 90% of chronic myeloid leukemia (CML). The c-*abl* proto-oncogene of chromosome 9 is moved near the breakpoint cluster region (bcr) proto-oncogene of chromosome 22. The two genes join to form a fusion protein, bcr-Abl,which has intrinsic tyrosine kinase activity.
How does the p53 tumor suppressor gene regulate the cell cycle?	If a cell sustains damage to its DNA, the level of p53 protein rises and prevents the cell from entering the S phase of the cell cycle until the damage is repaired by enzymatic processes inherent to the cell.
What is the result of two mutant p53 genes?	In the absence of at least one good copy of the p53 gene, cells will continue to cycle without allowing time for DNA repair and will undergo progressive mutation.

What are the 5 main types of cancer implicated by mutations of p53?	Colorectal, breast, small cell lung, hepatocellular, and astrocytomas
What is the genetic etiology of retinoblastoma (Rb)?	Two "hits" at the Rb tumor suppressor gene locus
What are the 3 major categories of carcinogens?	1. Chemical 2. Physical 3. Viral
What are the 4 stages of chemical carcinogenesis?	1. Initiation: a chemical induces a mutation in the DNA of a cell 2. Promotion: cellular proliferation "fixes" the mutation in a population of cells 3. Progression: more mutations are triggered 4. Cancer: autonomous proliferation of monoclonal cells with the potential for invasion and metastasis
Give 2 examples of direct carcinogens.	1. Alkylating agents (including chemotherapeutics) intercalate between the bases of DNA and increase the risk of developing acute leukemias. 2. Heavy metals (nickel, chromium, uranium) bind DNA and lead to lung and skin carcinoma.
How do most indirect carcinogens act?	Procarcinogens are metabolized by enzymatic pathways within the liver to carcinogens capable of damaging DNA.
What cancers are commonly associated with each of the following indirect carcinogens?	
Polycyclic hydrocarbons	Bronchogenic cancer (from cigarette smoke)
Vinyl chloride	Angiosarcoma of the liver
Alatoxin B1	Hepatocellular cancer
Nitrosamines	Gastrointestinal (GI) and brain cancer

Aromatic amines, aniline dyes, δ-naphthylamine	Transitional cell bladder cancer

Identify the purpose of the Ames test and describe how it works.

The Ames test is used to assess whether a chemical is a mutagen.
1. A suspected carcinogen is combined with a strain of *Salmonella* that lacks the capability to synthesize the amino acid histidine.
2. The cells are cultured on media, which lacks histidine.
3. The growth of cells on this deficient media signals a mutational event, which has given the strain the ability to synthesize histidine.

Name 3 physical carcinogens.

1. Ionizing radiation [ultraviolet (UV) light, X-rays, and gamma rays]
2. Asbestos
3. Foreign bodies

How does UV radiation lead to cancer?

UV rays cause the formation of bonds between pyrimidine bases of DNA called thymine dimers, leading to all forms of skin cancer (squamous cell, basal cell, or melanoma).

What are the effects of X-rays and gamma rays?

X-rays and gamma rays cause carcinoma by causing double-stranded DNA breaks.

What is the usual effect of X-rays and gamma rays in the following subpopulations?

Early radiologists	Skin cancer and leukemia
Uranium miners	Lung cancer
Survivors of atomic bombs	Acute and chronic myelocytic leukemia
Radium watch dial workers	Osteosarcoma
Patients who have received head and neck irradiation	Thyroid cancer

What are the 2 known effects of asbestos exposure?

1. Malignant mesothelioma. Often presents after a long latency period of > 20 years.
2. Bronchogenic cancer

How do foreign bodies lead to cancer?

Chronic inflammation predisposes the surrounding tissue to transformation.

How do DNA viruses cause cancer?

DNA viruses incorporate their genetic material into host DNA, and produce viral proteins that bind to and suppress the products of host tumor suppressor genes. This results in unregulated cell growth and division.

Identify the types of carcinoma that can result from infection with the following DNA viruses.

Epstein-Barr virus (EBV)

Burkitt lymphoma, nasopharyngeal cancer

Human papilloma virus (HPV) (especially strains 16 and 18)

Cervical cancer

Hepatitis B

Hepatocellular cancer

What is a retrovirus?

An RNA virus that replicates by forming DNA via reverse transcriptase.

Name 2 ways a retrovirus may cause cancer.

1. The virus carries nucleotide sequences called viral oncogenes (v-oncs) which, when expressed, lead to malignant transformation.
2. The insertion of a viral promoter in the region of a cellular oncogene (insertional mutagenesis)

Which retrovirus is felt to be the etiologic factor in each of the following cancers?

Adult T-cell leukemia or lymphoma

Human T-cell lymphotrophic virus, type 1(HTLV-1)

Hairy cell lymphoma

HTLV-2

Kaposi sarcoma, lymph-oma	Human immunodeficiency virus (HIV)

KINETICS OF TUMOR GROWTH

What 3 factors are important in determining the growth rate of tumors?	1. Growth fraction: the proportion of cells that continue to move through the cell cycle rather than remaining quiescent. 2. Duration of the cell cycle. 3. The balance between the death of cells and the production of new cells.
What is the clinical significance of the growth fraction?	Chemotherapeutic drugs act by killing dividing cells; therefore, tumors in which a large proportion of the cells are traversing the cell cycle will be more susceptible to treatment than a tumor with a small growth fraction.
What is meant by the "doubling time" of a neoplasm?	The time for a tumor to double in volume.
At what size does an internal tumor become clinically detectable?	Approximately 1 gram (1 cubic centimeter)
Name 3 factors involved in the death of malignant cells.	1. Apoptosis: genetically programmed cell death 2. Inadequate supply of blood or nutrients 3. Host defenses

EPIDEMIOLOGY

What percentage of deaths in the United States are caused by cancer?	20%–25%
What are the 3 most common types of cancer in American women (percent of all cancers)?	1. Breast (32%) 2. Colorectal (15%) 3. Lung (11%)
What are the 3 most common types of cancer in American men (percent of all cancers)?	1. Prostate (22%) 2. Lung (19%) 3. Colorectal (15%)

What type of cancer has made a remarkable increase in incidence and now accounts for the leading cause of cancer deaths in both men and women?

Lung cancer

Why has there been an increase in incidence?

The incidence of lung cancer mirrors the increased incidence of smoking in the population. Although the incidence of lung cancer remains lower than that of breast cancer, lung cancer has overtaken breast cancer as the leading cause of cancer deaths in women in the past 10 years.

What are the 3 leading causes of death from cancer in American women?

1. Lung (21%)
2. Breast (18%)
3. Colorectal (13%)

What are the 3 leading causes of death from cancer in American men?

1. Lung (34%)
2. Prostate (12%)
3. Colorectal (11%)

Which cancer has shown the fastest increase in incidence in the past 40 years?

Melanoma. Its incidence has tripled since 1950.

Smoking is a risk factor for which types of cancer?

Lung, esophagus (especially when combined with alcohol), larynx, oral, bladder, kidney, pancreas, cervical, and gastric cancers

What happens to the risk of developing lung cancer if one stops smoking?

The risk begins to drop immediately and falls to the level of non-smokers at 10 years post-cessation.

What important point is illustrated by the study of cancer incidence in Japanese immigrants to the United States?

Studies illustrate the importance of the environment in carcinogenesis. The incidence of gastric cancer is very high in Japan (133 cases per 100,000 people per year), but Japanese immigrants to the United States have an incidence that is much closer to the American population (39 cases per 100,000 people per year).

What are the recommenda-

1. Monthly self breast exams

tions for breast cancer screening?

2. Yearly office visit and exam
3. Mammography every 1–2 years for those 40–50 years of age, and every year in those over 50 years of age
   *Note: more aggressive screening for women at increased risk and/or with a family history of breast cancer in a first degree relative (e.g., mother, sister)

Name 5 risk factors for cervical cancer.

Age, HPV infection, low socioeconomic status, multiple sexual partners, and cigarette smoking

What are the screening recommendations for cervical cancer?

Annual Pap smear beginning at 18 years of age or with the onset of sexual activity. If the Pap smears are consistently normal, frequency may be decreased to every 2–3 years.

Excessive fat or calorie intake is implicated in which 5 cancers?

Colorectal, breast, pancreas, prostate, and uterine cancers

Name 6 risk factors of colorectal cancer.

Familial adenomatous polyposis, hereditary non-polyposis colon cancer syndrome, first degree relative with colon cancer, ulcerative colitis, high-fat/low-fiber diet, age

What are the screening recommendations for colorectal cancer?

1. Annual digital rectal examination beginning at 40 years of age
2. Annual fecal occult blood testing beginning at 50 years of age
3. Sigmoidoscopy every 3 years starting at 50 years of age

FAMILIAL CANCER SYNDROMES

Describe the "two hit theory" and its relationship to familial cancer syndromes.

Both copies of the tumor suppressor gene must be inactivated for abnormal cell growth and division to occur. Familial cancer syndromes are inherited in an autosomal dominant manner; one "hit" is inherited through the germline, the second "hit" is the result of a somatic mutation. With both genes turned off, unregulated cell division occurs and leads to neoplastic transformation.

What are the 6 character-istic findings in inherited cancer syndromes?

1. Present at an earlier age
2. Autosomal dominant (except the DNA repair syndromes)
3. Positive family history
4. Bilateral involvement of paired organs
5. Multiple primary foci within an organ
6. Multiple primary foci within tissues of the same embryologic origin

How do sporadic and familial retinoblastoma (Rb) differ?

Sporadic Rb: average age at presentation is 2 years, no family history, unifocal, and caused by two somatic mutations at the Rb locus.

Familial Rb: average age at presentation is 15 months, autosomal dominant, bilateral, multifocal, and only one third have a positive family history because most "first hits" at the Rb locus arise from a germline mutational event during meiosis.

What are the MEN syndromes?

Multiple Endocrine Neoplasia (MEN) syndromes consist of multiple primary tumors of endocrine tissues.

Name the 2 types of the MEN syndrome.

Type I, or Werner syndrome, and Type II, or Sipple syndrome

Name the 3 tumors of Type I, Werner syndrome.

Parathyroid hyperplasia
Pancreatic islet neoplasms
Anterior pituitary adenomas
(Think PPP.)

Name the 7 tumors of Type II, Sipple syndrome.

IIA. **M**edullary thyroid cancer
   Pheochromocytoma
   Parathyroid hyperplasia
   (Think MPP.)
IIB. Medullary thyroid cancer
   Pheochromocytoma
   Mucosal neuromas
   Marfanoid habitus

Describe familial adenoma-tous polyposis.

Multiple colonic polyps which inevitably degenerate into malignant lesions with increasing age; an autosomal dominant disease with high penetrance

What are 4 findings in Gardner syndrome?

Multiple colon polyps, desmoid tumors, osteomas of mandible and skull, sebaceous cysts

What is the Li-Fraumeni cancer syndrome?

An autosomal dominant syndrome, associated with the germline mutation of the p53 gene, which is characterized by early onset of multiple primary tumors of distant cell types, including soft tissue sarcomas, osteosarcomas, adrenocortical cancer, brain tumors, or breast cancer

What are the DNA repair syndromes?

Autosomal-recessive inherited defect in DNA repair mechanisms, which predisposes cells to DNA mutation and neoplastic transformation.

Name 4 of the DNA repair syndromes.

1. Xeroderma pigmentosum
2. Fanconi anemia
3. Bloom syndrome
4. Ataxia telangiectasia

Describe xeroderma pigmentosum.

A type of skin cancer wherein the defect is in "nucleotide excision repair," and results from the lack of the cellular machinery to repair thymine dimers.

For what type of malignancy are patients with Fanconi anemia at a higher risk?

Acute myelocytic leukemia (AML)

What is the defect in Bloom syndrome?

A defect in DNA ligase leads to a variety of cancers, facial telangiectasias, growth retardation, and impaired immunity.

GRADING AND STAGING

What are the 2 main purposes of grading and staging cancers?

1. To determine prognosis and predict clinical behavior
2. To aid in the formation of an appropriate treatment plan

Which better predicts the prognosis of a cancer, the grade or the stage?

Stage

How is the grade of a cancer determined?

Grades are assigned according to a system that classifies tumors based on the appearance of cells. The sample is evaluated for the degree of differentiation; poorly differentiated neoplastic

cells exhibit anaplasia marked by:
1. increased ratio of the nucleus to the cell size
2. variability in the size, shape, and/or staining of nucleus and cytoplasm (pleomorphism)
3. increased number of mitoses
Cancers usually are assigned grades from I-IV, where I is well-differentiated (better prognosis, low grade) and IV is anaplastic (worse prognosis, high grade).

How is the stage of a cancer determined?

Cancer staging follows a clinical scheme that classifies cancers based on the extent of disease. Determining factors are:
1. Size of the primary tumor
2. Extent of local invasion
3. Metastasis to local lymph nodes
4. Distant metastasis
A cancer usually is assigned stages I-IV, where I is local disease only (good prognosis) and IV is metastatic disease (poor prognosis).

What is the TNM system?

An international system that classifies cancer according to 3 parameters:
T: size of primary tumor
N: number of positive lymph nodes
M: presence or absence of metastasis

What staging system is used for colon cancer?

Astler-Coller modified Dukes classification scheme

Name the Astler-Coller modified Dukes classification stages.

A

Confined to the mucosa

B1

Invades muscularis propria

B2

Invades serosa

C1

Invades muscularis propria with metastases to local nodes (B1 + nodes)

C2

Invades serosa with metastases to local nodes (B2 + nodes)

D

Distant metastases

How does the staging of colon cancer impact prognosis and treatment?

A: Virtually always cured by surgical excision
B: 5-year survival rate with surgery is approximately 70%
C: Improved prognosis with both surgery and adjuvant chemotherapy; 5-year survival rate is approximately 35%
D: Incurable

Identify and describe the 2 systems for staging malignant melanoma.

Clark system and Breslow microstaging system

Describe the Clark system.

I

Lesion is confined to intraepidermal carcinoma in situ

II

Invades the papillary dermis

III

Expands the papillary dermis

IV

Invades the reticular dermis

V

Invades the subcutaneous tissues

Define the Breslow microstaging system.

Precise measurement of the maximum thickness of a lesion; depth of invasion predicts probability of metastasis.
<0.75 mm almost never metastasizes
>4.0 mm metastasizes in >60% of the cases

Which system better predicts prognosis for a malignant melanoma?

The Breslow system more accurately predicts the clinical course.

CLINICAL MANIFESTATIONS

What constitutional symptoms are associated with malignancy?

1. Fever
2. Anorexia, weight loss, cachexia
3. Shaking, chills, night sweats

What is a paraneoplastic syndrome?

Remote effects of malignancy not related to invasion or metastasis

Name the cancers associated with the following endocrine abnormalities.

Cushing syndrome	Small cell lung cancer
Syndrome of inappropriate secretion of antidiuretic hormone (SIADH)	Small cell lung cancer
Hypercalcemia	Squamous cell lung cancer and breast adenocarcinoma by release of parathyroid hormone-related protein (PRP) or myeloma and lymphoma by secretion of osteoclast-activating factor (OAF)
Hypocalcemia	Osteoblastic metastasis to bone
Hypoglycemia	Insulinomas

Name and describe 5 neurologic and myopathic syndromes associated with neoplasms.

1. Subacute motor neuropathy:slowly progressive lower motor neuron weakness
2. Amyotrophic lateral sclerosis (ALS): rapidly progressing ascending motor and sensory paralysis, 10% with ALS have underlying malignancy
3. Peripheral neuropathy: purely sensory, combined sensorimotor, or autonomic
4. Dermatomyositis/polymyositis: 5–7 times the risk of cancer
5. Eaton-Lambert syndrome: resembles myasthenia except muscle strength increases with exercise and exhibits a poor response with edrophonium, often associated with small cell lung cancer

How may cancer affect the coagulation system?

A hypercoagulable state is often manifested by
1. Venous thrombosis
2. Disseminated intravascular coagulation (common with acute myelocytic leukemia, M3 promyelocytic leukemia, and adenocarcinomas)
3. Nonbacterial thrombotic endocarditis

| What are the 3 primary modalities for treating cancer? | Surgery, chemotherapy, and radiation therapy |

POWER REVIEW

Name the following tumors:

Benign tumor of the glandular breast tissue	Breast adenoma
Benign tumor of bone	Osteoma
Malignancy derived from bile duct epithelium	Cholangiocarcinoma
Malignancy of bone	Osteosarcoma
A retired shipyard worker presents with shortness of breath and pleural effusion. What are the most likely neoplastic etiologies and why?	Asbestos exposure predisposes the patient to bronchogenic cancer (especially if patient has a smoking history), and malignant mesothelioma.
What historical information would lead you to strongly suspect thyroid cancer in a patient with an anterior neck mass?	History of neck irradiation
What test should be performed in a patient with Kaposi sarcoma?	HIV test
A female patient has bone metastasis. What is the most likely site of the primary neoplasm?	Breast
A patient has colon cancer that invades the muscularis propria and involves local lymph nodes. What stage is this? What is the appropriate therapy?	Modified Dukes classification stage C1. Patients with stage C colon cancer have increased survival if treated with both surgery and adjuvant chemotherapy.

A 50-year-old male patient presents with blood in his stool. Colonoscopy reveals a large fungating mass in the transverse colon, but an otherwise normal exam. Two of the patient's siblings and the patient's father died of colon cancer. What is the most likely diagnosis?

Hereditary, non-polyposis colorectal cancer (Lynch syndrome)

What is the Philadelphia chromosome?

Transformation 9:22—seen in 90% of patients with chronic myelogenous leukemia (CML)

How do UV rays lead to cancer?

DNA is damaged through the formation of thymine dimers.

What is the leading cause of cancer deaths in both men and women?

Lung cancer

What is p53?

A tumor suppressor gene. It is a protein product involved in halting DNA synthesis so DNA repair can take place. "Two hits" lead to unregulated progression through the cell cycle and the accumulation of mutations.

A patient presents with a hard, fixed, left supra-clavicular node. What diagnosis should be considered?

Virchow node, which is often secondary to occult GI malignancy

6

The Immune System

BASIC CONCEPTS

What are the 6 types of cells that constitute the immune system?

1. Neutrophils
2. Monocytes/macrophages
3. Lymphocytes
4. Mast cells
5. Basophils
6. Eosinophils

What is the major histocompatibility complex (MHC) and why is it important?

Polymorphic cell surface molecules divided into class I and II. The MHC is important in allograft rejection, antigen presentation, and lymphocyte signaling.

What 2 types of cells express class I?

All nucleated cells
Platelets

What kinds of antigen do the cells in class I present?

Degraded endogenous peptides 8–10 amino acids long

What cells express class II?

Antigen-presenting cells (macrophage series, including dendritic cells)
B cells
Activated T cells
Endothelial cells

What kinds of antigen do the cells in class II present?

Longer exogenous peptides (13–30 amino acids long) maintaining some prior structure

What is a granuloma?

Infectious or other foreign material that can't be degraded or removed and becomes enclosed in inflammatory tissue

What is the typical histopathology of granuloma formation?

Macrophage-derived epithelioid and multinucleated giant cells arise and enclose the area with cellular and connective tissue under continued T-cell stimulation.

CELLS OF THE IMMUNE SYSTEM

MONONUCLEAR PHAGOCYTES

List the most important mononuclear phagocytes in each of the following anatomic locations.

Circulating blood	Monocytes
Bone marrow	Macrophages
Liver	Kupffer cells
Lungs	Alveolar macrophages
Connective tissue	Histiocytes
Brain	Microglia

What are Langerhans cells?   The dendritic cells of the skin

What are the important functions of Langerhans cells?   Antigen presentation, engulfment of bacteria, and production and release of cytokines

To what cells do Langerhans cells present antigen?   To helper T cells associated with class II MHC

LYMPHOCYTES

What are lymphocytes?   Any of the mononuclear nonphagocytic leukocytes found in the blood, lymph, and lymphoid tissues

Name 3 classes of lymphocytes.
1. T cells
2. B cells
3. Natural killer (NK) cells

T CELLS

What are the 3 T-cell subsets?   Cytotoxic T cells, helper T cells, and suppressor T cells

What are the characteristics of each group?   Cytotoxic T cells represent 70%-80% of circulating blood lymphocytes.

Helper T cells are characterized by a T-cell receptor (TCR).

Suppressor T cells express pan-T markers including CD3, CD2, CD5.

What is the TCR?

The polymorphic antigen-binding molecule, analogous to surface immunoglobulin (Ig), that binds antigen (Ag) associated with MHC on other cells

What is the typical structure of the TCR?

Disulfide-linked alpha (α) and beta (β) chains noncovalently associated with CD3

What alternate T cell subset exists and what percent does it represent?

5% or less instead express gamma (γ) and delta (δ) chains and play a role in presenting hydrophobic antigens.

What are cytotoxic T cells?

Surface CD8+ cells integral to cell-mediated immunity and responding to MHC I antigens

How do cytotoxic T cells work?

They bind the MHC I antigens of cells and kill them, thus enacting cell-mediated immunity.

What are helper T cells and how do they work?

CD4+ cells that mediate humoral immunity via specific stimulation of B cells through their MHC class II-associated antigens.

What are suppressor T cells and how do they work?

CD8+ cells that exert an inhibitory effect on B-cell responses

What are the 3 primary functions of cell-mediated immunity?

Elimination of cells infected with virus, tumor cells, and cells infected with intracellular bacteria

What cells provide non-specific help in the elimination of these same infected or tumor cells?

Natural killer (NK) cells

What term is given to the immune system's ongoing patrol to destroy abnormal cells (particularly, neoplastic cells)?

Immune surveillance

B CELLS

What percent of blood lymphocytes do B cells represent?	About 15%
From what cells do B cells originate and where?	Lymphoid progenitor cells, thought to differentiate in fetal liver and spleen and adult bone marrow
In what 4 anatomic locations do B cells reside?	1. Blood 2. Lymph node cortex and germinal centers 3. Splenic white pulp and lymphoid follicles 4. Bone marrow
What are the 5 stages of development of B cells?	Pro-B, pre-B, immature B, mature B, and plasma cell.
What are the 2 possible termination cell types?	Memory or resting B cell, plasma cell

What are the important maturation events at each of the steps?

Pre-B cell	Cytoplasmic Ig heavy chain (only μ)is produced.
Immature B cells	A specific surface IgM is expressed.
Mature B cells	Isotype switching may occur to express IgA, E, or G instead.
Plasma cell differentiation	Immunoglobulins can be secreted.
What is the role of surface Ig?	It is the receptor for specific soluble antigen, to be internalized and presented with MHC II.

NATURAL KILLER (NK) CELLS

What makes NK cells different from other lymphocytes?	They lack traditional T or B markers, including TCR or surface Ig.

What is the function of NK cells?	They exert a killing function apparently not restricted to MHC molecules. Their killing is dependent upon cell-cell contact and is enhanced by interferon and interleukin 2 (IL-2).
What percent of lympho-cytes do NK cells typically represent?	15%–20%
What morphologically based name is also given to NK cells?	Large granular lymphocytes (LGLs)

LYMPHOKINES

Name the most appropriate lymphokine for each function listed.

Participates in B-cell development into plasma cells	IL-5
Stimulates stem cell differentiation	IL-3
Is a growth factor for B cells, mast cells, and activated T-cells as well as an up-regulator of B-cell MHC class II expression	IL-4
Is an important stimulant of T-cell growth and proliferation	IL-2
Is important in T and B cell maturation and in growth of precursor cells	IL-6
Is important for Ig class switching and maturation, activating macrophages, and increasing MHC II expression	IFN-γ

LYMPHOCYTE CELL MARKERS

What helper T marker molecule binds to MHC II-presented Ag?	CD4
Name a cytotoxic suppressor T and NK cell marker that is associated with MHC I Ag presentation.	CD8
Name a myeloid and lymphoid precursor marker.	CD34
Name a pan-T-cell marker associated with Ag recognition.	CD3
Name a T-cell marker that also identifies the B-1 B cell subset.	CD5
Name a pan-B-cell marker.	CD19
A pre-B cell marker and also the common acute lymphoblastic leukemia antigen (CALLA)?	CD10

THE IMMUNOGLOBULIN MOLECULE

Name the 5 immunoglobulin types.	IgM, IgG, IgA, IgD, and IgE
Identify the correct immunoglobulin for each description.	
A pentameric molecule that is formed when the initial Ig is expressed and secreted	IgM
A dimer associated with J chain and a secretory component as main Ig of secretions	IgA

A monomeric Ig that is the most abundant serum Ig	IgG
A monomer that binds basophil and mast cell Fc receptors and is important in parasite defense and allergy	IgE
A monomer on the surface of mature B cells with only a trace present in serum	IgD
In what form do all of these immunoglobulins appear as surface Ig?	As monomers
What are the light chain types and how are they distributed in humans?	The two light chain types are kappa (κ) and lambda (λ). In humans, two thirds of immunoglobulins express κ and one third express λ.
What is the basic structure of an immunoglobulin monomer?	Y-shaped symmetrical molecule with light chains each bound by a disulfide bond to a longer heavy chain. Identical heavy chains meet with a pair of disulfide bonds to make the base of the Y and the Fc "constant" portion of the molecule. In the Y "arms" (Fab portion), light and heavy chains each terminate to form the variable regions.
What forms the variable region of the heavy chain?	One of each of the polymorphic V, D, and J genes of chromosome 14.
What forms the variable region of the light chain?	One V and J region from either κ (chromosome 2) or λ (chromosome 22) alleles.
What enzyme can split the antibody into the Fc and 2 Fab fragments?	Papain
What enzyme can split the Ab into the Fc and an F(ab')$_2$?	Pepsin

What cells are "effector cells" (have Fc receptors)?	NK cells, neutrophils, eosinophils, mast cells, monocyte cells, and platelets
What cells express receptors for IgG (Fcγ)?	Macrophages, B cells, NK cells, and neutrophils
What cells express receptors for IgE (Fcε)?	Mast cells, basophils, eosinophils, and macrophages
What are the most important chemotactic factors for neutrophils?	C5a complement component and leukotriene B4

COMPLEMENT SYSTEM

How is the complement system organized?	Into classic and alternate pathways
How is each pathway activated?	The classic pathway requires all 9 parts, activated by C1-bound antibody. In the alternate pathway, C3 is activated directly.
How do both pathways culminate?	In formation of the membrane attack complex (MAC)
What is the classic pathway?	C1 binds IgM or IgG and cleaves C2 and C4 after activated to form the C4b2a complex (C3 convertase). This then splits C3 into C3a (causing release of vasoactive amines and lysosomal enzymes) and C3b (an opsonin that binds C4b2a to form C5 convertase).
What does C5 convertase do?	It cleaves C5 into C5b, then joins the MAC and the chemotactic C5a.
What are the steps of the alternate pathway?	C3 is activated to C3b by C3 priming convertase, then is deposited and acts with factor B and magnesium to form C3b,B, which activates the membrane attack sequence and feeds back with further C3 cleavage.
How is C3 activated in the alternate pathway?	Activated directly by endotoxin, aggregated immunoglobulins (IgA and some IgG), or snake (cobra) venom to be deposited on the activating surface as C3b

How can C3b be removed after deposition on these surfaces?	It cannot; it is not degraded once deposited.
What 2 cytotoxic cells contain receptors for opsonized C3b?	Macrophage series Neutrophils
What disease is associated with a deficiency of C1 esterase inhibitor?	Hereditary angioedema

CLINICAL HYPERSENSITIVITY

How many types of hyper-sensitivity reactions are there?	Four

TYPE I

What is it?	Immediate sensitivity
What are the clinical features of type I hyper-sensitivity?	Depending on severity: urticaria, wheal and flare skin reactions, hypotension, wheezing, and respiratory compromise
What are some examples?	Anaphylaxis, hay fever, food allergies, bee-sting allergy, asthma, and atopic dermatitis
What is an allergen?	A specific term for an antigen that induces IgE production and, therefore, sensitization
What is the mechanism for type I hypersensitivity?	Antigen cross-linking of IgE bound to basophil and mast cell membranes, leading to degranulation and mediator release
What are some of the most important mediators?	Histamine, leukotrienes, bradykinins, and prostaglandins

TYPE II

What is it?	Antibody-mediated hypersensitivity

What are some examples?	Autoimmune hemolytic anemias, hemolytic disease of the newborn, transfusion reactions, hyperacute graft rejection, myasthenia gravis, Goodpasture syndrome, and pemphigus
What causes type II hypersensitivity?	Antibodies (usually IgM or IgG autoantibodies) binding cell or protein surfaces
What is the mechanism of cell damage for type II hypersensitivity?	Complement deposition and cell lysis via the MAC, destruction of cells by cells homing to Fc receptors and opsonized C3b, and production of inflammatory mediators

TYPE III

What is it?	Immune complex disease
What are some examples?	Lupus nephritis, the Arthus reaction, serum sickness, some types of endocarditis, and polymyositis
What is the mechanism for type III hypersensitivity reactions?	Immune complex deposition with resultant inflammation and direct toxicity
What are 3 situations with significant complement formation?	1. Autoimmune disease 2. Chronic or persistent infection 3. Inhaled antigens
What is the Arthus reaction?	An acute inflammatory hemorrhagic reaction and localized dermal vasculitis induced by immune complex formation following injection of an antigen
What cells normally clear immune complexes?	The phagocyte series

TYPE IV

What is it?	Delayed-type hypersensitivity (DTH) (also known as cell-mediated hyper-sensitivity)
What are some examples of type IV hypersensitivity?	Chronic transplant rejection, purified protein derivative (PPD) reaction, and

chronic infectious diseases (particularly intracellular ones)

What is the mechanism of type IV hypersensitivity?

Certain helper T cells secrete cytokines, including IFN-γ, and activate macrophages after exposure to appropriate antigens.

What are the clinical features of type IV hypersensitivity reactions?

Progressive erythema, followed by induration and occasionally ulceration and necrosis at site of antigen exposure starting after 12–18 hours and usually reaching peak at 24–48 hours

What are the key immune cells for type IV hypersensitivities?

Antigen-specific helper T cells and macrophages

What is anergy?

Inability to mount a DTH reaction, such as in an intradermal PPD test

What is granulomatous hypersensitivity?

A very serious form of DTH

What is the cause?

Antigen, usually infectious, that is persistent within macrophages leading to characteristic granulomatous inflammation

What disease is an example of a granulomatous hypersensitivity?

Sarcoidosis

AUTOIMMUNE DISEASES

What are some theories of the pathogenesis of autoimmunity?

1. Increased or inappropriate helper T action
2. Antibody cross-reacting with self and foreign (usually microbial) antigens
3. Inappropriate production of autoantibodies
4. Antibody binding to self-antigens altered by drugs, chemicals, or microbes
5. Failure or decreased T-suppressor activity
6. Previously protected or hidden self-antigens recognized

7. "Superantigen" T-cell independent B-cell activation

Name the correct autoantibody for each of the following characteristics.

Sensitive but non-specific marker of autoimmunity; antibody pattern can be helpful	Antinuclear antibody (ANA)
Specific for systemic lupus erythematosus (SLE); present in about 50% of cases	Antibodies to double-stranded (ds) DNA
Sensitive but nonspecific autoantibody	Antibodies to single-stranded (ss) DNA
One of the nucleolar "antigens" very specific for scleroderma	Scl-70 autoantibody
5. RNA protein specific for Sjögren syndrome (present in 60%-70% of cases); antibody also binds Epstein-Barr virus (EBV) RNA	Sjögren syndrome B (SS-B) (La)
Associated with Sjögren syndrome, and also with SLE (in about one third of cases)	SS-A Φ
High titers in mixed connective tissue disease	Anti-ribonucleoprotein
Associated with polymyositis and dermatomyositis	JO-1
Specific for SLE, present in 25%–60% of cases	Smith (Sm)
Indicative of CREST syndrome variant of scleroderma	Anti-centromere

SYSTEMIC LUPUS ERYTHEMATOSUS (SLE)

What is it?	Multisystem disease of uncertain etiology with components of type II and III hypersensitivity
What epidemiological associations have been made?	Hormonal—predominantly strikes women of childbearing age. Genetic—linked to specific HLAs (DR2, DR3, A1, and B8), and deficiencies of complement C2 and C4 Environmental—may include infectious agents such as viruses, drugs, or environmental toxins
What organs may be involved?	Skin, kidneys, joints, heart, serosal membranes, vasculature, and the lymphoreticular system
Name the common clinical features of SLE by area of involvement.	
Systemic features	Fever, fatigue, and weight loss
Heart	Aseptic, small fibrinoid valvular vegetations involving mitral and tricuspid valves (Libman-Sacks endocarditis)
Chest	Serosa of pericardium and pleura is often inflamed, leading to exudative effusion. Inflammation may also involve lungs.
Vasculature	Vasculitis secondary to immune complex deposition
Skin	Complexes at dermoepidermal junction give rise to characteristic maculopapular erythematous lesions through degeneration of the dermal basal layer and vasculitis.
Joints	Exudative but non-erosive arthritis
Abdominal organs	Autoimmune hepatitis, peritoneal inflammation, splenomegaly, and lymph node enlargement

Hematologic features

Cytopenias of all three lineages by autoimmune etiology

What are the pathogenic mechanisms involved in SLE?

1. Autoantibodies—especially the ANA including dsDNA and ssDNA, RNA, Smith antigen, histones, nucleoli, and RNA-associated proteins
2. Immune complex accumulation—may be a key mechanism of autoantibody toxicity
3. Lymphocyte dysfunction (e.g., abnormal B-cell activation or decreased suppressor T action)—may contribute significantly

What are 2 common causes of mortality from SLE?

Kidney failure
Infectious complications

SCLERODERMA

What is it?

A poorly understood multi-system autoimmune connective tissue disease

What is the characteristic histopathology?

Fibrosis of skin and internal organs with small vessel destruction

What is the mechanism of scleroderma?

Endothelial damage and fibroblast proliferation (by an uncertain immune mechanism)

What autoantibodies are associated?

Antinucleolar antibodies, especially Scl-70, are very specific. Also ANA, rheumatoid factor (RF), and smooth muscle antibodies.

What are typical skin manifestations?

"Tightness" of skin is typical, beginning with dermal collagen buildup with lymphocytic infiltrates and edema near vessels, and progressing to hyalinization and sclerosis. Eventually, this leads to atrophy of the overlying epidermis.

What happens initially to the kidneys?

Benign periarteriolar intimal fibrosis and thickening occurs, progressing to fibrinoid necrosis and cortical ischemia.

What may result?

Acute renal failure and severe hypertension

Dysmotility caused by fibrosis of submucosal muscularis of the distal two thirds of the esophagus occurs in what percent of patients?	About 50%
What are the musculo-skeletal manifestations?	Early skeletal muscle perivascular mononuclear infiltrate and edema followed by intrafascicular fibrosis; also, mild inflammatory nonerosive synovitis that may involve tendon sheaths leading to carpal tunnel syndrome
What causes progressive dyspnea on exertion in patients with scleroderma?	Diffuse interstitial fibrosis as well as vessel thickening
What is the typical course?	Slowly progressive
What are signs of a particularly poor prognosis with scleroderma?	Malignant hypertension, cardiac, renal, and pulmonary manifestations
What is the CREST syndrome and what does it stand for?	This is a related, less severe variant of scleroderma and is characterized by **C**alcinosis, **R**aynaud syndrome, **E**sophageal dysmotility, **S**yndactyly, and **T**elangiectasias.
What antibody is strongly associated with CREST?	Anti-centromere antibodies

DERMATOMYOSITIS AND POLYMYOSITIS

What are characteristic features of these conditions?	Symmetrical proximal muscle weakness and inflammatory myopathy
What are associated antibodies?	Antibodies to nuclear antigens PM1 and JO-1's are very specific.
How are the 2 entities different?	Characteristic malar erythematous and scaling rash are present in dermatomyositis but are not found in polymyositis.

What other skin finding is pathognomonic for dermatomyositis?

A purplish red-tinted "heliotropic rash" of the upper eyelids

Describe the striated muscle histopathology of dermatomyositis?

Early edema and scarce mononuclear infiltrate progressing along with myofibril breakdown and interstitial fibrosis

What is the dermatologic histopathology of dermatomyositis?

Perivascular infiltrates, edema, and liquefaction of dermo-epidermal junction similar to SLE.

SJÖGREN SYNDROME

What are the primary clinical features?

Enlargement of salivary glands with xerostomia (dry mouth) and kerato-conjunctivitis sicca

With what other diseases is it associated?

Often occurs with other autoimmune diseases, especially rheumatoid arthritis and SLE.

What are the associated antibodies?

Antibody to the RNA protein SS-B is very specific and present in 60%–70% of cases. Also other antibody, including ANA and antibody to salivary duct cells.

What is the immunopathologic mechanism?

The idiopathic inflammation includes both CD4 and CD8 + T-cells and involves both type II and IV hypersensitivity.

What is the histopathology of Sjögren syndrome?

Salivary duct destruction surrounded by dense infiltrate of plasma cells and various lymphocytes occurs early, with progressive fibrosis, fatty replacement, and atrophy.

What malignancy is difficult to distinguish from Sjögren syndrome?

Lymphoma, particularly when infiltrate is dense

To what malignancy are patients with Sjögren syndrome predisposed?

Lymphoma

MIXED CONNECTIVE TISSUE DISEASE (MCTD)

What is it?	A disorder that combines features of SLE, scleroderma, and polymyositis
What autoantibodies are characteristic?	High levels of antibody to extractable nuclear ribonucleoprotein

IMMUNODEFICIENCY DISORDERS

What are the 4 conditions caused by major primary T-cell deficiencies?	1. Chronic mucocutaneous candidiasis 2. DiGeorge syndrome 3. MHC class II deficiency 4. Wiskott-Aldrich syndrome
What are the 4 primary B-cell disorders?	1. Isolated IgA deficiency 2. Bruton agammaglobulinemia 3. Transient hypogammaglobulinemia of infancy 4. Common variable immunodeficiency
What are 2 B- and T-cell disorders?	1. Severe combined immunodeficiency (SCID) 2. Hereditary ataxia-telangiectasia
What are some general features of the B cell antibody deficiency disorders?	Recurrent sinopulmonary infections Frequent infection with encapsulated bacteria Susceptibility to enteroviral infections Low serum and secretion antibody levels
What other hereditary immunodeficiency disorders exist?	Chronic granulomatous disease, myeloperoxidase deficiency, and Chédiak-Higashi syndrome
What do all of these disorders involve?	Monocyte/granulocyte dysfunction

ISOLATED IGA DEFICIENCY

What are the genetic causes?	The genetic defect is not clear.
What is the frequency of occurrence?	1 in 500 to 700 (most common immunodeficiency)

What are the symptoms?	Some recurrent infections, particularly URI's, otherwise it is generally asymptomatic.
What happens to IgG and IgM levels in these patients?	They are usually normal although 20% also lack an IgG isotype.
To what difficulty with blood transfusion are these patients predisposed?	Anaphylactic reaction to donor IgA molecules
What other diseases are associated?	Allergies, inflammatory bowel disease, celiac disease, and other autoimmune diseases

BRUTON AGAMMAGLOBULINEMIA

What is the typical age at presentation?	6 months, when maternal antibodies have waned
What is the clinical presentation?	Recurrent bacterial otitis, pharyngitis, skin infection, and bronchitis
What is the genetic inheritance pattern?	X-linked
What are the relevant laboratory findings?	Absent or very low Ig levels and no circulating mature B-cells
What is the immunologic defect?	B cell maturation defect after the pre-B cell stage
What are the anatomical pathological findings?	Absence of plasma cells and germinal centers in lymph nodes and splenic white pulp

COMMON VARIABLE IMMUNODEFICIENCY (CVID)

What is the typical presentation?	Recurrent infections
What is the usual age at presentation?	Can vary from infants to elderly, but presents most often in young adults
What is the genetic defect?	The association is not clear

What illnesses are associated with CVID?	Patients often suffer from gluten hypersensitivity (celiac disease) and giardiasis
What causes CVID?	Although several mechanisms are postulated, the cause is unknown.
What are the pertinent laboratory findings?	Hypogammaglobulinemia despite normal numbers of circulating B cells
What are the histopathologic findings?	Hypoplastic germinal centers and other B-cell areas; no plasma cells; occasionally, noncaseating granulomas in various organs

TRANSIENT HYPOGAMMAGLOBULINEMIA OF INFANCY

What is it?	Decreased Ig levels in infancy as maternal antibody declines
What causes it?	A delay of up to 36 months in antibody production due to a T helper defect

DIGEORGE SYNDROME

What is it?	Thymic aplasia leading to lack of T cells
What is the cause?	Failure of the 3rd and 4th pharyngeal pouches to descend in utero
What other anatomic defects are present?	Lack of parathyroid glands
What is the genetic defect?	Not genetically associated; thought to result from an early intrauterine growth defect
What is the typical clinical presentation?	Tetany due to hypocalcemia in infancy
Name an associated condition.	Hypoparathyroidism (absent gland)
How is DiGeorge syndrome treated?	Transplantation of fetal thymus or replacement of thymic hormone

CHRONIC MUCOCUTANEOUS CANDIDIASIS

What is it?	A selective T-cell defect
What are the typical clinical features?	Recurrent candidal infections of the mucous membranes and skin
What is the genetic inheritance pattern?	Autosomal recessive
What are some associated conditions?	Endocrinopathies, including hypo-parathyroidism, Addison disease, diabetes mellitus, hypothyroidism, and pernicious anemia

SEVERE COMBINED IMMUNODEFICIENCY (SCID)

What is it?	Nearly complete absence of T and B lymphocytes due to one of several stem cell defects
What is the clinical presentation?	Recurrent infections in infancy (e.g., thrush, chronic diarrhea, and pyogenic infections)
What is the genetic inheritance pattern?	X-linked or autosomal recessive
What causes the X-linked form?	A mutation in IL-2 receptor gene
What is the most common mechanism causing the recessive form?	Lack of adenosine deaminase leading to selective accumulation of toxic and inhibitory purine breakdown products in lymphoid cells
What are the histopatho-logic findings?	Lack of lymphoid tissue in spleen, lymph nodes, or thymus; thymus doesn't descend
Should patients receive prophylactic immunizations?	Yes; only killed vaccines should be used because live-attenuated viruses cause severe infections.
Can SCID be diagnosed prenatally?	Yes, by amniocentesis
How is it treated?	Bone marrow transplant or gene therapy

ACQUIRED IMMUNODEFICIENCY SYNDROME (AIDS)

What disease states are associated with acquired immunodeficiency?

Malnutrition, infections, malignancy, autoimmune diseases, aging, uremia, and immunosuppressive drugs or toxins

How is AIDS transmitted?

By blood, sexual contact, or transplacental transmission

What populations are at risk?

IV drug users, homosexual males, heterosexuals (particularly women) with infected partners, hemophiliacs and others who receive blood products frequently, and infants of infected mothers

How does the virus infect cells?

The viral coat glycoprotein GP120 is trophic for CD4 (on helper T and monocyte cells) and infects the CD4 by endocytosis.

How is the virus copied?

Viral reverse transcriptase incorporates RNA into host DNA to be replicated during host cell stimulation

How can disease progression be tracked?

By measuring viral loads, total CD4+ count, and CD4+/CD8+ ratios

What is the normal CD4+/ CD8+ ratio?

1:1 to 3:1

How is this ratio affected in a patient with AIDS?

It drops below 1:1, becoming "inverted"

What other infections can cause an "inverted" ratio of CD4+/CD8+?

Other viral illnesses, such as EBV, cytomegalovirus (CMV), and influenza A

What causes the change in ratio?

An increase in the CD8+ population

What occurs clinically in acute infection?

6–8 weeks after exposure, 60%–80% of patients with primary HIV infections get a mononucleosis-like syndrome. This syndrome is often not recognized.

How is AIDS defined?

HIV+ with either a CD4 count <200 or after a characteristic opportunistic infection

HIV-ASSOCIATED CONDITIONS

INFECTIONS

Give some examples of various types of infections seen with HIV.

Viruses	EBV, CMV, herpes simplex and herpes zoster viruses (HSV and HZV), hepatitis B virus (HBV), and human papilloma virus (HPV)
Fungi	*Histoplasma, Candida, Coccidioides, Aspergillus,* and *Cryptococcus*
Bacteria	*Mycobacterium tuberculosis* and *M. avium-intracellulare, Enterobacteriaceae,* and other pyogenic bacteria
Protozoans	*Pneumocystis, Cryptosporidium, Toxoplasma*

What symptoms are typically associated with HIV infection?

Mild malaise, fatigue, and fever in the context of mild CD4 decrease

Describe the histopathologic findings in the following stages of progression of HIV infection.

Early findings

Increased plasma cells and follicular hyperplasia

Later findings

Mixed pattern of both hyperplasia and depletion within follicles

Then still later, when the patient has the AIDS-related complex (ARC)?

Diffuse lymphoid depletion with follicular decay, medullary fibrosis, and vascular proliferation

What symptoms characterize ARC?

>3 months fever, diarrhea, and weight loss in the context of low CD4 count

KAPOSI SARCOMA

What is Kaposi sarcoma?

A typically mucocutaneous angioproliferative neoplasm to which

	patients infected with HIV are predisposed
What is the probable pathophysiology?	Endothelial cells proliferate due to high growth factors and incompetent immune surveillance
What is the gross appearance?	Multiple purple or red papular mucocutaneous nodules
What areas may be affected besides mucous membranes and skin?	Visceral organs and lymph nodes
What is the histopathology?	Clumps of pointed cells surrounding irregular, dilated vascular areas with thin endothelium and extravasated RBCs
What fraction of patients with AIDS develop Kaposi sarcoma?	About one third
In what other population is it typical?	Elderly males

HIV-ASSOCIATED LYMPHOMA

Besides Kaposi sarcoma, to what other neoplasms are patients with HIV predisposed?	Squamous cell carcinoma of the tongue, cloacogenic carcinoma of the rectum, non-Hodgkin lymphoma (and, to a lesser extent, Hodgkin lymphomas)
What are the typical cells of origin in HIV-associated lymphoma?	B cells
What virus is associated?	Epstein-Barr virus (EBV)

POWER REVIEW

What type or types of cells are best described by each of the following?	
Respond to completely degraded peptides	Cytotoxic T-lymphocytes
Antigen-presenting cells of the skin	Langerhans cells

Associated with Class II MHC	Helper T cell
IL-2 primarily stimulates these	T cells
Lymph node germinal centers	B cells
Have CD3 on their surface	T cells
Participate in cell-mediated immunity	CD8+ cytotoxic T-cells and NK cells
IL-6 is important in differentiation of these	Plasma cells
Have CD19 on the surface	B cells (Pan-B marker)
First express surface IgM	Immature B cells
Binds MHC with antigen, maintaining some higher structure	Helper T cells
Binds soluble antigen	Mature or memory B cells
What is the common acute lymphocytic leukemia antigen?	CD10
What lesion is caused by a histopathologic reaction to foreign undegradable matter?	Granuloma
What autoimmune disease is suggested by each of the following?	
Heliotropic rash	Dermatomyositis
Dry eyes	Sjögren syndrome
Libman-Sacks endocarditis	SLE

Often occurs with SLE and RA	Sjögren syndrome
Variant of scleroderma	CREST syndrome
Pleuritis and pericarditis	SLE
Predisposes to lymphoma	Sjögren syndrome
Mediated by endothelial damage and proliferation	Scleroderma
Autoimmune cytopenias	SLE
Esophageal dysmotility	Scleroderma or CREST syndrome
Malar rash	SLE or dermatomyositis
Skin "tightness"	Scleroderma
Immune complex damage is likely the key mechanism	SLE

Name the appropriate autoantibody for each description.

Specific for SLE?	DsDNA, smith Ag (Sm)
Associated with CREST syndrome?	Anti-centromere
Specific for scleroderma?	Scl-70
Sensitive general marker of autoimmunity?	Anti-nuclear antibodies
Associated with mixed connective tissue disease	Anti-smooth muscle
Associated with poly/ dermatomyositis?	Anti JO-1 and PM1
Specific for Sjögren syndrome?	SS-B
Name the common causes of mortality in SLE.	Renal failure and infection

Name the correct hyper-sensitivity syndrome for each of the following examples or characteristics.

PPD skin testing	Type IV
Solely antibody-mediated	Type II
Allergic reactions	Type I
Immune complex disease	Type III
ABO transfusion reactions	Type II
Delayed-type hyper-sensitivity	Type IV
The Arthus reaction	Type III
Immediate sensitivity	Type I

Name the correct immuno-deficiency for each of the following.

The most common	IgA deficiency
Associated with lack of a thymus	DiGeorge syndrome
Caused by lack of adenosine deaminase	Recessive form of SCID
Associated with endocrinopathies	Chronic mucocutaneous candidiasis
Associated with hypoparathyroidism	DiGeorge syndrome and chronic mucocutaneous candidiasis
A defect in IL-2 receptor gene	X-linked form of SCID
Also X-linked	Bruton agammaglobulinemia
Associated with celiac sprue	Isolated IgA deficiency and CVID

Successfully treated with gene therapy	SCID
Selectively lacking circulating mature B-cells	Bruton agammaglobulinemia
Without adequate antibody despite normal mature B numbers	CVID
Name some immunodeficiencies resulting from phagocytic defects.	Chronic granulomatous disease, myeloperoxidase deficiency, Chédiak-Higashi syndrome

7

Transplant Pathology

INTRODUCTION

Define the following.

Allograft	A graft from another member of the same species
Xenograft	A graft from another species
Autograft	A graft from the same individual (e.g., autologous bone marrow transplant)
Syngeneic graft	A graft from a genetically identical individual (e.g., monozygous twin)

What 2 important pathologic reactions can occur with transplantation?

1. Rejection
2. Graft versus host (GVH) disease

For which organ is ischemic time most critical?

Heart

For which solid organ is ischemic time least critical?

Kidney

Which is the most recently developed transplant?

Lung

Which organ is probably most susceptible to infection?

Lung

What cytokine is most important in lymphocyte proliferation and rejection?

Interleukin-2 (IL-2)

What cytokine induces greater MHC expression in the graft?

Interferon (IFN)-γ

HLA AND THE MHC

What is the HLA system?

The human leukocyte antigens (HLA) are the very polymorphous major histo-compatibility complex (MHC) markers integral in immune action and graft immunogenicity.

Where are the HLA genes located?

The short arm of chromosome 6

How are they organized?

The class I MHC, expressed on most cells and presenting antigen to CD8+ cytotoxic T lymphocytes, have 3 loci named A, B, and C each with many phenotypes. Class II, on B cells and antigen presenting cells (APCs), present antigen to CD4+ helper T cells.

What is the maximum number of MHC proteins a person can express?

12, including an A, B, C, DP, DR, and DQ from each parent

What is the structure of class I?

A transmembrane protein non-covalently associated with the shorter β-2-microglobulin protein

Class II?

Two non-covalently linked trans-membrane peptides

What CD molecule is associated with both?

CD3

What is Class III?

Genes for C2, C4, TNF-α, and factor B complement components

REJECTION

What are the 4 general categories of rejection of a graft or transplant?

1. Hyperacute rejection
2. Acute cellular rejection
3. Acute vascular rejection
4. Chronic rejection

HYPERACUTE REJECTION

What is it?

Reaction of donor tissue with preformed recipient antibodies

What type of hypersensitivity is it?	Type II
When does it typically occur?	Within the first 72 hours
What are the mechanisms of antibody damage?	Complement-mediated and antibody-dependent cell-mediated toxicity
How can antibody damage be avoided?	By crossmatch of donor lymphocytes and recipient serum prior to transplant
What is this crossmatch called?	Mixed lymphocyte reaction

ACUTE CELLULAR REJECTION

What is it?	Primarily T-cell mediated cytotoxic damage
What is seen microscopically?	Mononuclear infiltrate, primarily lymphocytic. With recruited macrophages, neutrophils and plasma cells are also seen.
From the picture, how does one determine severity?	By the density of the infiltrate and extent of parenchymal damage

ACUTE VASCULAR REJECTION

What is it?	Rejection targeted primarily at the vasculature of the graft
What are the 3 general stages?	1. Early 2. Intermediate 3. Severe
What type of immunity is causal in acute vascular rejection?	Both cell-mediated and humoral immunity
What are the pathologic changes in each stage?	
Early	Subendothelial inflammation and hypertrophy of endothelium
Intermediate	Moderate intimal proliferation with more significant wall inflammation

Severe	Significant fibrinoid necrosis and intimal proliferation

CHRONIC REJECTION

What is the dominant pathologic feature?	Fibrosis
What is the progression?	Chronic humoral or cellular rejection leads to increasing intimal fibrosis and micro-ischemia.

GRAFT VERSUS HOST (GVH) DISEASE

What is graft versus host disease?	An immune reaction of the host against a graft (e.g., organ)
In what 2 phases may GVH characteristically occur?	Acute or chronic phase
What 3 organs are prominently involved?	1. Liver 2. Intestines 3. Skin
In what type of transplant is GVH the greatest problem?	Bone marrow transplant (allogeneic)
Which solid organ transplant is most likely to cause problems with GVH, and why?	Lung, because of donor lymphoid tissue present in the graft
In what type of transplant can GVH be clinically helpful, and why?	In bone marrow transplant for malignancy; the graft versus tumor effect is therapeutic.

ACUTE GVH DISEASE

What organs show signs first?	Skin and GI tract
What condition do GI findings resemble?	Chemotherapy or radiation ileitis or colitis
What are the microscopic upper GI findings?	Individual cell necrosis in the stomach and small bowel

What are the microscopic colon findings?	Crypt cell necrosis progressing from individual cells to abscesses and, eventually, epithelial denudation
How is the skin involvement classified?	Grade I through IV

What are the findings of each stage?

Grade I	Dermal perivascular lymphocytic infiltrate also invading epidermis with basal cell vacuolation
Grade II	Occasional apoptotic keratinocytes
Grade III	Significant keratinocyte necrosis and basal layer damage
Grade IV	Bullae form and there is dermal-epidermal clefting.
Clinical laboratory findings with liver involvement?	Cholestatic picture with transaminase elevation
Histopathologic findings?	Cholestasis, some hepatocyte necrosis, and lymphocytic infiltrate within ducts showing cytoplasmic swelling, vacuolation and nuclear loss

CHRONIC GVH DISEASE

What is the general histologic change?	Loss of parenchymal structures
When does it occur?	Over 100 days post-transplant
Where does it strike cutaneously?	May be localized or generalized
What findings are typical?	Atrophied epidermis over prominent dermal fibrosis
Of what disease are the changes reminiscent?	Scleroderma
What are the histopathological stomach and intestine findings?	Fibrosis of serosa, submucosa, and lamina propria along with hyalinized vasculature

What is a typical finding in the esophagus?	A desquamative esophagitis
What hepatic microscopic findings are present?	Marked "bile duct drop-out," portal tract fibrosis, and cholestasis

RENAL TRANSPLANTS

What are the 3 modalities of renal transplants?	1. Living related donor 2. Living unrelated donor 3. Cadaveric transplants
What clinical indicator is used to follow possible rejection?	Plasma creatinine (as indicator of CrCl)
What type of rejection occurs most often?	Acute cellular rejection
What complication frequently occurs immediately post-transplant?	Primary nonfunction of the graft
How frequently does it occur and how long does it last?	It occurs in about one third of cases and the anuric period varies greatly.
What is the usual cause?	Harvest injury
What are other possible causes (differential diagnoses) of primary non-function?	Acute tubular necrosis (ATN), hyperacute rejection, infection, thrombosis, thrombotic angiopathy, pre- or post-renal state, or preexisting disease
Microscopic findings of harvest injury?	Tubular dilatation, epithelial vacuolation, or necrosis
What is the frequency of occurrence of harvest injury?	About 50% of cases show some signs
What are 2 possible causes?	Graft cold ischemic time and/or relevant intra-donor insults
In a failed transplant, what else must be considered in the differential with rejection?	Glomerulonephritis, recurrent disease, or cyclosporine (CSA) toxicity

GLOMERULONEPHRITIS

How frequently does primary glomerulonephritis occur?

Quite rarely

What are the most common causes?

1. Acute serum sickness
2. Membranous glomerulopathy
3. Anti-glomerular basement membrane (GBM) disease

RECURRENT DISEASE

How often does recurrent disease occur, and when?

Only in 2%-3% of cases, usually > 6 months post-transplant

How often does recurrent disease lead to graft loss?

About 50% of the time

How often is there (clinically silent) pathology in the donor kidney?

There are positive findings about 40% of the time and specific pathology in 15%.

CYCLOSPORINE (CSA) TOXICITY

What are the 4 different categories of CSA toxicity?

1. Tubular
2. Functional
3. Acute vascular-interstitial
4. Chronic vascular-interstitial

What are the mechanistic/ pathologic characteristics of each of the following.

Tubular toxicity

Epithelial damage is evident with isometric tubular vacuolation, prominent lysosomes, mitochondrial enlargement and calcification.

Functional toxicity

GFR and RPF are decreased without major pathologic changes.

Acute vascular-interstitial toxicity

Usually occurs soon after transplant; features are reminiscent of hemolytic uremic syndrome (HUS) (e.g., capillary occlusion by fibrin thrombi).

Chronic vascular toxicity

Slow decline of renal function and

	increasing hypertension, usually after many months of CSA
Microscopic findings of CSA toxicity?	Sclerosis of glomeruli and arterioles with some interstitial fibrosis, tubular atrophy, and fibrinoid arteriopathy
What must chronic vascular toxicity be distinguished from?	Hypertensive or diabetic arteriopathy

HYPERACUTE REJECTION

What is the time course and mechanism?	Usually occurs in first 72 hours due to preformed antibody
What are the microscopic findings?	Edema, interstitial hemorrhage, vascular damage and thrombosis, and capillary neutrophilia

ACUTE CELLULAR REJECTION

When does it usually occur?	In the first 3 months
What are the histopathological findings?	Interstitial and peritubular infiltrate (tubulitis) of neutrophils, monocytes, and lymphocytes. Occasional lymphocytic glomerulitis is seen as well.
How is it classified?	Graded as mild, moderate or severe
What is the prognosis?	It is usually responsive to immunosuppression.

ACUTE VASCULAR REJECTION

What is the mechanism?	Cellular and/or antibody-mediated damage
What is the time course?	Usually in the first 3 months
What is the prognosis?	Poor when rejection is moderate or severe because it is not well responsive to immunosuppression
What other conditions are associated?	Intravascular or glomerular immunoglobulin/complement deposits

How is it classified pathologically?	Mild (grade 1), moderate (grade 2), and severe (grade 3)

What are the histopathological characteristics of each stage?

Mild (grade 1)	Subintimal inflammatory infiltrate and endothelial hypertrophy
Moderate (grade 2)	More hypertrophy and mononuclear infiltrate with perivascular fibrinoid necrosis and occasional interstitial hemorrhage
Severe (grade 3)	More extensive grade 2 lesions

CHRONIC REJECTION

What is the overall histopathologic theme?	Fibrosis of various areas
What are the microscopic glomerular findings?	General sclerosis with capillary loops thickened and infiltrated by mesangium
What are these findings called?	Post-transplant glomerulopathy
What are the vascular microscopic findings?	Medial thickening and intimal fibrosis
What are the interstitial microscopic findings?	Tubular atrophy, membrane thickening, and fibrosis
What is the prognosis?	Poor

LIVER TRANSPLANTS

What are diseases that commonly lead to transplant?	Hepatitis B, C, hepatitis B/hepatitis D, primary biliary cholangitis, primary sclerosing cholangitis, and autoimmune hepatitis
Which of these are most likely to recur?	The hepatitis viruses
What is the differential diagnosis for cholestasis in a liver graft?	Functional cholestasis, anastomotic insufficiency, intrahepatic duct, and parenchymal ischemia

What is thought to be the cause of functional cholestasis?	"Harvest injury" from cold ischemia
How long does it typically last?	2–3 weeks post-transplant
What are the microscopic findings?	Hepatocellular edema and lobular cholestasis without inflammation

VASCULAR OCCLUSION

Which vessels are affected?	Can be the arteries or veins
When is it most likely to occur?	Initial occurrence is 2 months post-transplant
What is found microscopically in arterial occlusion?	Centrilobular necrosis
What is occlusion of the hepatic vein called?	Budd-Chiari syndrome
What is seen microscopically in venous occlusion?	Centrilobular hemorrhage

REJECTION

What type of acute rejection is most typical?	Cellular-mediated rejection
How is it characterized histopathologically?	A periportal inflammation or "ductitis" primarily of lymphocytes and eosinophils
How does chronic rejection often appear clinically?	Increased LFTs and hyperbilirubinemia (jaundice)
What is seen histopathologically?	Progressive loss of bile ducts (ductopenia) and microvascular narrowing from sub-intimal foam cells

BONE MARROW TRANSPLANT (BMT)

For what types of diseases is BMT used as therapy?	Malignancy, marrow aplasia, and dysfunctional marrow elements (e.g., sickle cell anemia)
What are the 2 most important complications?	1. GVH disease 2. Infection

What is seen in BMT rejection?	Disappearing marrow elements
What other nonspecific changes are seen micro-scopically?	Edema, hemorrhage, fat necrosis, micro-granulomas, and plasma cell/lymphocyte proliferation
How long does bone marrow reconstitution take post-transplant?	3–4 weeks in allogeneic BMT, slightly longer in autologous BMT
How can it be followed?	By microscopic observation

What are the characteristic findings of reconstitution at the following points of time?

1 week post-transplant	Isolated myelo- and erythroblasts
2 weeks post-transplant	Some precursors of all 3 lineages present, often with temporary dysplastic signs within erythroid line
3–4 weeks post-transplant	Precursor cells have reconstituted
What other temporary abnormalities are present?	Granulocyte abnormalities, including vacuolation, degranulation, and pseudo-Pelger-Huët nucleic anomaly
What percent of allogeneic BMT patients develop GVH disease?	33%–66%
What system is most often affected?	GI tract
What are the typical symptoms?	Abdominal pain, ileus, diarrhea, dyspepsia, nausea, and vomiting

HEART TRANSPLANTATION

What findings suggest ischemic injury (harvest injury)?	Substantial inflammation and necrobiosis of myocytes
How is rejection diagnosed?	Decreased function (i.e., ejection fraction) can suggest rejection clinically, but biopsy is diagnostic.

What are the characteristic findings?	Geographic necrosis with granulation tissue
What can complicate repeated biopsies?	"Prior biopsy effect" (i.e., altered tissue secondary to scarring)
What is the "quilty effect"?	A subendocardial lymphocytic infiltrate
With what is it associated?	The etiology is unknown; Epstein-Barr virus (EBV), early posttransplantation lymphoproliferative disorder (PTLD), and cyclosporine (CSA) toxicity are postulated.

REJECTION

How is acute cellular rejection characterized?	Mild, moderate, or severe
What are the characteristics of each?	
Mild	Some interstitial and perivascular lymphoid infiltrate but no myocyte destruction
Moderate	More significant infiltrates and some local myocyte destruction
Severe	Dense infiltrate also including granulocytes and extensive myocyte death
What are the specific signs of chronic rejection?	Variable fibrosis leading to coronary artery sclerosis and lipid-filled macrophage accumulation
What is another name given to this process?	Accelerated atherosclerosis
How soon does it begin to occur?	Usually 1–2 years post-transplant

LUNG TRANSPLANTS

What are the 3 operative options for lung transplant?	A heart-lung, single lung, or double lung transplant

What additional specific findings may accompany rejection of a lung transplant?	Lymphocytic bronchitis or bronchiolitis
From what condition must these be distinguished?	Obliterative bronchiolitis
What is obliterative bronchiolitis?	A progressive fibrosis of the bronchioles
What are the histopathologic findings of obliterative bronchiolitis?	Concentric, obliterative, or eccentric fibrosis of the airway submucosa
How is obliterative bronchiolitis characterized?	Active (with inflammation) or inactive (without)
What is the differential diagnosis of obliterative bronchiolitis?	Rejection, GVH disease, airway ischemia, or infection

REJECTION

How is acute rejection of a lung transplant classified?	Minimal, mild, moderate, or severe
What are the characteristics of each?	
Minimal acute rejection	Perivascular infiltrate of macrophages, lymphocytes and plasma cells visible under moderate magnification.
Mild acute rejection	More common, larger, perivascular infiltrates also including granulocytes
Moderate acute rejection	Still more neutrophilic infiltrate, also including alveolar spaces and septae
Severe acute rejection	Coalescing inflammation of interstitium and alveoli with some necrosis and hemorrhage
What are the typical histopathologic findings of chronic rejection of a lung transplant?	Intimal fibrosis leading to occlusion of the graft microvasculature

With what other complication of organ transplant do these changes correlate clinically?	Accelerated atherosclerosis in heart graft

IMMUNOCOMPROMISED INFECTIONS

What viruses are most often problematic?	HSV, CMV, HIV, and EBV
Name 2 common fungal infectious agents.	1. *Candida* 2. *Aspergillus*
Name some important parasitic agents.	Toxoplasmosis, *Pneumocystis carinii, Giardia, and* Coccidia
With what problem is EBV associated?	Post-transplant lymphoproliferative disorder (PTLD)
How should positive HIV status be viewed pre-transplant?	It usually is an absolute contraindication for harvest or receipt of an organ.

CYTOMEGALOVIRUS (CMV)

When is this infection most common?	Within the first few months post transplant
What organs are most often involved?	Lungs and GI tract (although nearly any may be involved)
What are the microscopic findings?	Enlarged cells with cytoplasmic and nuclear inclusions
What can be done diagnostically in the lab?	Immunohistochemistry or in situ hybridization for viral antigens or DNA
What patient type is particularly susceptible?	A previously seronegative recipient

HERPES SIMPLEX VIRUS (HSV)

What is the location?	Can be disseminated or localized
What organs or sites are involved?	May involve mucocutaneous surfaces, eyes, esophagus, CNS, and lungs
Characteristic microscopic findings?	Cowdry type A intranuclear inclusions and polykaryon nuclei

CANDIDAL INFECTION

When is candidal infection significant?	Quite often—it is frequently the first sign of an immunosuppressed individual.
What is the location?	It may be disseminated or local in various organs.
What are the microscopic findings?	Yeast and pseudohyphae invading tissue seen on silver stain

ASPERGILLOSIS

Where is *Aspergillosis* most significant?	In lung transplant recipients, particularly at anastomotic junctions
What complication may this cause?	Anastomotic graft dehiscence
What complication may result from parenchymal invasion?	Hematogenous dissemination

PARASITIC INFECTIONS

In what type of transplant is *Toxoplasma* most significant?	Heart
How does *Pneumocystis carinii* typically present?	As pneumonitis in significantly immuno-compromised patients
How can it be diagnosed definitively?	Lung biopsy
What are the microscopic findings?	Foamy alveolar exudate and cysts that stain black with methenamine silver
Where do *Giardia* and *Coccidia* frequently present?	With GI infection in BMT recipients

POST-TRANSPLANT LYMPHOPROLIFERATIVE DISORDERS (PTLDS)

How frequently do such disorders occur?	In 1%–2% of transplants
What cell type is usually involved?	B cells

What infection is typically associated?	Primary or reactivated EBV infection
What is the mechanism?	Lack of cell mediated immunity and lymphoproliferative EBV effect
What are the 2 types?	Monomorphous and polymorphous PTLD
Which is more severe?	Monomorphous PTLD has a poorer prognosis
What are the characteristics of polymorphous PTLD?	Heterogeneous B-cell populations of immunoblasts, lymphocytes, and plasma cells
What is the treatment and how does it work?	Decreased immunosuppression usually re-establishes immune surveillance and EBV control
What is the pathophysiology of monomorphous PTLD?	B-cell malignancy evolves out of the EBV-stimulated growth.
What neoplasm does the growth resemble?	Large cell lymphoma

POWER REVIEW

What chromosome are HLA loci located on?	6
How many HLA proteins does an individual usually express?	12
What are the names/MHC associations of the loci?	Class I: A, B, C Class II: DP, DR, DQ
Which MHC is associated with β-2 microglobulin?	Class I
Which is associated with CD3?	Both
Which binds helper T cells?	Class II
Which is primarily used by antigen-presenting cells?	Class II

Identify the type of organ transplant described.

Most likely to lead to graft versus host (GVH) disease	Bone marrow transplant
A solid organ with frequent GVHD on transplant	Lung
Most sensitive to *Toxoplasma*	Heart
Most prone to immuno-compromise	Bone marrow transplant
Aspergillus particularly problematic	Lung
Most sensitive to ischemic time	Heart
A solid organ, easiest to assess clinically for rejection	Kidney

How quickly will a bone marrow transplant typically repopulate the marrow?	3–4 weeks if allogenic, a little longer for autologous
What is seen in bone marrow transplant rejection?	Decreasing marrow elements
What organs are most affected in GVHD?	Skin, gut, and liver
What are the characteristics of chronic GVHD?	Parenchymal damage to affected organs >100 days post-transplant
What are the types of organ rejection?	Hyperacute, acute vascular, acute cellular, and chronic

What type of rejection corresponds to each of the following?

Fibrosis as pathologic feature?	Chronic rejection

Primarily T-cell mediated?	Acute cellular rejection
A form of immediate hypersensitivity?	Hyperacute rejection
Primarily lymphocytic infiltrate?	Acute cellular rejection
Humoral and cell-mediated immunity?	Acute vascular rejection
Most likely to form by day 3 post-transplant?	Hyperacute rejection
Causes damage from microvascular occlusion/ ischemia?	Chronic rejection
Obviated by pre-operative mixed lympho-cyte reaction?	Hyperacute rejection
Subendothelial prolifer-ation and endothelial hypertrophy?	Acute vascular rejection
What are the microscopic findings of HSV?	Polykaryon nuclei and Cowdry type A inclusions
How is *Pneumocystis carinii* pneumonia definitively diagnosed?	Lung biopsy
How is it diagnosed micro-scopically?	Foamy alveolar exudate and black cysts stained with methenamine silver
How is *Candida* recognized microscopically?	Pseudohyphae and yeast seen on silver stain
What is the frequency of post-transplant lympho-proliferative disorder?	1%–2% of transplants
What virus is associated with this disorder?	Epstein-Barr virus (EBV)
What is the originating cell type and the neoplasm it resembles?	B-cell, large cell lymphoma

8

Genetic Disorders

INTRODUCTION

How many chromosomes are contained in diploid cells?	46
What is aneuploidy?	A chromosome number that is not a multiple of 23
Name 2 causes of aneuploidy.	1. Nondisjunction 2. Anaphase lag
What is the most common cause of aneuploidy?	Meiotic nondisjunction
What is mosaicism?	2 cell lines in 1 individual
What is the usual result of polyploidy?	Spontaneous abortion
How many chromosomes are contained in tetraploid cells?	92
What is a chromosome inversion?	Reunion of a chromosome broken at two points, with the internal fragment reinserted in an inverted position
What term denotes exchange of chromosomal segments between non-homologous chromosomes?	Translocation
Describe the difference between reciprocal translocation and Robertsonian translocation.	Reciprocal translocation is a break in two chromosomes leading to an exchange of chromosomal material. No genetic material is lost, so it is often clinically silent. Robertsonian translocation is the joining of the long arms of two acrocentric chromosomes with a common centromere. The short arms are lost.

What is isochromosome formation?	The transverse division of 1 chromosome results in 2 new chromosomes, or 2 isochromes, each of which consists of 2 long arms or 2 short arms. Often, 1 of the 2 isochromosomes (usually short arm) is lost.
What is lyonization?	The process by which one X chromosome in each cell is randomly inactivated at an early stage of embryonic development
What is a Barr body?	A clump of chromatin in the interphase nuclei of all somatic cells in females, representing one inactivated X chromosome
What 2 groups lack Barr bodies?	1. Normal males (XY) 2. Individuals with Turner syndrome (XO)
How many Barr bodies does an XXX individual have?	2
Why are all normal females mosaics?	Females have 2 distinct cell lines, 1 with an active maternal X and 1 with an active paternal X.
Give 2 reasons why extreme karyotype deviations in the sex chromosomes are compatible with life.	1. X chromosomes may undergo lyonization 2. Y chromosomes carry minimal genetic information
What is the incidence of congenital anomalies?	2%
Genetic disorders account for what percentage of congenital anomalies?	25%

CHROMOSOMAL DISORDERS

ABNORMALITIES OF AUTOSOMAL CHROMOSOMES

What is the most frequently occurring chromosomal disorder?	Down syndrome

Down syndrome

What percentage of cases of Down syndrome are due to trisomy 21?	95%
What is the usual cause of this condition?	Maternal meiotic nondisjunction
What is the major risk factor for Down syndrome?	Increasing maternal age
What causes the familial form of this disorder?	Translocation between chromosome 21 and another chromosome. The fertilized ovum contains 3 copies of the chromosome 21 material. This accounts for 3%—5% of cases.
Does the familial form of Down syndrome have any relation to maternal age?	No
What is the usual translocation in Down syndrome?	14q;21q
What is the chance of a woman in her mid-30s having a child with Down syndrome?	1 in 1000
What is the chance of a woman older than 45 years having a child with Down syndrome?	1 in 30

Name the clinical manifestations of Down syndrome in the following categories:

Intelligence	Mental retardation
Face	Epicanthal folds; large forehead; broad nasal bridge; wide-spaced, upward slanting eyes; protruding tongue; small low-set ears; and Brushfield spots (speckled iris)
Extremities	Short, broad hands with curvature of the 5th finger; single palmar crease; and wide space between the 1st and 2nd toes

Body proportions	Microcephaly, short stature, flat occiput, and increased skin on the back of the neck
Muscles	Hypotonia
Name some complications of Down syndrome.	**Congenital heart disease—related (33%):** atrioventricular (AV) canal, ventral septal defect (VSD), atrial septal defect (ASD), patent ductus arteriosus (PDA), and tetralogy of Fallot **Other:** acute leukemia (20-fold increased risk), increased susceptibility to infection, atlantoaxial instability, early-onset Alzheimer disease, and gastrointestinal (GI) abnormalities (e.g., duodenal atresia or stenosis, imperforate anus, Hirschsprung disease)

Fragile X syndrome

What cytogenetic defect is characteristic of this syndrome?	A defect in the long arm of the X chromosome, leading to chromosome breakage in vitro
What genital abnormality is seen in males with fragile X syndrome?	Macro-orchidism
What is the most common clinical manifestation of this condition?	Mental retardation
Name 4 other clinical features associated with this disorder.	1. Increased head circumference 2. Facial coarsening 3. Joint hyperextensibility 4. Abnormalities of the cardiac valves

Cri du chat syndrome

What is cri du chat syndrome?	A disorder characterized by partial loss of the short arm of chromosome 5
Name some clinical manifestations of this condition in the following categories:	
Intelligence:	Severe mental retardation

Face:	Round face, hypertelorism, low-set ears, and epicanthal folds
Extremities:	Short hands and feet and transverse palmar crease
Gross features:	Microcephaly, unusual cat-like cry, and low birth weight
Cardiovascular:	Congenital heart disease

Edwards syndrome

What is Edwards syndrome?   A chromosomal abnormality caused by trisomy 18

What is the most frequent cause of this disorder?   Maternal meiotic nondisjunction

Name some clinical features of this disorder.
Intelligence: mental retardation
Face: prominent occiput, micrognathia, and low-set ears
Extremities: rocker-bottom feet and index finger overlapping 3rd and 4th fingers
Other: congenital heart disease and horseshoe kidney

Patau syndrome

What is the chromosomal abnormality involved?   Trisomy 13

Name some clinical characteristics of Patau syndrome.
Intelligence: mental retardation
Head: microcephaly, microphthalmia, cleft lip and palate, and brain abnormalities
Extremities: polydactyly and rocker-bottom feet
Other: congenital heart disease and polycystic kidneys

ABNORMALITIES OF SEX CHROMOSOMES

What is the name of the disorder characterized by a 47,XXY karyotype?   Klinefelter syndrome

What is the most frequent cause of Klinefelter syndrome?   Maternal meiotic nondisjunction

Name the clinical characteristics of Klinefelter syndrome in the following categories:

    Genitourinary: Atrophic testes with decreased testosterone production and infertility, and female escutcheon

    Intelligence: Mild mental retardation (extent correlates with number of X chromosomes)

    Other: Gynecomastia, tall stature, and high-pitched voice

When is the diagnosis of Klinefelter syndrome usually made?

At puberty

Why are persons with Klinefelter syndrome tall?

As a result of delayed fusion of the physeal plate

What are the 3 clinical manifestations of XYY syndrome?

1. Tall stature
2. Severe acne
3. Mild mental retardation

What percentage of persons with XYY syndrome display antisocial behavior?

2%

What is the most common cause of primary amenorrhea?

Turner syndrome

What is the most common karyotype in Turner syndrome?

45,XO

What is the most striking clinical change in Turner syndrome?

Female hypogonadism

Name the clinical features of Turner syndrome in the following categories:

    Genitourinary: Replacement of the ovaries by fibrous streaks, resulting in decreased estrogen production; infantile genitalia; and lack of secondary sex development

Body:	Short stature, webbed neck, low hairline, shield-like chest, wide carrying angle of the arms, and lymphedema of the neck and extremities
Other:	Coarctation of the aorta, horseshoe kidney, defective vision and hearing, increased risk of thyroid disease, and multiple pigmented nevi
What is the pattern of mental retardation in persons with multi-X chromosome abnormalities?	The degree of retardation increases with the number of additional X chromosomes.
What clinical abnormalities are associated with the XXX karyotype and other multi-X syndromes?	Usually no associated conditions are present, except for occasional mild mental retardation or menstrual irregularities.

INHERITED DISORDERS

MODES OF INHERITANCE

Which type of inheritance is characterized by equal distribution of the phenotype in both sexes and a 50% chance of inheriting the gene?	Autosomal dominant
In autosomal recessive inheritance, what percentage of the offspring will phenotypically manifest the disorder?	25%
In autosomal recessive inheritance, what percentage of offspring will inherit the gene?	75%
Which type of inheritance pattern is characterized by a lack of male-to-male transmission?	X-linked inheritance

If the female parent is a heterozygous carrier for an X-linked recessive trait and the male parent is genotypically normal, what are the 4 possible outcomes?	1. Heterozygous female carrier 2. Affected male 3. Normal male 4. Normal female
Tell how X-linked dominant inheritance differs from X-linked recessive inheritance.	Heterozygous females and hemizygous males phenotypically manifest X-linked dominant disorders. (Only males phenotypically manifest X-linked recessive traits.)
What is unique about mitochondrial inheritance?	Transmission is exclusively maternal.

AUTOSOMAL DOMINANT DISORDERS

What is the most frequently occurring hereditary renal disorder?	Adult polycystic kidney disease
What is the pathophysiology of adult polycystic kidney disease?	Numerous bilateral cysts replace and ultimately destroy renal parenchyma.
At what age does adult polycystic kidney disease become manifested clinically?	30–50 years
What is the genetic defect in familial hypercholesterolemia?	Anomaly of low-density lipoprotein (LDL) receptor
How does an abnormal LDL receptor cause problems?	Decreased transport of LDL cholesterol into cells causes hypercholesterolemia and increased incidence of atherosclerosis.
What are the raised yellow lesions filled with lipid-laden macrophages seen in the skin and tendons?	Xanthomas
What is the rare disorder characterized by telangiectasias of the skin and mucous membranes, which appears with increased frequency in Mormons in Utah?	Hereditary hemorrhagic telangiectasia (Osler-Weber-Rendu syndrome)

What is hereditary spherocytosis?

Presence of spheroidal erythrocytes. The erythrocytes are sequestered and destroyed in the spleen, resulting in hemolytic anemia.

Where is the chromosomal defect in Huntington disease?

4p

What is the pathophysiology of Huntington disease?

Progressive degeneration and atrophy of the caudate nuclei, putamen, and frontal cortex occurs.

What is the typical age of onset of Huntington disease?

30–40 years

Name 3 clinical manifestations of Huntington disease.

1. Progressive dementia
2. Extrapyramidal or choreiform movements
3. Emotional disturbances

What test can diagnose Huntington disease before symptoms appear?

Restriction fragment length polymorphism

What disorder is caused by a defect in connective tissue due to deficient fibrillin, a glycoprotein constituent of microfibrils?

Marfan syndrome

What are the clinical manifestations of Marfan syndrome?

Musculoskeletal

Tall stature, thin body habitus, abnormally long legs and arms, arachnodactyly, and hyperextensible joints

Ocular

Dislocation of the ocular lens (ectopia lentis)

Vascular

Aneurysm of the proximal aorta, aortic valvular insufficiency, risk of dissecting aortic aneurysm, and mitral valve prolapse

What is a Lisch nodule?

Pigmented iris hamartoma

What is the phenotypic expression of neurofibromatosis (von Recklinghausen disease)?

Multiple neurofibromas; café au lait spots; Lisch nodules; skeletal disorders (e.g., scoliosis, bone cysts); and increased incidence of other tumors (e.g., pheochromocytoma, Wilms tumor, rhabdomyosarcoma, leukemia)

What is a neurofibroma?

A benign tumor of peripheral nerve of Schwann cell origin

What are the characteristics of type II neurofibromatosis?

Bilateral acoustic neuromas, which may be accompanied by meningiomas, gliomas, schwannomas, neurofibromas, or juvenile posterior lenticular opacity

Where are the genetic defects in neurofibromatosis types I and II?

Type I: chromosome 17
Type II: chromosome 22

What pathologic lesions are seen in the cerebral cortex in tuberous sclerosis?

Glial nodules and distorted neurons

What are 3 common clinical manifestations of tuberous sclerosis?

1. Mental retardation
2. Seizures
3. Adenoma sebaceum

What tumors are associated with tuberous sclerosis?

Hamartomas of the brain, retina, and viscera
Rhabdomyomas of the heart
Renal angiomyolipomas

What are the characteristics of von Hippel-Lindau disease?

Hemangioblastoma or cavernous hemangioma of the cerebellum, brainstem, or retina
Adenomas
Cysts of the liver, kidney, pancreas, and other organs

What type of cancer has a marked increased incidence in von Hippel-Lindau disease?

Renal cell carcinoma

What is the defective gene in von Hippel-Lindau disease?

Chromosome 3p

AUTOSOMAL RECESSIVE DISORDERS

What are lysosomal storage diseases?	Disorders characterized by deficiency of a specific single lysosomal enzyme, resulting in accumulation of abnormal metabolic products
Which disorder occurs primarily in descendants of Ashkenazi Jews?	Tay-Sachs disease
What enzyme is deficient in Tay-Sachs disease?	Hexosaminidase A
What accumulates in Tay-Sachs disease, causing central nervous system (CNS) degeneration?	G_{m2} ganglioside
What are the 3 clinical characteristics of Tay-Sachs?	1. Severe motor deterioration 2. Severe mental deterioration 3. Blindness
What ocular finding is seen in individuals with Tay-Sachs disease?	Cherry-red spot in the macula
What is the prognosis in Tay-Sachs disease?	Death before 4 years of age
Which autosomal disorder is characterized by a deficiency of glucocerebroside?	Gaucher disease
What is a Gaucher cell?	An enlarged histiocyte with a distinctive "wrinkled tissue paper" cytoplasmic appearance
Differentiate the 3 types of Gaucher disease.	1. Type I (adult): accounts for 80% of cases; characterized by hepatosplenomegaly, erosion of the femoral head and long bones, and mild anemia; possibly normal life span 2. Type II (infantile): marked by severe CNS involvement; death before 1 year of age 3. Type III (juvenile): less severe than type II; involvement of brain and

viscera; onset usually in early
childhood

What enzyme is deficient in Niemann-Pick disease?

Sphingomyelinase

What cells are seen in Niemann-Pick disease?

Foamy histiocytes that contain sphingomyelin

What are the 5 clinical manifestations in Niemann-Pick disease?

1. Hepatosplenomegaly
2. Anemia
3. Fever
4. Possible neurologic deterioration
5. Cherry-red spot in macula (50% of cases)

What is the prognosis in Niemann-Pick disease?

Death by 3 years of age

What is Hurler syndrome?

A mucopolysaccharidosis caused by a deficiency of α-L-iduronidase, resulting in accumulations of the mucopoly-saccharides heparan sulfate and dermatan sulfate in the heart, brain, liver, and other organs

What are the clinical features of Hurler syndrome?

Hepatosplenomegaly
Dwarfism
Gargoyle-like facies, stubby fingers, and
    corneal clouding
Progressive mental retardation

What is the prognosis in Hurler syndrome?

Death by 10 years of age

For the 4 primary glycogen storage diseases, name the deficient enzyme associated with each condition.

Von Gierke disease

Type 1 glycogenosis: glucose-6-phosphatase

Pompe disease

Type 2 glycogenosis: α-1,4-glucosidase

Cori disease

Type 3 glycogenosis: amylo-1,6-glucosidase

McArdle syndrome

Type 5 glycogenosis: muscle phosphorylase

Which glycogen storage disease that can also be classified as a lysosomal storage disease results in accumulation of glycogen in liver, heart, and skeletal muscle, causing cardiomegaly, muscle hypotonia, and splenomegaly?

Pompe disease

What causes death in Pompe disease?

Cardiorespiratory failure

Which glycogen storage disease produces painful muscle cramps and weakness following exercise?

McArdle syndrome

What are the consequences of von Gierke disease?

Accumulation of glycogen, primarily in the liver and kidney, causes hepatomegaly and hypoglycemia.

Which glycogen storage disease results from a deficient debranching enzyme and is characterized by stunted growth, hepatomegaly, and hypoglycemia?

Cori disease

What is the defect in classic galactosemia?

A deficiency of galactose 1-phosphate uridyltransferase, causing buildup of galactose-1-phosphate

What are 4 clinical manifestations of classic galactosemia?

1. Failure to thrive
2. Infantile cataracts
3. Mental retardation
4. Progressive hepatic failure, leading to cirrhosis and death

How might the symptoms of galactosemia be prevented?

Early removal of galactose from the diet

What is the other type of galactosemia?

Galactokinase-deficiency galactosemia, which is much less frequent than the classic form. This disorder often is marked only by infantile cataracts.

What disorder of amino acid metabolism is characterized by mental deterioration, seizures, hyperactivity, decreased pigmentation (i.e., blond hair and blue eyes), and mousy body odor?

Phenylketonuria (PKU)

What causes PKU?

A deficiency in phenylalanine hydroxylase, which leads to failure of conversion of phenylalanine to tyrosine in the liver

Why is a phenylalanine-free diet necessary in individuals with PKU?

High serum concentrations of phenylalanine are neurotoxic and cause progressive cerebral demyelination.

What metabolites are found in large amounts in the urine in children with PKU?

Phenylpyruvic acid and phenylacetic acid

What may be the consequences of PKU screening before the 3rd day of life?

False-negative results

What disorder results from a deficiency of homogentisic oxidase?

Alkaptonuria

What are the 4 clinical consequences of alkaptonuria?

1. Urine that turns black on standing
2. Ochronosis (dark pigmentation of fibrous tissues and cartilage)
3. Arthritis
4. Cardiac valvular disease

What is the most common lethal genetic disease in Caucasians?

Cystic fibrosis

What gene is mutated in cystic fibrosis?

The cystic fibrosis transmembrane conductance regulator (CFTR) gene codes for a membrane protein involved in transport of chloride and other ions across membranes.

On which chromosome is the CFTR gene located?

7q

What mutation accounts for 70% of cases of cystic fibrosis?	Delta 508
What is the carrier frequency of the CFTR gene in Caucasians?	1 in 25
Describe the mechanism of disease causation in cystic fibrosis.	Defective transport of chloride and other ions across cell membranes results in an inability to hydrate secretions so that they are abnormally viscous.
What are the clinical manifestations of cystic fibrosis?	**Pulmonary:** chronic pulmonary disease, with severe chronic bronchitis; bronchiectasis; and lung abscesses **GI:** chronic pancreatitis, pancreatic insufficiency, meconium ileus, and secondary biliary cirrhosis **Genitourinary:** sterility
What test is used to detect the presence of cystic fibrosis?	The sweat chloride test
How does the sweat chloride test work?	It detects increased sodium and chloride concentrations in sweat, which are due to impaired reabsorption by sweat ducts.

X-LINKED RECESSIVE DISORDERS

What is Hunter syndrome?	A lysosomal storage disease caused by a deficiency of L-iduronosulfate sulfatase, resulting in accumulations of heparan sulfate and dermatan sulfate
What are some clinical characteristics of Hunter syndrome?	Hepatosplenomegaly, micrognathia, retinal degeneration, joint stiffness, mild mental retardation, and cardiac lesions
What lysosomal storage disease results from α-galactosidase A deficiency?	Fabry disease
What substance accumulates in Fabry disease?	Ceramide trihexoside
What skin lesion is characteristic of Fabry disease?	Angiokeratoma (over the lower trunk)

What other clinical features are seen in Fabry disease?

Febrile episodes, severe burning pain in the extremities, multiple cardiac anomalies, and cerebrovascular accidents

What is the cause of death in Fabry disease?

Renal failure

What is the mutated gene and resultant deficient protein in hemophilia A (classic hemophilia)?

Mutation of the F8 gene on the tip of Xq leads to a deficiency of coagulation factor VIII.

What 4 problems do individuals with hemophilia encounter?

1. Hemorrhage from minor wounds and trauma
2. Bleeding from oral mucosa
3. Hematuria
4. Hemarthroses

Which X-linked recessive disorder is caused by a deficiency of hypoxanthine—guanine phosphoribosyl-transferase?

Lesch-Nyhan syndrome

What metabolic pathway is impaired in Lesch-Nyhan syndrome?

Purine metabolism, resulting in excess uric acid production

What are the clinical manifestations of Lesch-Nyhan syndrome?

Gout, mental retardation, choreoathe-tosis, spasticity, self-mutilation, and aggressive behavior

What enzyme deficiency is characteristic of Duchenne muscular dystrophy?

Dystrophin

What is the clinical course of Duchenne muscular dystrophy?

Weakness around the pelvic and shoulder girdles becomes evident about 3—4 years of age, and this condition progresses, making patients wheelchair-bound by 10 years. They are usually bedridden by 15 years of age and die from respiratory insufficiency or cardiac arrhythmia.

What causes pseudohyper-trophy of the calves?

Fibrofatty replacement of muscle tissue

What disorder predisposes individuals to episodes of hemolysis on exposure to certain medicines, infections, and fava beans?	Glucose-6-phosphate dehydrogenase (G6PD) deficiency
In which 3 populations is G6PD deficiency most common?	1. Kurdish Jews 2. West African blacks 3. Mediterranean populations
How does G6PD deficiency cause hemolysis?	Erythrocytes lacking G6PD are less resistant to oxidation, so hemoglobin denatures under stress and precipitates as Heinz bodies on the erythrocyte membrane. The red blood cells (RBCs) are then phagocytized in the spleen.

POLYGENIC DISORDERS

Describe the etiology of a polygenic disorder.	Polygenic disorders are caused by abnormalities regulated by two or more genes. Environmental factors are also involved in modulation of the genetic defects.
Name some medical conditions thought to be polygenic in origin.	
Cardiovascular:	Ischemic heart disease, hypertension, and congenital heart disease
Neurologic:	Schizophrenia and bipolar disorder
GI:	Pyloric stenosis and Hirschsprung disease
Developmental:	Neural tube defects and cleft lip and palate
Musculoskeletal:	Gout, ankylosing spondylitis, and congenital hip dislocation
Other:	Psoriasis, hypospadias, diabetes mellitus type II

DISORDERS OF SEXUAL DIFFERENTIATION

What determines genetic sex?	Presence or absence of a Y chromosome

What determines gonadal sex?	Presence of ovaries or testes. The gene responsible for development of testes (H-Y gene) is found on the Y chromosome.
What is a true hermaphrodite?	An individual who has both ovarian and testicular tissue with ambiguous external genitalia
What is a pseudohermaphrodite?	An individual who has gonads of one sex but ambiguous external genitalia
List 4 possible causes of pseudohermaphroditism in males.	1. Testicular feminization (tissue resistance to androgens) 2. Defects in testosterone synthesis 3. Maternal intake of hormones during pregnancy 4. Chromosomal abnormalities (46XY/45X mosaicism)
List 3 possible causes of pseudohermaphroditism in females.	1. Increased androgenic hormones from congenital adrenal hyperplasia 2. Androgen-secreting adrenal or ovarian tumor in the mother 3. Hormones administered to the mother during pregnancy

POWER REVIEW

What is the most common form of Down syndrome?	Trisomy 21
What is the most common cause of aneuploidy?	Meiotic nondisjunction
What is mosaicism?	2 cell lines in one individual
What is a Robertsonian translocation?	Joining of the long arms of two acrocentric chromosomes, with loss of the short arms
Define lyonization.	Process by which all X chromosomes but one are randomly inactivated early in embryonic development
What is the most common genotype of Turner syndrome?	45,XO

What is a Barr body?	Clump of chromatin representing one inactivated X chromosome
What leads to the familial form of Down syndrome?	Translocation involving chromosome 21
What genetic defect is responsible for cri du chat syndrome?	Deletion of short arm of chromosome 5
What chromosomal abnormality causes Edwards syndrome?	Trisomy 18
What chromosomal abnormality causes Patau syndrome?	Trisomy 13
What disorder is characterized by a 47,XXY karyotype?	Klinefelter syndrome
Describe the phenotypic characteristics of Klinefelter syndrome.	Atrophic testes, tall stature, gynecomastia, and mild mental retardation
What syndrome is characterized by replacement of ovaries by fibrous streaks?	Turner syndrome
What is the second most common genetic cause of mental retardation after Down syndrome?	Fragile X syndrome
What are the characteristics of Marfan syndrome?	Tall stature, slender build, abnormally long arms and legs, arachnodactyly, hyperextensible joints, ectopia lentis, mitral valve prolapse, and aneurysm of proximal aorta
What are the clinical manifestations of neurofibromatosis?	1. Café au lait spots 2. Multiple neurofibromas 3. Bone cysts 4. Scoliosis 5. Pigmented nodules in iris

Which autosomal dominant disorder is characterized by adenoma sebaceum, brain tubers, seizures, and mental retardation?	Tuberous sclerosis

What enzymes are deficient in the following autosomal recessive disorders?

Tay-Sachs disease	Hexosaminidase A
Gaucher disease	Glucocerebrosidase
Niemann-Pick disease	Sphingomyelinase
Hurler syndrome	α-L-iduronidase
Von Gierke disease	Glucose-6-phosphatase
Pompe disease	α-1,4-glucosidase
McArdle syndrome	Muscle phosphorylase
Galactosemia	Galactose 1-phosphate uridyltransferase
PKU	Phenylalanine hydroxylase
What is the most common lethal genetic disease in Caucasians?	Cystic fibrosis
What are 4 clinical manifestations of cystic fibrosis?	1. Chronic pulmonary disease 2. Pancreatic insufficiency 3. Meconium ileus 4. Cirrhosis
How does a mutation in the CFTR gene cause disease?	Abnormal transport of chloride and other electrolytes across cell membranes causes increased viscosity of mucus.
What is Hunter syndrome?	This X-linked recessive lysosomal storage disease results from a deficiency of L-iduronosulfate sulfatase. Heparan sulfate and dermatan sulfate accumulate.
What is missing in hemophilia A?	Factor VIII

What disorder results from deficient hypoxanthine—guanine phosphoribosyl-transferase?   Lesch-Nyhan syndrome

What type of inheritance is seen in Duchenne muscular dystrophy?   X-linked recessive

9   Environmental Pathology

What is environmental pathology?	The study of disease states resulting from environmental causes
What are the main categories of environmental factors?	Physical conditions, chemicals, drugs of abuse, air pollutants, and therapeutic drugs

PHYSICAL INJURY

Name 4 mechanisms of physical injury.	1. Mechanical injury 2. Thermal injury 3. Electric injury 4. Radiation injury

MECHANICAL INJURY

Name 5 terms that are used to describe mechanical injuries?	Abrasion, laceration, incision, puncture, and contusion

Define each:

Abrasion	Superficial loss of epidermal cells
Laceration	Jagged tear, often with stretching and damage of underlying tissue
Incision	Clean cut by a sharp object
Puncture	Deep tubular wound by a sharp, thin object
Contusion	Bruise caused by disruption of underlying small blood vessels, often with damage to internal organs

Name some of the various causes of death due to mechanical injury.

Hemorrhage, fat embolism, ruptured viscera, secondary infection, and renal shutdown

How is a fat embolism most likely to occur?

It could develop up to several days after a long bone fracture.

How does renal shutdown occur?

The process usually takes place as a result of acute tubular necrosis, especially when it is associated with myoglobin casts arising from a crush injury of skeletal muscle.

Abdominal traumas may lead to what kinds of injuries?

Contusion, splenic rupture, hepatic rupture, and intestinal rupture

What serious complication can result from hepatic and splenic rupture?

Internal hemorrhage

What serious complication can result from intestinal rupture?

Peritonitis

What serious conditions can result from thoracic trauma?

Rib fracture, hemothorax, and pneumothorax

Rib fracture can lead to what complications?

Penetrations into the lungs or into thoracic vessels

How do the entry and exit wounds of a gunshot injury differ in terms of size?

The entry wound is usually smaller than the exit wound.

Under what circumstances is the entry wound of a gunshot injury larger than the exit wound?

In a gunshot wound that occurs at point-blank range, the expanding gases disrupt the skin, especially over unyielding surfaces such as the skull.

What is a coup injury?

An injury to the brain at the point of external trauma

What is a contrecoup injury?

An injury to the brain opposite the point of external trauma, due to oscillation of the brain after impact

What often causes severe complications in head trauma?	Tearing of blood vessels and white matter tracts in the brain

THERMAL INJURY

What is hypothermia?	A generalized condition in which the body temperature is below normal
What persons are especially prone to hypothermia?	Elderly individuals
What is frostbite?	Localized freezing of body tissue, usually exposed areas
What pathologic manifestations may result from severe, prolonged frostbite?	Intracellular ice crystals, intravascular thrombosis, and possible gangrene
What terminology has replaced first-, second-, and third-degree burns?	First- or second-degree burns are referred to as partial-thickness burns, and third-degree burns are referred to as full-thickness burns.
How do partial-thickness and full-thickness burns differ in terms of the extent of skin damage?	In partial-thickness burns, epidermal damage varies, but no significant injury to the underlying dermis occurs. In full-thickness burns, the epidermis, dermis, and dermal appendages are injured.
Compare the treatments for partial-thickness burns and full-thickness burns.	Partial-thickness burns generally heal without intervention, whereas full-thickness burns warrant skin grafting.
Name several complications of full-thickness burns.	Hypovolemia, shock, infection, ulcers, and pulmonary damage from smoke and fumes
Shock is common with burns covering what percent of the body surface?	> 20% of the body surface area
What is the most common cause of death in burn patients who go into shock?	Sepsis from *Pseudomonas aeruginosa*
What is a Curling ulcer?	An acute gastric ulcer associated with severe burns

What is heat stroke?

Inability to dissipate body heat

In what 2 groups does heat stroke occur?

1. Febrile patients
2. Dehydrated patients exposed to prolonged elevated temperatures

Describe the pathophysiology of heat stroke.

Physiologic cooling processes are overwhelmed and become inactive.

What is the clinical appearance of patients with heat stroke?

Affected persons are dry and hot to the touch.

What are complications of heat stroke?

Generalized vasodilation, decreased effective blood volume, cellular hypoxia, and eventually life-threatening hyperkalemia

ELECTRIC INJURY

When can fatal electric injury occur?

When current passes through the brain or heart, causing cardiopulmonary arrest or arrhythmias

Which is more dangerous— alternating or direct current?

Alternating, because it causes strong muscular contractions. This often does not allow the victim to let go of an electric wire.

RADIATION INJURY

Name 3 sources of ionizing radiation.

1. X-rays
2. Radioactive waste
3. Nuclear disasters

Briefly describe the 2 theories that explain the mechanism of cellular damage by ionizing radiation.

1. Indirect action theory: Toxic free radicals damage vital cell components such as DNA, enzymes, and membranes.
2. Direct actions theory: Direct hits disrupt molecules such as DNA.

What does the latency period concept state?

That the biologic effect of radiation damage may not be apparent for many years—even decades.

What theory of radiation damage is best supported by the latency period phenomenon?

The indirect action theory

What rule of thumb helps predict the sensitivity of cells to radiation damage?	Cells are affected in direct proportion to both normal rate of mitotic activity and reproduction but in inverse proportion to level of specialization.
Classify specialized cells into 3 groups according to their degree of radiosensitivity.	
Radiosensitive	Lymphoid, hematopoietic, germ, and gastrointestinal (GI) mucosal tissue, and rapidly dividing tumor cells
Somewhat radiosensitive	Fibroblasts; cells of the endothelium, elastic tissue, salivary glands, and eye
Radioresistant	Cells of bone, cartilage, muscle, central nervous system (CNS), kidney, liver, and most endocrine glands
In the following systems, what conditions are caused by localized ionizing radiation?	
Skin	Dermatitis, ulceration, and skin malignancies
Lungs	**Acute changes:** adult respiratory distress syndrome (ARDS) **Chronic changes:** septal fibrosis, bronchiolar metaplasia, and hyaline thickening of blood vessel walls
GI tract	Inflammation and ulceration
Hematopoietic	Bone marrow depression and leukemia
Severe, generalized radiation causes what 3 serious conditions?	1. CNS injury due to capillary damage 2. GI mucosal denudation 3. Acute bone failure (pathologic fractures)
What type of radiation causes sunburn?	Ultraviolet (UV) light
UV light is associated with what skin lesions?	Premalignant actinic keratosis as well as malignant squamous and basal cell carcinomas and melanoma

Actinic keratosis is a pre-malignant precursor to what malignant skin lesion?	Basal cell carcinoma
Therapeutic radiation causes tumors. For the following irradiated sites, name the tumors that develop along with the years of delay in appearance.	
Skin	Squamous cell carcinoma (8–50 years) Lymphomas and leukemias (5–20 years)
Tumors of head, neck, and mediastinum	Thyroid cancer (5–20 years)
Soft tissue and bone	Sarcoma (most commonly malignant fibrous histiocytoma and osteosarcoma) [5–20 years]

CHEMICAL INJURY

METHANOL

In what substances is methanol (methyl alcohol) found?	Solvents, paint removers, and antifreeze
Methanol is toxic to what cells?	Retina, optic nerve, and CNS neurons
What classic outcome is most feared with cases of high-dose methanol poisoning?	Blindness

CARBON TETRACHLORIDE (CCL₄) AND POLYCHLORINATED BIPHENYLS (PCBs)

Carbon tetrachloride (CCl_4) causes what hepatic conditions?	Centrilobular necrosis and fatty change in the liver
PCBs cause what symptoms?	Chloracne, impotence, and visual changes

CARBON MONOXIDE (CO)

What is the mechanism of injury in CO poisoning?	Hypoxic injury occurs because CO displaces oxygen on its hemoglobin

carrier. The affinity of CO for hemoglobin is 200 times greater than its affinity for oxygen.

What cells are most vulnerable to injury?

Neurons of the brain, specifically foci of neuronal necrosis in the basal ganglia, lenticular nuclei, and cortical gray areas

What classic sign is associated with CO poisoning?

Cherry-red color of the lips, skin, blood, viscera, and muscles

ORGANOPHOSPHATE INSECTICIDES

What clinical scenario is typical of organophosphate insecticide poisoning?

A farmer who presents in mid-spring with twitching and paralysis

What mechanism is involved in organophosphate insecticide poisoning?

Inhibition of acetylcholinesterase, causing muscle twitching, flaccid paralysis, and cardiac arrhythmias

What is the antidote for organophosphate insecticides?

Early treatment with pralidoxime

CYANIDE

What mechanism is involved in cyanide poisoning?

Cyanide inhibits intracellular cytochrome oxidase by binding with ferric iron, thereby preventing cellular oxidation.

What clinical signs are apparent in cyanide poisoning?

Generalized petechial hemorrhages and the odor of bitter almonds on the patient's breath or at autopsy. The blood and viscera are also cherry-red, as in CO poisoning.

What is the antidote to cyanide poisoning?

Nitrite (given promptly)

LEAD

Name 2 methods of lead intake.

1. Ingestion, usually from lead paint
2. Inspiration, particularly from automotive emissions

What lead level in the blood is considered toxic?

>30 μg/dl

How is lead poisoning manifested clinically in the following organs/systems?

Red blood cells (RBCs)

Basophilic stippling and microsomic microcytic anemia

CNS

Encephalopathy with irritability and sometimes with seizures and coma (especially in children, who have a less well developed blood—brain barrier)

Peripheral nervous system

Peripheral neuritis, causing wrist drop and foot drop (more common in adults)

Kidney

Fanconi syndrome (renal tubular acidosis)

GI tract

Lead colic, a poorly localized abdominal pain

What causes the microcytic, hypochromic anemia of lead poisoning?

Lead causes deficiency of heme synthesis, especially by blocking aminolevulinic acid (ALA) dehydratase. This results in increased ALA in the urine as well as increased copropoporphyrin in the stool.

What classic oral sign is helpful in the diagnosis of lead poisoning?

Lead lines, which are mucosal deposits of lead sulfide at the junction of the teeth and gums

What radiographic sign is useful in the diagnosis of lead poisoning in children?

Increased radiodensity along epiphyseal lines of long bones

CHEMICALS OF ABUSE

TOBACCO SMOKING

Smoking causes how many premature deaths per year in the United States?

About 350,000

What fraction of the total deaths in the United States are caused by smoking?

One-sixth

What are the chances that a chronic smoker will die from a smoking-related disease?

45%

Cigarette smoking increases the risk of what cancers?

1. Bronchogenic: small cell and squamous
2. Oral and laryngeal
3. Esophageal
4. Gastric
5. Pancreatic
6. Renal cell carcinoma
7. Bladder, transitional cell carcinoma
8. Lymphoma

Cigarette smoking is strongly associated with what medical diseases?

1. Myocardial infarction (MI)
2. Congestive heart failure
3. Atherosclerosis
4. Stroke and cerebrovascular accident
5. Chronic bronchitis and emphysema
6. Peripheral vascular disease
7. Peptic ulcer disease

ALCOHOL

What pathologic findings are common in chronic alcoholism?

1. Acute fatty liver and hepatomegaly
2. Alcoholic hepatitis and cirrhosis, leading to portal hypertension, esophageal varices, and late-developing hepatocellular cancer
3. Pancreatitis
4. Gastritis (acute and chronic)
5. Oral and pharyngeal carcinoma
6. Alcoholic cardiomyopathy
7. Aspiration pneumonia
8. Peripheral neuropathy due to myelin sheath degeneration
9. Cerebral dysfunction [e.g., thiamine deficiency-mediated Wernicke-Korsakoff syndrome (alcoholic encephalopathy)]
10. CNS trauma

What common comorbid conditions accompany chronic alcohol use?

Nutritional deficiencies, drug abuse, and infections

MARIJUANA, HEROIN, AND COCAINE

Name 3 clinical consequences of long-term use of marijuana?	1. Chronic bronchitis 2. Cancer 3. Amotivation syndrome
Name some complications of heroin use.	Think PAID: **P**hysical dependence **A**RDS **I**nfection from intravenous drug abuse (IVDA) [human immunodeficiency virus (HIV), hepatitis B and C, or right-sided infective endocarditis] **D**eath (from respiratory or cardiac arrest or acute pulmonary edema)
What are the effects and complications of cocaine use?	1. Mood elevation followed by irritability, anxiety, depression, and possible suicidality 2. Acute cocaine toxicity from sympathomimetic and dopaminergic effects (tachycardia, hypertension, hyperthermia, arrhythmias, psychosis), which can be followed by seizures, brainstem depression, and cardiovascular collapse 3. Acute death due to coma, stroke, or MI 4. Hypertension with possible cerebral hemorrhage 5. Nasal ulceration or septal perforation from "snorting" 6. Infection resulting from IVDA (HIV, hepatitis B and C, right-sided infective endocarditis) 7. Coronary artery disease

AIR POLLUTANTS—PNEUMOCONIOSES

What is the definition of a pneumoconiosis?	A disease that involves inflammation and fibrosis of the lungs caused by inorganic dusts
What size of particles are implicated in pneumoconioses?	1–5 μ. Smaller particles can exit with expired air, and larger particles are trapped in the major bronchi.
What is the body's last line of defense against particles that collect in the alveoli?	Pulmonary alveolar macrophages

Which type of lung disease results from pneumo-conioses—-restrictive or obstructive?	Restrictive
What are the most common pneumoconioses?	Asbestosis, silicosis, and coal worker's pneumoconiosis (CWP)

ASBESTOSIS

What persons are occupationally at risk for asbestosis?	Shipyard, roofing, brake lining, and insulation workers
What other risk factors are considered potential risks for asbestosis?	The risk associated with exposure to old buildings is unproven.
Does asbestos exposure increase the risk of lung cancer?	Yes. Bronchogenic carcinoma is 4–5 times more likely to occur in asbestos-exposed workers. Mesothelioma is 100 times more likely in asbestos-exposed workers.
Does cigarette smoking increase the risk of bron-chogenic lung cancer in asbestos-exposed workers?	Yes; the likelihood that these workers will develop this type of lung cancer is 50–90 times that of the general population.
Does cigarette smoking increase the risk of meso-thelioma in asbestos-exposed workers?	No
What other cancers have an increased asbestos-related incidence?	GI lymphomas as well as gastric, colonic, and renal adenocarcinomas
What is the classic micro-scopic sign of asbestosis?	"Asbestos bodies"

SILICOSIS

What persons are occupa-tionally at risk for pure silicosis?	Sand blasters, miners, glass workers, metal grinders and polishers, and cement workers
What is the pathogenesis of silicosis?	Alveolar macrophages phagocytose the silica dust and die after rupture of silica-

laden phagolysosomes, and the cycle repeats. Silica may also be fibrogenic by directly stimulating release of fibroblast growth factor from macrophages.

What is the classic sign of chronic silicosis?

"Eggshell" radiographic appearance

Silicosis increases the risk for what 2 diseases?

1. Pulmonary tuberculosis (TB)
2. Caplan syndrome [rheumatoid arthritis (RA) with lung nodules]

Is lung cancer increased with silicosis?

No

COAL WORKER'S PNEUMOCONIOSIS (CWP)

CWP is also known as what disease?

"Black lung disease"

What causes CWP?

Inhalation of coal dust that contains both carbon and silica

What defines simple CWP?

Radiographic opacities that are ≤ 1 cm in diameter

What are the sequelae of simple CWP?

Simple CWP may cause only chronic bronchitis but occasionally develops into progressive massive fibrosis (PMF).

Define PMF.

It is the endpoint of CWP, characterized by regions of black scars > 1 cm in diameter radiographically (or 2 cm pathologically).

Name 3 complications of PMF.

1. Right ventricular hypertrophy, with pulmonary hypertension and cor pulmonale
2. TB
3. Caplan syndrome

What percentage of patients with PMF develop TB?

40%

What is Caplan syndrome?

The association of RA and pulmonary nodules in persons with pneumoconioses

CWP and PMF increases the risk for what cancer?	Gastric carcinoma (not lung cancer)

ANTHRACOSIS

What is the definition of anthracosis?	Accumulation of carbon dust in the lungs
What 2 groups of people are most likely to develop anthracosis?	1. City dwellers 2. Tobacco smokers
How serious is pure anthracosis?	By itself, pure carbon dust is usually inconsequential

BERYLLIOSIS

What persons are occupationally exposed to beryllium?	Electronic, aerospace, ceramic, and nuclear industry workers
Is the incidence of bronchogenic carcinoma increased?	Yes, by twofold

THERAPEUTIC AGENTS

Name 3 adverse effects of antibiotics.	1. Development of drug-resistant organisms 2. Overgrowth syndromes (pseudomembranous colitis and thrush) 3. Rare fatal aplastic anemia caused by chloramphenicol
Pseudomembranous colitis is classically associated with which antibiotic?	Clindamycin
What are the adverse effects of sulfonamides?	Polyarteritis nodosa, renal stones, bone marrow failure, and hemolytic anemia in glucose-6-phosphate dehydrogenase (G6PD) deficiency
What are the adverse effects of aspirin (acetylsalicylic acid)?	Gastritis or gastric ulcer, Reye syndrome, and allergic reactions

Define Reye syndrome.	Condition that occurs in children following an acute febrile illness, almost always in association with aspirin uptake, which is characterized by microvesicular fatty change in the liver and CNS encephalopathy
What are the presenting symptoms of an allergic reaction?	Urticaria, asthma, nasal polyps, angioneurotic edema, and anaphylaxis
What toxic effects are associated with cancer therapeutic agents?	Hair loss, GI erosions and ulcerations, bone marrow failure, acute leukemias, and other cancers

POWER REVIEW

Name the classic pathologies or signs of pathologies associated with the following injuries.

Long bone fracture	Fat embolism
Skeletal muscle crush injury	Renal shutdown
Hepatic or splenic rupture	Internal hemorrhage
Intestinal rupture	Peritonitis
Head trauma	Coup and contrecoup injury and vessel and white matter tearing
Prolonged cold exposure	Hypothermia and frostbite
Full-thickness burn	Shock, *Pseudomonas* sepsis, and Curling ulcer
Prolonged heat exposure	Heat stroke and hyperkalemia
Electrocution	Cardiopulmonary arrest and arrhythmia
UV radiation	Skin cancer
Ionizing radiation	Various cancers

**Name the classic patholo-
gies or signs of pathologies
associated with the
following chemicals.**

Methanol	Blindness
PCBs	Impotence
CO	Hypoxic injury and cherry-red lips
Organophosphate insecticides	Muscle twitching and paralysis and cardiac arrhythmias
Cyanide	Inhibition of cellular oxidation and cherry-red blood
Lead	Basophilic stippling, microcytic anemia, encephalopathy, peripheral neuritis, and "lead lines" on gums

**Name the classic patholo-
gies or signs of pathologies
associated with the following types of chemical abuse.**

Tobacco smoking	Bronchogenic carcinoma, heart disease, and stroke
Alcohol	Cirrhosis, CNS trauma, and Wernicke-Korsakoff syndrome
Heroin	Infection
Cocaine	Acute death and infection

**Name the classic patholo-
gies or signs of pathologies
associated with the
following environmental
pollutants.**

Inorganic dusts	Pneumoconioses
Carbon dust	Anthracosis
Silica	Silicosis and "eggshells" on radiography

Coal dust (carbon and silica)	Simple CWP, PMF, TB, and Caplan syndrome
Asbestos	"Asbestos bodies," bronchogenic carcinoma, and mesothelioma
Which inhaled dust is more fibrogenic—carbon or silica?	Silica

Name the classic pathologies or signs of pathologies associated with the following therapeutic agents.

Antibiotics	Drug-resistant organisms
Chloramphenicol	Aplastic anemia
Clindamycin	Pseudomembranous colitis
Aspirin	Gastritis and Reye syndrome

TABLE 9–1
Summary of Pneumoconioses

Type	Pathologic Features	Comments
Silicosis	Upper lobe nodules, eggshell calcification	Increased TB, no increase in mesothelioma
CWP	Small upper lobe nodules, emphysema	No increase in lung cancer
PMF	2–10 cm nodules	Increased TB, no increase in lung cancer
Caplan syndrome	Pulmonary nodules and rheumatoid arthritis	Can occur in silicosis, CWP, or PMF; must be distinguished from TB
Asbestosis	Finely nodular radiograph and pleural plaques	Need not be present for risk of mesothelioma
Asbestos exposure	Essentially normal lungs	Increased mesothelioma and lung cancer
Berylliosis	Hypersensitivity reaction, with granulomas in finely nodular radiograph	Bronchial biopsy helfpul; increased lung cancer

CWP = coal worker's pneumoconiosis; PMF = progressive massive fibrosis; TB = tuberculosis.

10   Nutritional Disorders

MALNUTRITION: MARASMUS AND KWASHIORKOR

Tell how marasmus and kwashiorkor differ.

Marasmus is a deficiency of calories (usually most nutrients are lacking), whereas kwashiorkor is caused by a protein deficiency.

What individuals typically suffer from marasmus?

Non—breast-fed infants who do not eat a sufficient amount

What other nutritional disorders occur with marasmus?

Various vitamin deficiencies

Is loss of subcutaneous fat characteristic of marasmus?

Yes, individuals lose muscle, organ, and subcutaneous tissue; they are emaciated.

Does marasmus cause edema or ascites?

No, these are common symptoms of kwashiorkor.

Do children with kwashiorkor ingest sufficient calories?

Yes, but they lack sufficient protein.

What individuals typically develop kwashiorkor?

Children who are no longer breast-fed

What do children with kwashiorkor typically eat?

Starches

Do children with kwashiorkor grow well?

No. Kwashiorkor and marasmus both cause growth retardation.

Name 4 abnormalities found in children with kwashiorkor but not marasmus.

1. Fatty liver
2. Severe edema
3. Anemia
4. Malabsorption due to atrophy of the small intestinal villi

Is hepatosplenomegaly found in marasmus or kwashiorkor?	Kwashiorkor
What causes the edema of kwashiorkor?	Hypoalbuminemia

Describe the following features of children with kwashiorkor.

Hair	Fine and brittle
Skin	Dry and thickened
Which is typically found in kwashiorkor—diarrhea or constipation?	Diarrhea, because of atrophy of the small intestinal villi.
In kwashiorkor, what often happens to the liver?	Cirrhosis develops.

OVEREATING

The overall death rate in obese persons is how much higher than it is in normal individuals?	50%
Name 5 diseases associated with obesity.	1. Atherosclerosis 2. Hypertension 3. Diabetes mellitus 4. Gallbladder disease 5. Some carcinomas
What percentage of the elderly suffer from diabetes mellitus type II?	About 10%
Type II diabetes mellitus shows strong correlation with consumption early in life of what substance?	Fat

VITAMINS

WATER-SOLUBLE VITAMINS

Name the water-soluble vitamins.	B complex vitamins (thiamine, riboflavin, niacin, pyroxidine, B_{12}), folic acid, and vitamin C

Name 3 physical examination findings common to the B complex vitamin deficiencies.	1. Glossitis 2. Dermatitis 3. Diarrhea
Which exhibits the most striking evidence of B complex deficiencies—metabolically active or inactive tissues?	Metabolically active tissues, because B complex vitamins are involved in the release and storage of energy

Thiamine

What is another name for thiamine?	Vitamin B_1
What 3 syndromes result from thiamine deficiency?	1. Dry beriberi 2. Wet beriberi 3. Wernicke-Korsakoff syndrome
In Asia, what individuals typically develop thiamine deficiency?	People who eat polished rice
In the United States, what 2 groups of individuals typically develop thiamine deficiency?	1. Alcoholics 2. Persons on fad diets
Peripheral neuropathy is characteristic of which syndrome of thiamine deficiency?	Dry beriberi; muscular atrophy follows.
High-output cardiac failure occurs as part of which syndrome of thiamine deficiency?	Wet beriberi
What causes high-output cardiac failure in wet beriberi?	Dilatation of arterioles and capillaries leads to arteriovenous shunting and hypervolemia, just as in warm shock.
What happens to the heart in wet beriberi?	It dilates.
What conditions constitute the Wernicke triad?	1. **C**onfusion 2. **O**phthalmoplegia 3. **A**taxia "**COA**"

Does memory loss occur in Wernicke-Korsakoff syndrome?	Yes, with confabulation
Which part of the brain demonstrates pathology in Wernicke-Korsakoff syndrome?	Degenerative changes occur in the brainstem and diencephalon, with involvement of paramedian masses of gray matter and mammillary bodies.

Riboflavin

What is another name for riboflavin?	Vitamin B_2
What 2 groups of individuals typically develop riboflavin deficiency?	1. Alcoholics 2. People in developing countries
What organ system is usually affected in riboflavin deficiency?	The skin
Name the characteristic problems in riboflavin deficiency.	Cheilosis, glossitis, corneal vascularization, and seborrheic dermatitis (face, scrotum, and vagina)

Niacin

What are other names for niacin?	Vitamin B_3, nicotinic acid
What amino acid can synthesize niacin?	Tryptophan. Niacin deficiency cannot occur if tryptophan intake is adequate.
Niacin deficiency usually presents as what condition?	Pellagra
What are the 4 "Ds" of pellagra?	**D**ementia, **d**ermatitis (exposed areas), **d**iarrhea, and **d**eath
Does corn have sufficient tryptophan and nicotinic acid to prevent pellagra?	No

Pyridoxine

What is another name for pyridoxine?	Vitamin B_6

Name 3 risk factors for pyridoxine deficiency.	1. Pyridoxine-deficient infant formula 2. Chronic alcoholism 3. Therapeutic drugs that inactivate pyridoxine
Infants with pyridoxine deficiency usually present with what condition?	Generalized seizures
Adults with pyridoxine deficiency usually present with what conditions?	Polyneuritis and anemia
What 2 drugs are known to inactivate pyridoxine?	1. Isoniazid 2. Penicillamine
Name 2 syndromes that increase dietary needs for vitamin B_6.	1. Homocystinuria 2. Pyridoxine-responsive anemia (a microcytic anemia with reduced heme synthesis)

Vitamin B_{12}

What is another name for vitamin B_{12}?	Cobalamin
What 3 groups of individuals typically develop vitamin B_{12} deficiency?	1. Persons with pernicious anemia 2. Strict vegetarians 3. Persons with small bowel disease (especially of the ileum)
Why might a Japanese person become deficient in vitamin B_{12}?	The fish tapeworm, *Diphyllobothrium latum,* competes with the small bowel for vitamin B_{12}. This tapeworm is often found in sushi.
What characterizes blood cells in pernicious anemia?	Presence of megaloblasts (i.e., ineffective erythropoiesis) and hypersegmented neutrophils
How is the central nervous system (CNS) affected by vitamin B_{12} deficiency?	Degeneration of the dorsal and lateral columns (long and myelinated) of the spinal cord occurs.
What neuropathy affects vitamin B_{12}—deficient individuals?	Subacute combined degeneration of the spinal cord

Name 4 clinical manifestations of subacute combined degeneration of the spinal cord.	1. Paresthesias 2. Slowed reflexes 3. Weakness 4. Ataxia

Folate

Name 5 causes of folate deficiency.	1. Diet 2. Alcoholism 3. Pregnancy 4. Methotrexate 5. Phenytoin
Does folate deficiency cause neuropathy?	No, but it does cause megaloblastic anemia.

Vitamin C

What is another name for vitamin C?	Ascorbic acid
What is vitamin C deficiency, or "the sailor's disease," also known as?	Scurvy
Name 6 findings of scurvy.	1. Pain (muscles, joints, bones) 2. Swollen, bleeding gums 3. Subperiosteal hemorrhage 4. Perifollicular petechial hemorrhage 5. Conjunctival hemorrhage 6. Impaired wound healing
Vitamin C deficiency impairs the synthesis of which 2 amino acids?	1. Hydroxyproline 2. Hydroxylysine
Which connective tissue element is affected by scurvy?	Collagen
Which bone element is affected by scurvy?	The osteoid matrix

FAT-SOLUBLE VITAMINS

What are the fat-soluble vitamins?	Vitamins A, D, E, and K

What disorders lead to deficiency of fat-soluble vitamins?	Disorders of fat absorption, including general malabsorption syndromes, pancreatic exocrine insufficiency, and biliary obstruction

Vitamin A

What foods contain vitamin A?	Animal products
What causes vitamin A deficiency?	Diet and malabsorption
What is the relationship between beta-carotene and vitamin A?	Beta-carotene is a precursor of vitamin A.
What foods contain beta-carotene?	Carrots and green leafy vegetables
In general, vitamin A deficiency affects which type of epithelium?	Mucous-secreting epithelium
Name 3 clinical manifestations of vitamin A deficiency.	1. Night blindness (rods) 2. Squamous metaplasia (hyperkeratosis) 3. Xerophthalmia (extreme dryness of conjunctiva and cornea, leading to ulceration and infection)
Development of hypervitaminosis requires how many units of vitamin A?	> 50,000 units/day
What are 2 presenting signs of hypervitaminosis in children?	1. Alopecia 2. Radiologic evidence of new periosteal bone formation
What are 2 presenting signs of hypervitaminosis in adults?	1. Hepatic injury 2. Portal hypertension with ascites

Vitamin D

What is the name of the active form?	Calcitriol $[1,25\text{-}(OH)_2D_3)]$

In which organ does the first step in the formation of vitamin D take place?	7-dehydrocholesterol is converted into cholecalciferol (vitamin D_3) in the skin.
In which organ does the conversion from cholecalciferol (vitamin D_3) to 25-hydroxyvitamin D_3 take place?	The liver
In which organ does the conversion from 25-hydroxyvitamin D_3 to the 1,25-dihydroxyvitamin D_3 take place?	The kidney
What childhood disease results from vitamin D_3 deficiency?	Rickets
What adult illness results from vitamin D_3 deficiency?	Osteomalacia
How does 1,25-dihydroxyvitamin D_3 affect the following structures?	
Intestines	Increases the absorption of calcium and phosphorus
Renal tubules	Stimulates parathyroid hormone-mediated reabsorption of calcium
Bones	Enhances calcification

Vitamin E

What biochemical property makes vitamin E useful as a supplement in patients at risk for heart attack?	It is an antioxidant.
Which portion of the cell is maintained in part by vitamin E?	The membrane
Which organ system may be affected by vitamin E deficiency?	CNS

Vitamin K

What age group is notorious for its vitamin K deficiency?

Premature infants, who are yet to be colonized by vitamin K—synthesizing organisms and do not eat green and yellow vegetables

Vitamin K is essential for what class of biochemical reaction?

Carboxylation

What condition results in development of vitamin K deficiency in adults?

Fat malabsorption or alterations in the intestinal flora due to antibiotics

What is a presenting feature of vitamin K deficiency?

Hemorrhagic diathesis (abnormal bleeding)

What clotting factors are affected by vitamin K deficiency?

Factors II, VII, IX, and X, as well as protein C

Is an excess of vitamin K harmful?

No

ESSENTIAL TRACE ELEMENTS

Which 4 ions are critical for neuromuscular excitation?

1. Sodium
2. Potassium
3. Chloride
4. Magnesium

Name 5 manifestations of zinc deficiency.

1. Growth failure
2. Hypogonadism
3. Poor wound healing
4. Anemia
5. Hepatosplenomegaly

Zinc is found in what foods?

Animal proteins

Which element is deposited in the liver, brain, and cornea in Wilson disease?

Copper

What is the characteristic finding in the cornea of patients with Wilson disease?

Kaiser-Fleischer rings

Describe the blood cells in iron deficiency anemia.	Microcytic and hypochromic

POWER REVIEW

A person who eats too few calories will develop what condition?	Marasmus
A person who eats too little protein will develop which condition?	Kwashiorkor
Name 3 striking features of kwashiorkor.	1. Edema 2. Protuberant abdomen (ascites) 3. Hepatosplenomegaly
Name 3 characteristic features of marasmus.	1. Loss of subcutaneous fat 2. Muscle wasting 3. Atrophy of most organs
Pancreatic insufficiency typically causes a deficiency of which vitamins?	Vitamins A, D, E, and K, because they are absorbed with lipids
Name 3 salient results of vitamin A deficiency.	1. Hyperkeratosis 2. Xerophthalmia (in children) 3. Night blindness (in adults)
What diseases due to vitamin D deficiency affect the following groups?	
Children	Rickets
Adults	Osteomalacia
How is deficiency of vitamin K manifested?	Bleeding
Which vitamins may present with dangerous syndromes of excess?	Vitamins A and D
Most water-soluble vitamins are used for what purpose in the body?	As coenzymes

Thiamine (vitamin B$_1$) deficiency results in what condition?	Beriberi
Riboflavin (vitamin B$_2$) deficiency results in what abnormalities?	Skin and mucous membrane changes
Niacin (vitamin B$_3$) deficiency results in what disorder?	Pellagra
The presence of which amino acid may prevent niacin deficiency?	Tryptophan
Which individuals are predisposed to niacin deficiency?	Persons who eat a corn-only diet; who have prolonged diarrhea, alcoholism, or cirrhosis; who have carcinoid syndrome; or who are taking isoniazid
Name the four Ds of pellagra.	**D**ermatitis, **d**iarrhea, **d**ementia, and **d**eath
Which individuals develop pyridoxine (vitamin B$_6$) deficiency?	Infants who are fed pyridoxine-deficient formula, patients on isoniazid or penicillamine (which inactivate the vitamin), and chronic alcoholics
What are the effects of pyridoxine deficiency in the following groups?	
Children	Generalized seizures
Adults	Polyneuritis and anemia
Vitamin B$_{12}$ deficiency occurs primarily in individuals who lack which factor?	Intrinsic factor
Name 2 clinical syndromes associated with vitamin B$_{12}$ deficiency	1. Pernicious anemia 2. Subacute combined degeneration of the spinal cord
Name 3 causes of folic acid deficiency.	1. Insufficient intake (alcoholism, poor diet)

2. Defective absorption (small bowel disorders)
3. Increased utilization (pregnancy)

Vitamin C deficiency   Scurvy
results in what disorder?

11 ___

Forensic Pathology

What is forensic pathology?

A subspecialty of anatomic pathology practiced primarily in a medical examiner's or coroner's office. It generally involves performing autopsies to determine the cause of death.

What is an autopsy?

An examination of the organs of a dead body to determine the cause of death or to study the pathologic changes present.

What components comprise an autopsy?

History of the event
Past medical history
Diagrams and photographs
Complete examination of chest, abdomen, brain, and neck
Histology
Toxicology

What types of cases go to the medical examiner?

Trauma, poisonings, drug intoxication, police custody deaths, postoperative death, sudden unexpected deaths

What 4 types of evidence are used to determine the time of death?

History as given by witnesses, physicians, or police, including when the person was last seen alive
Rigor mortis
Lividity
Body temperature

Define rigor mortis.

Muscle stiffness caused by depletion of ATP. Actin myosin filaments bind and stiffen muscle.

What muscles show rigor mortis first?

Small muscles (e.g., jaw muscles), then neck, then arms, then legs

When is rigor mortis first seen?

Between 2–8 hours after death

How soon does rigor mortis begin to subside?

This varies widely with temperature. After 24 hours at room temperature;

within less than 6 hours above 120° F, or
after several days below 40° F.

**What is postmortem
lividity?**

A postmortem phenomenon due to
gravity, wherein blood pools to
dependent skin after death and creates a
purple discoloration

**How is body temperature
used to estimate time of
death?**

After death, body temperature changes to
reach the environmental temperature.
The difference between the body
temperature and the environmental
temperature can be used to help estimate
the time of death.

GUNSHOT WOUNDS

**What are the character-
istics of a gunshot entrance
wound?**

A perforation with an abrasion collar;
gunpowder stippling

What is an abrasion collar?

The edges of the entrance wound,
abraded by the friction of the bullet
passing through the tissue

**What are the character-
istics of a gunshot exit
wound?**

An irregular tear in the skin

**What is gunpowder
stippling or tattooing?**

Partially burned gunpowder penetrates
the skin and appears as tiny specks of
discoloration around an entrance wound

**What is the importance of
noting gunpowder
stippling?**

It determines which wound is the
entrance wound and helps determine the
distance the firearm was from the victim.

**At what proximity to the
firearm will gunpowder
stippling be seen?**

Less than 2–4 feet

**What, in addition to the
pellets, can be found in a
shotgun wound fired at
close range?**

Plastic or cardboard wadding

**How do bullet wounds
cause so much internal
organ damage?**

Cavitation—a temporary cavity deforms
tissue and makes the injury many times
the actual diameter of the bullet

Why do skull gunshot wounds cause black eyes?	Shock wave from bullet fractures the orbital plates and blood tracks down and causes periorbital ecchymosis

STAB WOUNDS

What is a stab wound?	A wound caused by a sharp instrument
What are hesitation marks?	Superficial incised wounds seen in almost all self-inflicted wrist or other cuts as the person tries to figure out the amount of pressure needed to cut through the skin
What skin characteristics are seen in a stab wound by a knife with one sharp edge?	Stab wound with one squared off end and one sharp end
What are defense wounds in a case of stabbing or slashing?	Wounds on the hands or forearms as the patient attempts to block or grab the knife to defend the rest of the body

ASPHYXIA

Define asphyxia.	Impaired or absent exchange of oxygen and carbon dioxide; it occurs when a physical or chemical mechanism disrupts the delivery of oxygen
What are typical autopsy findings with homicidal strangulation?	Skin of neck may show bruises, ligature marks, fingernail abrasion, muscles of neck may show hemorrhage, hyoid bone may be fractured, petechiae may be seen
What are petechial hemorrhage?	Pinpoint bleeding
Where are petechial hemorrhages most commonly seen after strangulation?	Conjunctiva

MISCELLANEOUS

What is a coup head injury?	A brain injury at the point of impact
What is a countercoup injury?	Brain injury opposite to the point of impact

What chemicals are inhaled in a house fire?

Carbon monoxide, cyanide, HCl

Is there always an electro-thermal burn in fatal electrocutions?

No

What are the autopsy findings with drowning?

Foam in mouth, larynx, trachea, and bronchi
Pulmonary congestion and edema
Water swallowed into stomach
Hemorrhage into middle ear
Water aspirated into sinuses (sphenoid sinus)

Section II

Systemic Pathology

12

Vascular System

What are the 4 classes of arteries?

1. Large elastic (conducting)
2. Muscular (distributing)
3. Small
4. Arterioles

Describe the classes of arteries.

Large elastic arteries include the aorta and its branches. Muscular arteries supply blood to specific organ systems and are often named for the organ they supply (e.g., gastric artery). Small arteries (i.e., < 2 mm in diameter) are usually within organs. Arterioles immediately precede a capillary bed.

Where does the autonomic nervous system exert most of its control over the vascular system?

In the arterioles (think autonomic arteries are arterioles)

Which classes of arteries have 3 histologic layers?

Large elastic arteries and muscular arteries

What are the 3 layers?

Tunica intima, tunica media, tunica adventitia

What supplies blood to the cells that compose arteries?

Vaso vasorum (vessels of the vessels)

Where are the vaso vasorum located?

Tunica adventitia

ARTERIOSCLEROSIS

Define arteriosclerosis.

An arterial disease characterized by thickening of arterial walls with resulting luminal narrowing and sclerosis

How might your patients describe arteriosclerosis?

Hardening of the arteries

What are the 3 types of arteriosclerosis?

1. Atherosclerosis: formation of plaques (atheromas)
2. Monckeberg arteriosclerosis (medial calcific sclerosis): the formation of calcified bands within arteries
3. Arteriolosclerosis: proliferation of the vascular endothelium and fibromuscular tissue

Atherosclerosis

Where do atheromas form?

In the intima

What countries have the highest incidence of atherosclerosis?

The United States, Great Britain, Canada, Finland, and Northern Europe (i.e., "westernized" countries). This is most likely due to the diet of these populations, but genetics also may be a factor.

What makes up an atheroma?

A core of cholesterol, cholesterol esters, macrophages (foam cells with engulfed lipids), calcium, and necrotic tissue; with a fibrous subendothelial cap of smooth muscle, fibrin, collagen, and extracellular matrix material

Describe the effects of atherosclerosis.

It narrows channels (decreasing flow and causing ischemia in tissues downstream), damages the tunica media (predisposing to aneurysm, rupture, and dissection), and may calcify or ulcerate (often leading to arterial thrombosis and occlusion, as in unstable angina pectoris and myocardial infarction).

What are the 13 risk factors for atherosclerosis?

1. Dyslipidemia [decreased high-density lipoprotein (HDL), increased low-density lipoprotein (LDL) and triglycerides]
2. Hypertension
3. Smoking
4. Diabetes mellitus
5. Elevated homocysteine levels
6. Increasing age (especially males > 45 and females > 55)

7. Male gender or postmenopausal female
8. Lp(a) lipoprotein
9. Elevated uric acid levels in the blood
10. Sedentary lifestyle
11. Type A personality (angry form)
12. Oral contraceptives (progesterone component only)
13. Family history

Of these, what are considered the 4 major risk factors?

Dyslipidemia, hypertension, smoking, and diabetes mellitus

Patients with these risk factors are prone to what 5 types of diseases?

1. Coronary artery disease (angina pectoris, myocardial infarction, ischemic cardiomyopathy)
2. Cerebrovascular disease (transient ischemic attacks, strokes)
3. Peripheral vascular disease (claudication, gangrene)
4. Mesenteric ischemia (ischemic bowel, gangrene)
5. Renal artery stenosis (secondary hypertension, ischemic kidney)

Is the pathogenesis of atherosclerosis known?

No, but there are 4 theories.

Name the 4 theories, and describe their mechanisms.

Lipid infiltration (insudation)

Lipid is deposited in the vessel wall due to increased influx, decreased breakdown, or both.

Smooth muscle (monoclonal)

Abnormal growth, in a neoplastic manner, of clonal smooth muscle cells, or simple foci of proliferation at areas of stress (e.g., branch points)

Thrombogenic (encrustation)

Multiple episodes of intramural thrombosis leading to organization and formation of atheromatous lesions

Reaction to injury

Proliferation of smooth muscle due to release of the breakdown products of vessel injury, including platelet-derived growth factor (PDGF)

Why might vitamin E help slow or prevent this process?

Vitamin E is an antioxidant, which reduces lipid oxidation and thus absorption by macrophages. It has reduced the rate of nonfatal myocardial infarction (MI) in patients with proven symptomatic coronary atherosclerosis.

Give 3 reasons why macrophages are important in atherosclerosis formation.

1. Macrophages have receptors that facilitate the uptake of LDL and other lipids.
2. Macrophages release growth factors that stimulate smooth muscle proliferation.
3. Macrophages release chemotactic factors that attract leukocytes and contribute to inflammation and lipid oxidation.

Name and describe the 4 lesions of atherosclerosis.

Fatty streaks

Lipid-containing cells (foam cells) with some extracellular matrix in the tunica intima causing raised lesions in the aorta

Intimal pad

Smooth muscle cells and extracellular matrix accumulation in the tunica intima at branch sites and ostia

Atheromas

Smooth muscle cells, fibrous tissue, necrotic tissue, lipids, and lipid-containing cells

Complicated plaques

Atheromas that have undergone calcification, ulceration, thrombosis, or bleeding within the atheroma (intraplaque hemorrhage)

Where are these lesions usually found?

Fatty streaks

Thoracic aorta and coronary arteries

Intimal pads

Arterial branch points and ostia

Atheromas

Arterial branch points and ostia

Complicated plaques

Coronary and cerebral arteries, aorta

So, where are the most common sites of atherosclerosis?

Proximal coronary arteries, large branches off the carotid, circle of Willis, large lower extremity vessels, renal and mesenteric arteries

Monckeberg arteriosclerosis

Also known as?

Medial calcific sclerosis

What is sclerosis?

Rigidity; loss of elasticity

Where is Monckeberg arteriosclerosis formed?

The tunica media of medium and small muscular arteries (think **M**onckeberg **M**edial calcific sclerosis in the **M**edia of **M**uscular arteries), most often the radial and ulnar arteries

When does it occur?

After age 40 to 50

Describe the lesions.

Circumferential calcification is confined to the tunica media; therefore, the patency of the vessel lumen is preserved and blood flow is not hindered.

What is another name for vessels affected by this disease?

Pipestem arteries

What can these lesions progress to?

They can ossify, producing bone and bone marrow in the arterial media.

What misleading sign due to Monckeberg shows up on routine physical exam?

Falsely elevated systolic blood pressure caused by the blood pressure cuff's difficulty compressing a sclerosed brachial artery

What is the relationship between Monckeberg and atherosclerosis?

They may coexist, but are not related.

Arteriolosclerosis

What vessels are involved?

Small arteries and arterioles (think **arteriolo**—sclerosis)

What are the pathological lesions?

Fibromuscular and endothelial proliferation

What do the lesions cause?

Sclerosis and destruction of small vessels

Name a risk factor for development of arteriolosclerosis.	Hypertension
What group of patients can be normotensive, yet develop arteriolosclerosis?	Diabetic patients
What are the 2 forms of arteriolosclerosis?	Hyaline and hyperplastic
What does the hyaline look like with hematoxylin and eosin (H&E) staining?	Pink and acellular
Who gets hyaline arteriolosclerosis?	Older people with a long history of hypertension, diabetes mellitus, or both
In what organ system does hyaline arteriolosclerosis commonly manifest itself clinically?	Renal
Name the common condition hyaline arteriolosclerosis causes in the kidney, and describe how it develops.	Nephrosclerosis. Malignant hypertension leads to hyperplastic changes and development of malignant nephrosclerosis.
What vegetable is often associated with hyperplastic arteriosclerosis?	Onions, because its onionlike layers thicken the arterial walls
What vessels does hyperplastic arteriolosclerosis affect?	Arterioles, of course
Who gets hyperplastic arteriolosclerosis?	People with malignant hypertension
What is malignant hypertension?	Elevated blood pressure that rapidly causes vascular compromise and symptomatic disease in the brain, heart, or kidney
Name some of the signs and symptoms of malignant hypertension.	Hypertensive encephalopathy, hypertensive retinopathy, papilledema, renal failure, and acute left ventricular dysfunction

What is necrotizing arteriolitis?

Hyperplastic arteriolitis with inflammation and necrosis (death) of the arterial wall, and deposition of fibrin (a scar)

Lipids

Do all patients with atherosclerosis have hyperlipidemia?

No. The disease can be caused by the other risk factors mentioned, and it has a genetic component.

How do lipids circulate in the blood?

The electrochemically neutral lipids are embedded in a complex of polar lipids and apoproteins to form lipoproteins.

What are the neutral lipids?

Cholesterol esters and triglycerides

Which lipids are polar?

Cholesterol and phospholipids

What are apoproteins?

The protein components of lipoprotein molecules. They are the only part of the molecules that are genetically determined.

Why do we need cholesterol?

Cholesterol is a key component of cell membranes, bile acids, and steroid hormones.

Why should one give cholesterol-lowering medicines at night?

To coincide with the body's diurnal surge of cholesterol production

Elevation of triglycerides (hypertriglyceridemia) can cause what disease besides atherosclerosis?

Pancreatitis

How are lipoproteins classified?

Based on density

Name the 5 classes of lipoproteins.

1. Chylomicrons
2. Very low-density lipoprotein (VLDL): mostly triglycerides
3. Intermediate-density lipoprotein (IDL)
4. LDL ("bad cholesterol"): about 25% of total serum cholesterol
5. HDL ("good cholesterol"): about 75% of total serum cholesterol

What are the major apoproteins of each?

Chylomicrons?   C, A1, A2, B48

VLDL?   C, E, B48

IDL?   E, B100

LDL?   B100

HDL?   A1, A2

What levels of cholesterol are considered normal?
In general, for those without a history of cardiac disease, total cholesterol should be < 200, LDL < 130, and HDL > 35.

What is the Friedwald formula for calculating LDL, total cholesterol, HDL, and triglycerides?
LDL = total cholesterol − HDL − triglycerides/5

If your cholesterol level is > 250, lowering it 1% reduces the risk of coronary disease by how much?
Each 1% reduction in serum cholesterol gives you a 2% reduction in risk of coronary disease (think a two-for-one deal).

What may be better indicators of risk for atherosclerosis than measurements of LDL and HDL?
The levels of apoproteins B100 and A1

What is Lp(a)?
A lipoprotein whose structure closely resembles plasminogen (the precursor of plasmin, the body's endogenous clot dissolver). It equals LDL as a risk factor for atherosclerosis.

Name 2 ways in which Lp(a) lipoprotein might exert its effects.
1. It may interfere with clot lysis by saturating plasminogen receptors and competitively inhibiting plasmin generation.
2. It accumulates in the intima, where it may promote lipid oxidation and uptake.

What can lower LDL cholesterol levels?
Diet, exercise, and medications (e.g., resins and HMG co-reductase inhibitors)

What can raise HDL cholesterol levels?	Smoking cessation, weight loss, exercise, moderate alcohol consumption (red wine), and certain medications (e.g., niacin)
Describe the following types of familial hyperlipidemia.	
Type I	Deficient lipoprotein lipase levels lead to elevated chylomicrons and triglycerides.
Type II	Elevated LDL levels lead to early atherosclerosis and very high risk of coronary artery disease and death in childhood.
Type III?	Increased IDL and VLDL and moderate elevation of triglycerides
Type IV?	Elevated VLDL and triglycerides
Type V?	Elevated VLDL and chylomicrons
Which type of familial hyperlipidemia is most common?	Type IV
What are 3 superficial clinical manifestations of familial hyperlipidemias?	1. Endon xanthomas 2. Premature corneal arcus 3. Xanthelasma (represents deposition of lipid-laden cells)
Serum cholesterol levels are normal in which forms?	Types I and IV

FIBROMUSCULAR DYSPLASIA

What is fibromuscular dysplasia?	A rare thickening of muscular arteries without evidence of inflammation or a known etiology
What can it cause?	Secondary hypertension (due to stenosis of renal vasculature), loss of the involved kidney, and dissecting aneurysms
Who usually gets fibromuscular dysplasia?	Women in their 30s and 40s

Name 4 clinical signs besides hypertension and renal failure.	1. Abdominal bruit 2. Delayed intravenous pyelogram 3. Small kidney on ultrasound 4. Abnormal renal arteriogram

VASCULITIS

Define vasculitis.	Diffuse inflammation of blood vessels, often with an immune-mediated process
Name 3 forms of arteritis.	Polyarteritis nodosa (PAN), giant cell arteritis, and thromboangiitis obliterans
Name and describe 5 disorders associated with necrotizing vasculitis.	1. Wegener granulomatosis: granulomas of the sinuses and lung associated with glomerulonephritis 2. Systemic lupus erythematosus (SLE) 3. Rheumatoid arthritis (RA) 4. Hypersensitivity (leukocytoclastic) vasculitis including Henoch-Schönlein purpura and serum sickness-like disorders 5. Churg-Strauss syndrome (allergic granulomatosis): associated with eosinophilia, asthma, and vascular granulomas (especially of the lung)
What are the characteristic serum markers for the following disorders?	
Wegner granulomatosis?	c-ANCA
SLE?	ANA, anti-ds DNA, anti-Sm, anti-SS
RA?	Rheumatoid factor (RF)
Churg-Strauss?	Eosinophils
What are 2 typical skin findings of systemic vasculitis?	1. Palpable purpura rash, especially in the extremities 2. Nonblanchable petechiae
What is the usual treatment for vasculitic disorders?	Glucocorticoids and other anti-inflammatories

Polyarteritis nodosa (PAN)

What is PAN?	A group of immune-mediated necrotizing vasculitides of the small and medium

vessels in multiple organ systems. It usually involves renal and visceral vessels and spares the lung.

With what is PAN associated?

Hepatitis B infection in 30% of cases, and occasionally hairy cell leukemia

What lesions does PAN often form?

Microaneurysms

What are the clinical manifestations?

Nonspecific symptoms: fever, weight loss, malaise, kidney dysfunction

How is PAN diagnosed?

Through a biopsy, usually of the kidney

Giant cell arteritides

What are the 2 giant cell arteritides?

Takayasu arteritis and temporal arteritis

What cell type is usually present?

Multinucleated giant cells

What vessels does temporal arteritis affect?

Branches of the carotid artery, especially the temporal artery

Can temporal arteritis affect other vessels?

Yes, any medium or large artery

Who gets temporal arteritis?

Women > 50

With what disorder is temporal arteritis associated?

Polymyalgia rheumatica

What are the clinical signs and symptoms of temporal arteritis?

Headache, intermittent claudication of the jaw, tenderness of the temporal region on palpation, elevated erythrocyte sedimentation rate (ESR), fever, and weight loss

How is it diagnosed?

By history and physical exam. Definitive diagnosis is by temporal artery biopsy.

What is the most effective treatment?

Steroids

What is the big danger of temporal arteritis?

Ophthalmic artery involvement and blindness

How sensitive and specific is a biopsy for temporal arteritis?

Extremely sensitive, but not very specific due to skip lesions of the temporal artery

What 2 types of giant cells are seen in temporal arteritis?

Foreign body type and Langhans type

What is the difference between foreign body type and Langhans type?

Distribution of the nuclei. Nuclei are randomly positioned in foreign body type, but peripherally located in Langhans type.

What is another name for Takayasu arteritis?

"Pulseless disease" because of the associated weakness and loss of upper extremity pulses, or "aortic arch syndrome"

What vessels does Takayasu arteritis affect?

The aortic arch and proximal segments of the great vessels originating from it. The main pulmonary artery is involved in 50% of patients.

What is the lesion?

Irregular thickening of the artery

What are the symptoms and signs of Takayasu arteritis?

Dizziness, syncope, paresthesias, visual disturbances, palpitations, shortness of breath, chest pain, heart failure, and weakening of upper extremity pulses with increased lower extremity blood pressure. (Think of what happens if blood flow through the great vessels is hindered and the heart's work is increased.)

What is the characteristic clinical finding?

Lack of radial pulse

What are the 3 microscopic findings?

1. Both types of giant cells
2. Monocytes and PMNs in the vaso vasorum and adventitia
3. Monocytes invading the tunica media

Where does Takayasu arteritis begin?

At the junction of the adventitia and media

Where does temporal arteritis begin?

Tunica media

Who typically gets Takayasu arteritis?	Young Asian women

Thromboangiitis obliterans

What is another name for thromboangiitis obliterans?	Buerger disease
Where does it usually occur?	In medium-sized vessels, especially the radial and tibial arteries
What else can it affect?	Adjacent nerves and veins
What is the characteristic pathological process?	Recurrent thrombosis of medium-sized vessels
What is the greatest risk factor?	Cigarette smoking. The disease is almost exclusive to smokers.
Who gets thromboangiitis obliterans?	Usually young (age 25 to 50 years) male smokers. Incidence is increased among Jewish persons.
What are the clinical signs and symptoms?	
In arteries?	Pain, ulcerations, and gangrene in the extremity secondary to ischemia
In veins?	Thrombophlebitis
Why are these patients in pain?	The pain is caused by ischemia, much like a progressive coronary lesion.
How can the body itself relieve the pain?	Recanalize the obstructed area and restore flow.
What is seen microscopically?	Thrombus with microabscesses, fibrosis and inflammation spreading out from the artery, and eventual fibrous encasement of the artery, nearby veins, and nerves
What are the 3 fates of the thrombus?	Embolize; organize; form microabscesses

Kawasaki disease

What is Kawasaki disease?	A systemic vasculitis of children < 4 years of age

Signs and symptoms?	High fever, scleral injection, erythematous rash (including desquamation of the fingers), mucocutaneous involvement, lymphadenopathy, and irritability
What vessels are affected?	Small and medium-sized vessels, including the coronary arteries
What is used to treat Kawasaki disease?	Aspirin and intravenous (IV) immunoglobulin G
What are the potentially fatal complications?	Involvement of coronary arteries, aneurysm formation, thrombosis, myocarditis, and pericarditis

Behçet syndrome

What is Behçet syndrome?	A syndrome of oral aphthous ulcers, genital ulcers, ocular inflammation, and leukocytoclastic venulitis involving various organ systems including the central nervous, gastrointestinal (GI), and cardiovascular systems
What is the cause?	Unknown

FUNCTIONAL VASCULAR DISORDERS

What is Raynaud disease?	Recurrent vasospasm (etiology unknown) of small arteries and arterioles. It often occurs in the extremities, is bilateral and symmetrical, and causes tissue ischemia and pain.
What precipitates an exacerbation of Raynaud disease?	Exposure to cold, emotional stimuli, and stress
Who gets it?	Young women. Onset is usually in the teens.
What is Raynaud phenomenon?	The symptoms and signs of recurrent vasospasm of small vessels, secondary to another disorder such as SLE, scleroderma, and other connective tissue diseases

What are the characteristic color changes of both disorders?

White to blue to red: white due to loss of perfusion, blue due to cyanosis, and red due to reperfusion

What are 3 treatment options for these conditions?

1. Avoid cold exposure
2. Calcium channel blockers
3. Surgery with sympathectomy procedures

ANEURYSMS

Define aneurysm.

An abnormal dilatation of a blood vessel or of the heart

Which are the most common?

Arterial aneurysms

List the 5 causes of aneurysms.

1. Atherosclerosis
2. Idiopathic cystic medial necrosis
3. Syphilis
4. Arteriovenous (AV) malformation
5. Mycotic infection

What is the most common cause?

Atherosclerosis

Atherosclerotic aneurysms

Where do atherosclerotic aneurysms most commonly occur?

In the abdominal aorta below the origin of the renal arteries (infrarenal). The common iliac arteries often are involved.

At what size do most abdominal aortic aneurysms (AAA) warrant surgical repair?

At 5 cm diameter or larger, the statistical risk of rupture is higher than the risk of surgery.

What area of the artery is destroyed by atheromas, weakening the vessel wall and leading to aneurysm formation?

Atheromas in the tunica intima progress to involve the tunica media, which supplies much of the elasticity and strength to the arterial wall.

Name 4 complications of atherosclerotic aneurysms.

1. Dissection
2. Thrombosis and occlusion of flow, usually from mural thrombi
3. Cholesterol emboli
4. Rupture

Syphilitic (luetic) aneurysms

What stage of syphilis is associated with aneurysms?

Tertiary

Name 4 blood tests for syphilis.

VDRL, FTA, RPR, MHA-TP (Venereal Disease Research Laboratory test, fluorescent treponemal antibody, rapid plasmin reagin, microhemagglutination-*Treponema pallidum*)

Describe the 4 stages of syphilis.

Primary: involvement at the site of infection and chancres
Secondary: disseminated with lymphadenopathy, condylomata lata (10%), and a maculopapular rash
Latent: a variable asymptomatic period
Tertiary: obliterative endarteritis and gumma formation

Where do syphilitic aneurysms usually occur?

In the ascending aorta and transverse thoracic aorta

What is the pathological process leading to aneurysm formation?

Proliferative endarteritis of the vaso vasorum with plasma cell infiltration and gumma formation. This causes ischemia of the tunica media of the aortic wall, weakening of the wall, and aneurysm formation.

A syphilitic aorta is often called?

"Tree-bark aorta"

Name 4 complications arising from the position of syphilitic aneurysms.

Aortic insufficiency, heart failure, cardiac ischemia, and myocardial infarction

Syphilitic aneurysms affect the following anatomic structures. What are the symptoms?

Lungs

Respiratory compromise due to airway obstruction

Esophagus

Dysphagia due to obstruction

Recurrent laryngeal nerve

Cough, hoarseness

Vertebrae	Backache
Aortic valve	Incompetence, regurgitation
Coronary arteries	Angina, MI due to occlusion

Cirsoid aneurysms

What are cirsoid aneurysms?	Aneurysms resulting from AV fistulas
What is an AV fistula?	An abnormal direct connection between an artery and a vein, producing a shunt that bypasses a capillary bed
What are the 2 most common causes of an AV fistula?	Congenital defects and trauma
What finding on cardiac exam is associated with AV malformations of the GI tract?	Aortic insufficiency
What are the possible effects of cirsoid aneurysms?	Rupture, bleeding, and strain on the heart due to the shunting of blood (high-output failure)

Anatomic forms of aneurysms

Describe the 4 anatomic forms of aneurysms.	1. Saccular: to one side 2. Fusiform: spindle shaped 3. Cylindrical: distinct borders 4. Berry: 0.5 to 2.0 cm
Which 3 forms predispose to thrombus formation?	Saccular, fusiform, and cylindrical
Where are berry aneurysms usually found?	In small cerebral arteries and the circle of Willis. They are usually at the bifurcations of these vessels and are associated with congenital weakness of the media.
Why are berry aneurysms worrisome?	They can rupture and cause life-threatening subarachnoid hemorrhage.
Which 3 anatomic forms of aneurysms are associated with atherosclerosis?	Saccular, fusiform, and cylindrical

Mycotic aneurysms

What causes mycotic aneurysms?

Invasion and weakening of the vessel wall by bacteria or fungi

Where do they occur?

In the aorta and cerebral, mesenteric, splenic, and renal arteries

Name 3 complications of mycotic aneurysms.

Septic emboli; bacteremia; rupture

AORTIC DISSECTION

Aortic dissection is a concern in which patients?

Any patient with chest or upper back pain

What risk factors are associated with aortic dissection?

Chest trauma, motor vehicle accident, Marfan syndrome, syphilis, history of vascular disease, and hypertension

What is the major complication with aortic dissection?

Aortic rupture, which is often lethal. Immediate medical management is needed to lower the blood pressure and prevent further damage. Urgent surgical intervention is indicated.

How would one look for aortic dissection on physical exam?

Measure the blood pressure in both arms. Dissection can obstruct blood flow to one arm (usually the left) and cause a disparity between pressures.

What common radiograph can pick up an aortic dissection?

Chest x-rays show a widened mediastinum.

What is the usual plane of dissection?

Between the outer one third and the inner two thirds of the tunica media

Where does rupture usually occur and what does it cause?

Through the aventia of the aorta (the plane is closer to the outside), often into the pericardial sac, where it causes tamponade and death if not immediately recognized and treated.

What occurs if it ruptures toward the inside of the vessel?

A "double-barrel aorta" is created if the plane extends into the intima.

What is seen microscopically?	Areas of decreased or absent elastic tissue with metachromic acid mucopolysaccharides

IDIOPATHIC CYSTIC MEDIAL NECROSIS

What is damaged in idiopathic cystic medial necrosis?	The tunica media of the aorta
What can bleeding within this layer cause?	Longitudinal dissection
What is the cause of idiopathic cystic medial necrosis?	Unknown; the disease is idiopathic.
Describe the signs and symptoms.	Usually absent until dissection occurs. Then, one sees chest pain (expanding mass and obstruction of the coronaries), renal obstruction with failure and hematuria, and vertebral artery obstruction with sensory and motor abnormalities.

HYPERTENSION

How does the World Health Organization (WHO) define hypertension?	Sustained blood pressure elevation with systolic blood pressure > 160, diastolic blood pressure > 90, or both.
What is essential hypertension?	Elevated blood pressure with no known cause
Essential hypertension accounts for what percentage of hypertension?	$> 90\%$
What are the risk factors for essential hypertension?	Family history, high dietary sodium, smoking, stress, obesity, and sedentary lifestyle
What can essential hypertension do?	Routinely causes end-organ damage to the retina, heart, and kidneys. It is associated with left ventricular hypertrophy, cardiac ischemia, atherosclerosis, arteriolosclerosis, stroke, and nephrosclerosis.

What are small hemor-rhagic strokes in the brain caused by hypertension called?

Charcot-Buchard aneurysms or lacunar infarcts

What is secondary hyper-tension?

Elevated blood pressure caused by a known entity

What are 11 causes of secondary hypertension?

1. Renal parenchymal disease
2. Renal artery stenosis
3. Cushing disease
4. Conn disease
5. Acromegaly
6. Pheochromocytoma
7. Hyperthyroidism
8. Brain tumors
9. Coarctation of the aorta
10. Drugs
11. Toxins

Does bilateral renal artery stenosis produce secondary hypertension?

No, but unilateral stenosis does.

Name the 2 major causes of renal artery stenosis.

Atherosclerosis; fibromuscular dysplasia

How does renal disease produce hypertension?

Through improper activation of the renin-angiotensin system (RAS)

What is a good treatment for renal-induced hyper-tension?

Administration of angiotensin-converting enzyme (ACE) inhibitors, because they act on the RAS. (Use with caution in patients with renal failure.)

What is characteristic of malignant hypertension?

An accelerated course with multiple organ damage

What is a "flea-bitten" kidney, and what accounts for that name?

A kidney with malignant nephrosclerosis due to malignant hypertension. Petechiae on the surface of the diseased kidneys account for the name.

Who most often gets malignant hypertension?

Young black males

Who can develop malignant hypertension?

Anyone with hypertension can progress to malignant hypertension.

VEINS

What do large veins have that arteries do not?	Valves formed from endothelial folds
What do arteries have that veins do not?	Well-defined and developed layers
What is a consequence of this on veins?	Veins are more easily compressed, dilated, and penetrated (e.g., by neoplasms) than arteries.

VENOUS THROMBOSIS

Name and describe 3 different types.	1. Thrombophlebitis: thrombosis with inflammation 2. Phlebothrombosis: thrombosis alone 3. Deep venous thrombosis (DVT): thrombophlebitis of deep veins
What is Virchow's triad?	A famous pathologist's list of risk factors for venous thrombosis: stasis; endothelial damage; hypercoagulability
Where do venous thrombi usually form?	In deep veins of the lower extremities, often near valves
What is the greatest risk factor?	Immobility, such as lying in a hospital bed for a prolonged period
Name 5 fates of a thrombus.	1. Travel: embolize 2. Die: dissolved by body's intrinsic heparinization system or exogenous heparin 3. Grow older: organize 4. Change its mind: recanalize 5. Put on weight: grow larger
What is the most significant clinical consequence of a DVT?	Embolization to the pulmonary vasculature, causing pulmonary infarction [pulmonary embolism (PE)]
How is DVT detected clinically?	Physical exam is notoriously unreliable, but one can see unilateral leg edema, erythema, palpable venous cords, tenderness, or a positive Homans' sign. Other tests include Doppler ultrasound and venograms.

What is a positive Homans' sign?

Pain with dorsiflexion of the foot

What other kinds of emboli can go to the lungs?

1. Fat
2. Bone marrow
3. Tumor
4. Gas/air
5. Septic

What is the main clinical feature of superficial thrombophlebitis?

Tender, erythematous venous cords, usually without edema

What laboratory findings are associated with DVTs and PEs?

An elevated D-dimer and a low fibrinogen level are often present due to consumption of clotting factors.

Describe a skin manifestation of venous occlusion.

"Stasis dermatitis" with violaceous and erythematous edema and ulceration

VARICOSE VEINS

What are varicose veins?

Abnormally dilated and tortuous superficial veins

Where are they usually found?

In the superficial veins of the lower extremities

What is the cause?

Increased intraluminal pressure and loss of structural support, owing to valvular incompetence or absence, weakening of venous walls, or prolonged standing

What are 5 risk factors for developing varicose veins?

1. Older women with a positive family history of the disorder
2. People who spend a great deal of time on their feet
3. Obesity
4. Pregnancy
5. Positive history of thrombophlebitis

What are the clinical features?

At first, they are a cosmetic defect, but can progress to edema, aching pain, stasis dermatitis, ulceration, and cellulitis.

Other than the lower extremities, where do clinically significant varicose veins occur?

In the esophagus and the hemorrhoidal venous plexus

What is the major cause of these varices?	Portal hypertension secondary to cirrhosis of the liver
What is phlebosclerosis and where is it found?	Vein rigidity caused by calcification. It is often found in long-standing varicose veins of larger vessels and can show on x-ray.
Name 2 therapies for varicose veins of the lower extremities.	1. Elastic hose (provide structural support to veins) 2. Surgical vein stripping
What are some therapies for varices of the esophagus and hemorrhoidal venous plexus?	Banding, sclerotherapy, vasopressin injections, and shunting procedures to decrease the high pressure to these veins

PHLEBITIS

What is phlebitis?	Inflammation of veins
Name some of the causes.	The same risk factors as for venous thrombosis: infection, heart failure, stasis from immobility, pregnancy, post-operative, and cancer
What can it cause?	Injury to the vessel wall, thrombosis, and pain

LYMPHATICS

What is the function of lymphatics?	They return extravasated fluid from the interstitial spaces to the vascular system, and play a role in the immune system.
Describe their structure.	Endothelial canals with loose cellular connections. Larger vessels have valves and some smooth muscle. Fluid in the canals is moved by the action of adjacent skeletal muscle groups.
What is a primary disorder of the lymphatic system?	Very uncommon inherited or congenital defects in the lymphatics, which manifest as dilation and eventual fibrosis
Name 3 primary disorders of the lymphatic system.	1. Lymphedema praecox usually appears in women in their teens and 20s as severe lower extremity edema, and eventually extends up the body.

2. Milroy disease (heredofamilial lymphedema) can occur in one limb due to inherited failure of its lymphatics to develop.
3. Simple congenital lymphedema is a malformation of lymphatic formation during development, usually in a single limb.

What is a secondary disorder of the lymphatic system?

Disruption of lymphatic structure caused by something extrinsic to the system

What is more common, primary or secondary disorders?

Secondary disorders

Name 5 causes of secondary disorders.

1. Radiation
2. Surgery
3. Soft tissue infections
4. Neoplasms metastasizing through lymphatics
5. Filaria parasites

What is the most common infection of lymphatics (lymphangitis)?

Group A β-hemolytic streptococci (*Streptococcus pyogenes*)

What women commonly get secondary lymphedema of the upper extremities?

Those with breast cancer treated by surgery or radiation

What are the clinical features of lymphatic system disorders?

As in varicose veins, stasis dermatitis, edema, ulcerations, and cellulitis

What caused the Elephant Man's problem?

Filiariasis

What general type of cancers commonly metastasize through the lymphatic system?

Adenocarcinomas

What kind of edema does not pit, and why?

Lymphedema is not associated with pitting because the fluid extravasates into the interstitial compartment, and then cannot travel out effectively due to the obstructed lymphatics.

TUMORS OF THE VASCULAR SYSTEM

Name 3 benign vascular tumors.	Angiomas (hemangiomas), lymphangiomas, and glomangiomas
Name 3 malignant vascular tumors.	Angiosarcomas, lymphangiosarcomas, and hemangiopericytoma
What are 2 types of angiomas?	Cavernous hemangiomas and capillary hemangiomas
What is the most common tumor of infancy?	Angiomas causing port-wine stain "birthmarks"
What are cavernous hemangiomas and where are they usually found?	Benign tumors of cavernous channels, which form violaceous lesions on the skin, mucosal membranes, brain, liver, spleen, and pancreas
What are capillary hemangiomas and where are they usually found?	Benign tumors of loose capillaries forming red or bluish lesions on the skin, mucosal membranes, liver, spleen, and kidneys
What can capillary hemangiomas do clinically?	They can bleed if disrupted.
What is von Hippel-Lindau disease?	An autosomal dominant disorder characterized by multiple cavernous hemangiomas
Those with von Hippel-Lindau disease are at increased risk for what carcinoma?	Renal cell carcinoma
What is Sturge-Weber syndrome?	Port-wine stains of the face, in trigeminal nerve distribution, with ipsilateral cavernous hemangiomas in the retina and leptomeninges
Name 3 other clinical findings associated with Sturge-Weber syndrome.	Mental retardation; seizures; hemiparalysis
What is another name for cavernous lymphangiomas?	Cystic hygromas

Where are they usually found?	On the neck and axilla
Why are they difficult to treat?	They invade surrounding tissues, making complete surgical excision difficult.
How are capillary hemangiomas distinguished from capillary lymphangiomas microscopically?	By the presence of red blood cells (RBCs)
What is another name for glomangiomas?	Glomus tumors
What is a glomus body?	A neuromyoarterial group of cells that function in temperature regulation
Name the 4 places glomangiomas are usually found.	1. Subungual 2. Soft tissue 3. Wall of the stomach 4. Central nervous system (CNS)
What is the primary symptom?	Pain. These tumors are heavily innervated.
What are telangiectasias?	Abnormal dilatations (aneurysms) of small vessels
In what 2 clinical situations are they often seen, and why?	Pregnancy and liver disease; most likely due to increased estrogen levels
What is a spider telangiectasia?	A central, abnormally dilated vessel surrounded by small capillaries radiating outward
Name 3 skin manifestations of alcoholic liver disease.	Jaundice, palmar erythema, and spider telangiectasia
What is Osler-Weber-Rendu disease (hereditary hemorrhagic telangiectasia)?	An autosomal dominant disorder characterized by multiple telangiectasias. These can cause epistaxis and GI bleeding.
What is an angiosarcoma?	A malignant tumor of vascular tissue usually found in the skin, musculoskeletal system, breast, or liver
What are some risk factors?	Chemical exposures, such as arsenic, and certain radioactive agents

What is a risk factor for development of liver angiosarcoma?	Polyvinyl chloride (PVC) exposure
What is Kaposi sarcoma?	A rare malignant vascular tumor derived from endothelial cells, and characterized by painful purple or brown lesions
What 2 populations have a high incidence of Kaposi's sarcoma?	1. Ashkenazi Jewish men 2. HIV-infected homosexual men

POWER REVIEW

What accounts for 50% of all deaths in the United States?	Atherosclerotic disease and its complications
Where in the artery does one find atherosclerosis?	In the intima
What does Monckeberg arteriosclerosis do to blood flow?	It has no effect on blood flow.
Where in the artery does one find Monckeberg?	Monckeberg **M**edial calcific sclerosis in the **M**edia of **M**uscular arteries
Where in the vasculature system is most thermoregulatory control exerted?	Arterioles. They are autonomic arteries.
What are the 4 big risk factors for atherosclerosis?	1. Dyslipidemia 2. Hypertension 3. Smoking 4. Diabetes mellitus
What is the major modifiable risk factor for atherosclerosis?	Smoking
Which early pathological lesions of atherosclerosis correlate best with the location of advanced atherosclerosis?	The intimal pads
What is the major lipoprotein of the serum cholesterol?	LDL accounts for 75%.

What are the 2 key apo-proteins of LDL and HDL?

Apo B100 and A1, respectively

Which type of familial hyperlipidemia is most associated with early death from atherosclerotic disease?

Type II

What are the 2 risk factors for arteriolosclerosis?

Hypertension and diabetes mellitus

Where does arteriolosclerosis usually show itself?

In the kidneys, where it causes nephrosclerosis

Who gets fibromuscular dysplasia?

Women in their 30s or 40s

With what infection is PAN associated?

Hepatitis B

Where does PAN hit?

It can strike any muscular vessel.

What is the major complication of temporal arteritis?

Blindness, caused by involvement of the ophthalmic artery

Where does Takayasu arteritis exert its effects?

The aorta and proximal segments of the great vessels

Describe the pulses in Takayasu.

Upper extremity pulses are diminished or absent, and lower extremity pulses are increased.

What is the potentially lethal complication of Kawasaki disease?

Involvement of the coronary arteries

Who gets Buerger disease?

Young male smokers, especially those of Jewish descent

What is the usual cause of Raynaud phenomenon?

Connective tissue diseases

What is the usual cause of Raynaud disease?

The cause is unknown.

What is the most common cause of aneurysms?

Atherosclerosis

Where do atherosclerotic aneurysms occur?

The abdominal aorta, usually below the renal arteries (infrarenal)

Where do luetic aneurysms occur?

The ascending and transverse thoracic aorta

The destruction of what layer of the arterial wall predisposes to aneurysm formation?

The tunica media

What type of aneurysm is described as a "tree-bark aorta"?

Syphilitic

Name 2 disorders associated with idiopathic cystic medial necrosis.

Hypertension; Marfan disease

What is the plane of dissection in aortic dissections?

Between the outer one third and the inner two thirds of the tunica media

What is a cirsoid aneurysm?

An aneurysm that develops from an AV fistula

What anatomic form of aneurysm is usually found in the brain?

Berry

What is hypertension according to the WHO?

Sustained systolic BP > 160 and/or diastolic BP > 90

Who in the United States has a higher chance of developing accelerated or severe hypertension?

African Americans

What is the cause of most hypertension?

Over 90% of cases are classified as "essential," and are thus without a known cause.

What kind of renal artery stenosis causes secondary hypertension?

Unilateral, through activation of the RAS

What causes "flea-bitten" kidneys?

Malignant nephrosclerosis secondary to malignant hypertension

What makes malignant hypertension malignant?

End-organ damage to the brain, retina, heart, and kidneys

What predisposes to DVT?

Virchow's triad of stasis, endothelial damage, and hypercoagulability

Where are the most clinically significant DVTs found?

In the deep veins of the lower extremities

What is the dangerous complication of DVT?

Pulmonary embolism

What predisposes to varicose veins?

Anything that increases the intraluminal pressure

What is Milroy disease?

A primary disorder of the lymphatic system, which manifests as the failure of lymphatics to develop in one limb

What kind of tumors like the lymphatic system?

Adenocarcinomas

What is PVC a risk factor for?

Liver angiosarcoma

13 Anemia

What is anemia?

Technically, a decrease in whole body red blood cell (RBC) mass; practically, a drop in hemoglobin or hematocrit

What are 2 main causes?

1. Decreased production of RBCs
2. Increased loss of RBCs

Name 3 mechanisms of decreased RBC production.

1. Bone marrow suppression due to drug effects
2. Radiation
3. Infection

Name 2 mechanisms of increased RBC loss.

1. External blood loss (trauma)
2. RBC destruction (hemolytic anemia)

What lab test distinguishes hemorrhage from hemolysis?

Serum haptoglobin is decreased in hemolysis, but not in hemorrhage.

How does the body compensate for RBC loss?

Reticulocytosis and erythroid hyperplasia of the bone marrow

What are the classic symptoms of anemia?

Pallor, fatigue, tachycardia, palpitations, dizziness, and shortness of breath

What is peculiar about the anemia of pregnancy?

It is not a true anemia. The decrease in hematocrit is due to the dilutional effect of increased plasma volume.

What is myelophthisic anemia?

Blunted erythropoiesis due to infiltration of the bone marrow by neoplastic cells or fibrotic tissue

ACUTE POSTHEMORRHAGIC ANEMIA

What is the cause of initial symptoms?

Hypovolemia

What are typical lab values acutely?

Often, hemoglobin and hematocrit are normal in the first few hours due to the loss of plasma and RBCs.

183

IRON DEFICIENCY ANEMIA

What is the mechanism?

Impaired heme synthesis

In which three populations is it more common?

1. Infants (especially preemies)
2. Preadolescents
3. Pregnant women

How long will a newborn's iron stores last without supplementation?

6 months

What is the major cause in adults?

Chronic blood loss due to menorrhagia or gastrointestinal (GI) bleeding

What is present on the peripheral smear?

Hypochromic, microcytic RBCs

What are the 5 classic lab values?

1. Decreased hemoglobin
2. Decreased hematocrit
3. Decreased serum iron
4. Decreased serum ferritin
5. Increased total iron binding capacity (TIBC)

What are some clinical findings in extreme states of iron deficiency anemia?

Glossitis, gastritis, Plummer-Vinson syndrome (esophageal web), and koilonychia

MEGALOBLASTIC ANEMIA

What is the cause?

Deficiency of vitamin B_{12} or folate

How do these deficiencies lead to anemia?

Both vitamin B_{12} and folate are necessary for DNA synthesis. Decreased DNA synthesis subsequently leads to decreased RBC production.

What is a megaloblast?

An erythroid precursor cell found in the bone marrow

What are typical lab findings?

Pancytopenia, decreased vitamin B_{12}, decreased folate

What is seen on histology?

Oval macrocytosis, hypersegmented neutrophils (> 5 lobes), and megalo-blastic hyperplasia of bone marrow

VITAMIN B$_{12}$ DEFICIENCY

What is the most common cause?	Pernicious anemia
Define pernicious anemia.	An autoimmune disorder with failure of production of intrinsic factor (IF) due to anti-IF antibodies
How is IF related to vitamin B$_{12}$?	IF is essential for the absorption of vitamin B$_{12}$ in the distal ileum.
What are the 4 clinical findings of pernicious anemia?	1. Yellow skin 2. Stomatitis 3. Glossitis 4. Subacute combined degeneration of the spinal cord
How does subacute combined degeneration of the spinal cord manifest?	Ataxic gait, hyperreflexia, and impaired vibratory and positional sensation
What abnormal antibodies are found?	Anti-IF and antiparietal cell antibodies
What are the results of a Schilling test?	Decreased vitamin B$_{12}$ absorption corrected by adding IF
What type of gastritis is present?	Chronic fundal gastritis (Type A)
What feared entity may Type A gastritis progress to?	Gastric cancer
What are some other causes of vitamin B$_{12}$ deficiency?	Intestinal bacterial overgrowth, gastric resection, vegetarian diet, intestinal malabsorption, *D. latum* infestation
What are 2 causes of excess bacteria in the intestine?	Broad-spectrum antibiotics and blind-loop syndrome

FOLATE DEFICIENCY

What are some causes of folate deficiency?	Poor diet, pregnancy, sprue, drug effects, and *Giardia lamblia* infection

In which populations is diet-related folate deficiency often found?	Chronic alcoholics and fad dieters
What drugs are associated with decreased folate?	Phenytoin, oral contraceptives, and methotrexate
How does hemolytic anemia cause a relative deficiency of folate?	The compensatory accelerated erythropoiesis uses up the body stores of folate.

ANEMIA OF CHRONIC DISEASE

What is the cause of anemia of chronic disease?	As the name implies, this condition results from several underlying systemic pathologies, including renal disease, rheumatoid arthritis, and chronic infection.
How common is anemia of chronic disease?	Among anemias, second only to iron deficiency
What does the peripheral blood smear look like?	Usually normochromic and normocytic

APLASTIC ANEMIA

What is most often the cause?	Toxic exposure to radiation, chemicals, or drugs
What are some drugs associated with aplastic anemia?	Chloramphenicol, alkylating agents, sulfonamides, gold salts, and anti-malarials
What chemical may be a cause?	Benzene
What does the peripheral blood smear show?	Pancytopenia
What is the appearance of the bone marrow?	Marked hypocellularity. The bone marrow may be completely occupied by fat.
What 2 viral infections may be responsible?	Parvovirus; hepatitis C virus

HEMOLYTIC ANEMIA

List 3 lab abnormalities in hemolytic anemia.	1. Increased unconjugated bilirubin 2. Decreased serum haptoglobin 3. Decreased hemoglobinuria

What are some clinical effects of hyperbilirubi-nemia?	Jaundice and pigment-containing gallstones
What usually causes intra-corpuscular hemolytic anemia?	Genetic defects in the RBC, leading to their destruction.
What is the most frequent cause of extracorpuscular hemolytic anemia?	Acquired changes in the RBC environ-ment, which lead to their destruction (e.g., circulating antibodies, enlarged spleen)

IMMUNE HEMOLYTIC ANEMIAS

What is the most common type?	Warm antibody autoimmune hemolytic anemia (WAIHA)
What class of antibody mediates WAIHA?	IgG autoantibodies
How do the antibodies cause anemia?	They bind to RBC surface antigens at an optimum temperature of 37°C, making the RBCs susceptible to destruction in the spleen.
Name 3 diseases associated with WAIHA.	1. Systemic lupus erythematosus (SLE) 2. Hodgkin lymphoma 3. Non-Hodgkin lymphoma
What abnormality in RBC structure may be found on peripheral smear in WAIHA?	Spherocytosis, due to loss of RBC mem brane protein after circulation through the spleen
What is the result of a direct Coombs test in WAIHA?	Positive, due to IgG-RBC binding

COLD AGGLUTININ DISEASE

What class of antibody mediates cold agglutinin disease?	IgM
At what temperature are the antibodies active?	Below 30°C
Against what antigen are the antibodies often directed?	I blood group antigen

Acute cold agglutinin disease is often a complication of what 2 diseases?	Mononucleosis and mycoplasma pneumonia
What 2 diseases are associated with the chronic form of cold agglutinin disease?	Lymphoid neoplasms and Raynaud phenomenon

HEMOLYTIC DISEASE OF THE NEWBORN

What is another name for this condition?	Erythroblastosis fetalis
What is the cause?	Maternal antibodies against fetal RBC antigens cross the placenta, resulting in fetal hemolytic anemia.
Specifically, what is the antibody directed against?	Rh locus D of erythrocytes
How might ABO incompatibility be the cause?	Mother is blood group O, and fetus is blood group A or B.
How can Rh incompatibility be prevented?	Administration of anti-D IgG antiserum to Rh$^-$ mother at the delivery of an Rh$^+$ child prevents maternal alloimmunization.
Aside from anemia, what are some other consequences to the fetus?	Hydrops fetalis, kernicterus, fetal heart failure, postnatal rise in unconjugated bilirubin
What 2 common abnormalities of cord blood may help in diagnosis?	1. Direct Coombs test positive 2. Presence of immature RBC precursors
How do you treat acute Rh incompatibility?	Exchange transfusion of the newborn infant
Define kernicterus.	Neurologic damage caused by high levels of unconjugated bilirubin in the central nervous system (CNS), especially the basal ganglia

PAROXYSMAL NOCTURNAL HEMOGLOBINURIA

What is it?	An uncommon acquired intracorpuscular defect of RBCs
What is the cause?	A somatic mutation results in an abnormal bone marrow stem cell.

What is the typical presentation?	Morning urine contains hemoglobin and appears darker than normal due to complement-induced red cell lysis.

HEREDITARY SPHEROCYTOSIS

What is hereditary spherocytosis?	The most common inherited intra-corpuscular hemolytic anemia in Caucasians. It is characterized by spherical RBCs.
What is its mode of inheritance?	Autosomal dominant
What causes the anemia?	The abnormally shaped cells are trapped and destroyed in the spleen.
Why are the RBCs shaped like spheres?	Molecular defects in cytoskeletal proteins in the RBC (e.g., spectrin, ankyrin, and protein 4.2) cause the deformity.
What is the diagnostic test?	Increased erythrocyte osmotic fragility to hypotonic saline
What other abnormalities may contribute to the diagnosis?	
In lab values?	Reticulocytosis, increased mean corpuscular hemoglobin concentration (MCHC), and unconjugated hyper-bilirubinemia
On physical exam?	Acholuric jaundice and splenomegaly

HEREDITARY ELLIPTOCYTOSIS

What is it?	A condition characterized by elongated, oval RBCs, which may cause anemia
How is it inherited?	Autosomal dominant
What abnormality may be found on physical exam?	Splenomegaly

GLUCOSE-6-PHOSPHATE DEHYDROGENASE (G6PD) DEFICIENCY

What is it?	The most common enzyme-deficiency

hemolytic anemia. It is characterized by acute self-limited episodes of anemia.

What triggers the episodes of anemia?

Oxidative stress to the RBCs

What are some causes of oxidative stress?

Infection, sulfonamides, nitrofurantoin, antimalarials, and fava beans

How is it inherited?

X-linked, with incomplete dominance

In which populations is it most frequently found?

African Americans (10% carry the gene) and Mediterranean populations

PYRUVATE KINASE DEFICIENCY

What is it?

A chronic form of hemolytic anemia due to a deficiency of the enzyme pyruvate kinase

How is it inherited?

Autosomal recessive

How is this anemia different than G6PD deficiency?

The anemia is chronic and nonepisodic.

SICKLE CELL ANEMIA

What is it?

The homozygous form of hemoglobin S (Hb S), leading to severe lifelong hemolytic anemia

What is Hb S?

An abnormal hemoglobin structure due to a point mutation in codon 6 of the β-globin gene, with substitution of valine for glutamic acid

What percent of African Americans carry this mutation?

7%

What is a benefit of carrying the Hb S gene?

Resistance to malarial infection

How does the anemia develop?

At low oxygen tension, Hb S polymerizes and distorts the RBC to a sickled shape with stiffened membranes; the sickled cells may obstruct small vessels and are more susceptible to hemolysis.

Describe 3 diagnostic tests.	1. Sickled RBCs on peripheral smear 2. In vitro sickling of RBCs on exposure to reducing agents (positive sickle cell prep) 3. Electrophoresis demonstrating homozygous Hb S
What are associated clinical features of the disease?	Painful vaso-occlusive events, repeated splenic infarcts leading to autosplenectomy, stroke, cholelithiasis, hematuria, chronic leg ulcers, and aplastic crises
What is an aplastic crisis?	A sudden drop in hemoglobin
What is sickle cell trait?	Heterozygous Hb S, usually without clinical consequence; sickle cell prep is positive.
Name 2 other hemoglobinopathies.	Hb C disorders, Hb E disorders
How does Hb C cause disease?	If homozygous or heterozygous with another abnormal hemoglobin
What characterizes Hb C disease?	Mild hemolytic anemia, splenomegaly, target cells, intraerythrocytic crystals
In which population is Hb C found?	African Americans
In which 2 regions is Hb E found?	In southeast Asia and some urban areas of the United States

THALASSEMIAS

What are the 3 types of thalassemias?	β thalassemia major β thalassemia minor α thalassemia

β THALASSEMIA MAJOR

What are 2 other names for this disease?	Cooley anemia; Mediterranean anemia
Genetically, what causes it?	Double heterozygosity or homozygosity of defective β-globin genes; may be a point mutation or deletion.

What portions of the genes are defective?	The abnormality may be in the promotor sequence, introns, or coding regions.
Where is the β-globin gene located?	On chromosome 11
Geographically, where is the disease commonly found?	As with all thalassemias, it is prevalent in the Mediterranean, and in southeast Asia, Africa, and India.
What causes the anemia?	Aggregation of insoluble α-chains leads to early RBC destruction, decreased hemoglobin production, ineffective erythropoiesis, and relative folate deficiency.
What are some other features of the disease?	Splenomegaly, distortion of bones (e.g., skull, face, extremities) due to marrow expansion, microcytosis, hypochromia, increased hemoglobin F, hemosiderosis

β THALASSEMIA MINOR

Genetically, what causes it?	Heterozygous inheritance of a defective β-globin gene
How does it manifest clinically?	Anemia with minimal microcytosis and hypochromia
What is the diagnostic lab value?	Increased Hb A_2
What is sickle cell thalassemia?	Coinheritance of thalassemic β-globin gene (double heterozygous) and Hb S. The disease is similar to sickle cell anemia, although less severe.

α THALASSEMIA

What is the cause genetically?	Deletion of one or more of the 4 α-globin genes
Where are the α-globin genes located?	On chromosome 16
How does it manifest?	
One deletion?	No clinical consequences

Two deletions?	Mild to moderate thalassemic state
Three deletions?	Mild to moderate thalassemic state
Four deletions?	Intrauterine death

POWER REVIEW

What is the most common cause of anemia?	Iron deficiency
What condition is characterized by episodic anemia brought on by oxidative stress?	G6PD deficiency
What disease is present if oval macrocytes, hypersegmented neutrophils, and few platelets are seen on peripheral smear?	Megaloblastic anemia
What genetic mutation results in production of Hb S?	Point mutation at position 6 of the β-globin gene, with substitution of valine for glutamic acid
How is hereditary spherocytosis inherited?	Autosomal dominant
What would be the expected reticulocyte count after a hemorrhagic event?	Elevated
What causes subacute combined degeneration of the spinal cord?	Vitamin B_{12} deficiency
What leads to autosplenectomy in patients with sickle cell anemia?	Repeated splenic infarcts due to sickling of RBCs
What anemia is associated with decreased serum haptoglobin?	Hemolytic anemia
Which anemia is mediated by IgM antibodies specific for erythrocyte antigens?	Warm antibody autoimmune hemolytic anemia

Deletions in chromosome 16 may result in what disease?   α thalassemia

To what form of anemia has benzene been linked as a cause?   Aplastic anemia

14

Neoplastic and Proliferative Disorders of the Hematopoietic and Lymphoid Systems

LEUKEMIA

What is leukemia?	A group of malignancies originating from lymphoid or hematopoietic cell lines
Where in the body are the leukemic cells found?	In the bone marrow, liver, spleen, lymph nodes, and meninges
What results from bone marrow infiltration by leukemic cells?	Aplastic marrow with depletion of normally functioning white blood cells (WBCs), red blood cells (RBCs), and platelets
What characterizes acute leukemia?	A predominance of blasts in bone marrow and peripheral blood
What is the natural history of acute leukemia?	Death in 6 to 12 months
Which cells predominate in chronic leukemia?	More mature lymphoid or hematopoietic cells

ACUTE LYMPHOBLASTIC LEUKEMIA (ALL)

Which cells predominate in ALL?	Lymphoblasts, with 80% of B-cell origin
In what population is ALL found?	Children

What are some presenting symptoms?	Fatigue, weakness, lymphadenopathy, excessive bleeding, easy bruisability, bone pain, and joint pain
What is the prognosis?	With current treatment, 5-year survival rates are close to 80%.
How are the subgroups classified?	Based on morphology and cell-surface markers

ACUTE MYELOBLASTIC LEUKEMIA (AML)

Which cells predominate in AML?	Myeloblasts and early promyelocytes
What abnormal granule may be present in blasts?	Auer rods
In what population is it found?	Adults
What are some abnormalities on physical exam?	Petechiae, lymphadenopathy, hepatosplenomegaly, and thickened gums
What is the response to therapy?	Not as good as ALL; about 50%
How are the subgroups classified?	Based on morphology and cytochemical characteristics
What subtype is associated with a better prognosis?	Acute promyelocytic leukemia (APML)
What complication often arises in APML?	Disseminated intravascular coagulation (DIC)

CHRONIC LYMPHOCYTIC LEUKEMIA (CLL)

Which cells predominate in CLL?	Neoplastic lymphoid cells (98% are B cells), which closely resemble normal mature lymphocytes
Can the leukemic cells differentiate into antibody-producing plasma cells?	No
In what age group does CLL occur?	People > 60

Which sex is more affected?   Men

What are "smudge cells"?   Mechanically disrupted leukemic cells; seen in peripheral blood. They are common in CLL.

What is a typical WBC count?   50,000 to 200,000/μL. The majority are leukemic cells.

What is the natural history?   Slowly progressive disease, which is relatively benign

What is the mean survival?   3 to 7 years

How effective is treatment?   It may relieve symptoms, but has little effect on survival.

What are some complications?   Warm antibody autoimmune hemolytic anemia (WAIHA) and bacterial infection secondary to hypogammaglobulinemia

HAIRY CELL LEUKEMIA

What is hairy cell leukemia?   A low-grade clonal proliferation of a B lymphocyte

What are hairy cells?   Lymphoid cells with prominent cytoplasmic projections found on peripheral smear

Who is most often affected?   Middle-aged men

What are some presenting symptoms?   Fatigue, weakness, infection, and easy bruisability

How is it treated?   With splenectomy and interferon alfa

MYELOPROLIFERATIVE SYNDROMES

What are myeloproliferative syndromes?   Neoplastic clonal proliferations of myeloid stem cells

In what age group do they occur?   Middle-aged to elderly persons

What lab abnormalities are found?   Increased basophils and increased serum uric acid

On physical exam, what organ is often significantly enlarged?   The spleen

What are the 4 myeloproliferative disorders?	1. Chronic myelocytic leukemia 2. Polycythemia vera 3. Myeloid metaplasia 4. Essential thrombocytopenia

CHRONIC MYELOCYTIC LEUKEMIA (CML)

What is CML?	A myeloproliferative disorder with clonal proliferation of myeloid stem cells
Which cells predominate?	Myelocytes, metamyelocytes, bands, and segmented neutrophils
What is a typical WBC count?	50,000 to 200,000/μL (similar to CLL)
What do normal myeloid cells develop into?	RBCs, granulocytes, and platelets
What chromosomal abnormality is diagnostic?	The Philadelphia chromosome, a reciprocal translocation between chromosomes 9 and 22
What is the *bcr-abl* gene?	It is formed by transposition of the c-*abl* proto-oncogene of chromosome 9 onto an area of chromosome 22. The resultant hybrid codes for a protein with tyrosine kinase activity.
In what age group is it commonly found?	Persons 35 to 50 years old
What are some common symptoms?	Fever, splenomegaly, and fatigue
What is a blastic crisis?	An accelerated phase of the disease with increased blasts and promyelocytes. It precedes death in many cases.
What is the leukocyte alkaline phosphatase activity?	Often reduced

POLYCYTHEMIA VERA

What are the clinical characteristics?	Marked erythrocytosis, leukocytosis, thrombocytosis, splenomegaly, and decreased erythropoietin

What complications may the high hematocrit cause? Thrombotic or hemorrhagic disorders

What is the median survival? 10 to 20 years

What is the late phase of disease? Anemia with bone marrow fibrosis, extramedullary hematopoiesis, and increased WBC. It may be difficult to distinguish from CML.

What distinguishes it from secondary polycythemia? Low erythropoietin levels

What conditions are associated with secondary polycythemia? Chronic hypoxia, tumors producing erythropoietin, endocrine abnormalities

MYELOID METAPLASIA

What is myelofibrosis? Non-neoplastic fibrous tissue proliferating within the bone marrow cavity

Why are the liver and spleen enlarged? Because of profound extramedullary hematopoiesis

What is thought to be the primary abnormality? Megakaryocytic proliferation. Peripheral blood thrombocytosis and bone marrow megakaryocytosis are prominent.

What are some clinical features? Anemia, splenomegaly, teardrop-shaped erythrocytes

ESSENTIAL THROMBOCYTHEMIA

Where are the neoplastic cells? In peripheral blood (thrombocytosis) and in the bone marrow (megakaryocytosis)

What is the platelet count? Commonly greater than 1 million/μL

What are some complications? Bleeding and thrombosis

INFECTIOUS MONONUCLEOSIS

What is infectious mononucleosis? A benign, self-limited illness caused by the Epstein-Barr virus (EBV)

Which lymphocytes are affected?	B cells
How does it present clinically?	Sore throat, fever, fatigue, lymphadenopathy, and hepatosplenomegaly
Name 3 diagnostic features.	1. Circulating atypical lymphocytes 2. Anti-EBV antibody 3. Heterophil antibodies
What are some other causes of nonmalignant lymphadenopathy?	Toxoplasmosis (posterior cervical adenopathy), syphilis (inguinal adenopathy), cat-scratch disease (axillary adenopathy), AIDS, tuberculosis, and sarcoidosis

MULTIPLE MYELOMA

What is multiple myeloma?	A malignant plasma cell tumor
From what cell is the neoplastic clone derived?	B lymphocytes
How is the bone affected?	The malignant cells secrete excess osteoclast-activating factor, which causes lytic bone lesions.
What is found on radiographic exam of the bone?	Punched-out lesions and osteopenia (demineralization)
What is characteristically found on electrophoresis of immunoglobulins?	Identical molecules, called M protein, cause a sharp spike on electrophoresis.
What is the M protein?	A monoclonal IgG or IgA immunoglobulin of either κ or λ light chain specificity
What is the Bence-Jones protein?	Excess free immunoglobulin light chains found in the urine
Why is total protein increased?	Because serum immunoglobulins are markedly increased (hyperglobulinemia)
How does hyperglobulinemia affect RBCs?	It causes them to stack on top of one another in a rouleau formation.
Why are patients with multiple myeloma more susceptible to infection?	Normal Ig production is impaired due to clonal proliferation of the M protein.

What are some other clinical characteristics?	Anemia, hypercalcemia, increased erythrocyte sedimentation rate (ESR), amyloidosis, renal insufficiency with azotemia
What is the characteristic renal lesion?	Tubular casts of Bence-Jones protein, metastatic calcification, and infiltration of neoplastic cells

WALDENSTRÖM MACROGLOBULINEMIA

What is it?	Proliferation of IgM-producing plasmacytoid lymphocytes, an intermediate-stage cell between B lymphocytes and plasma cells
Where are the neoplastic cells found?	In the blood, bone marrow, lymph nodes, and spleen
In what population does it commonly occur?	Men over 50 years old
Do patients have M proteins?	Yes, due to the IgM (specific for either κ or λ) produced by the neoplastic cells
What percent of patients have Bence-Jones proteinuria?	10%
What complication may result from increased IgM?	Hyperviscosity syndrome
What is the natural history of the illness?	A slowly progressive course

MONOCLONAL GAMMOPATHY OF UNDETERMINED SIGNIFICANCE (MGUS)

What is MGUS?	A benign condition, usually without clinical consequence
In what percent of otherwise healthy elderly individuals does it occur?	5% to 10%
What are the defining characteristics?	A monoclonal M protein spike < 3g/dL, < 5% plasma cells in the bone marrow, and absence of Bence-Jones proteinuria

LYMPHOMA

HODGKIN DISEASE

What is Hodgkin disease?	A malignant neoplasm often occurring in young adults
What illness does it often resemble?	An inflammatory disorder with fever, leukocytosis, pruritus, and inflammatory cell infiltrates
What are the characteristic malignant cells?	Reed-Sternberg cells
How do these cells appear microscopically?	Binucleated or multinucleated giant cells with eosinophilic nucleoli
What are the 4 types of disease defined by the Rye classification?	1. Lymphocyte predominant 2. Mixed cellularity 3. Nodular sclerosis 4. Lymphocyte depleted
How is the number of Reed-Sternberg cells related to prognosis?	It is an inverse relationship. Lymphocyte-predominant (few Reed-Sternberg cells) disease has the best prognosis, and lymphocyte-depleted (abundance of Reed-Sternberg cells) disease, the worst.
Which type of Hodgkin disease is most common?	Mixed cellularity
Which type is least common?	Lymphocyte predominant
Which type occurs more frequently in women?	Nodular sclerosis
What are lacunar cells?	A variant of Reed-Sternberg cells present in nodular sclerosing Hodgkin disease
What portion of patients achieve cure with current therapies?	80%
What predicts prognosis of disease better than the histopathologic type?	Clinical staging (i.e., Ann Arbor classification) based on dissemination, presence of disease in extralymphatic sites, and systemic signs

How does the disease typically spread through the body?	In a step-by-step fashion to contiguous lymph node regions
Which systemic symptoms are associated with a poor prognosis?	Fever, chills, pruritus, and weight loss

NON-HODGKIN LYMPHOMA

What is non-Hodgkin lymphoma?	A malignant neoplasm of lymphoid cells
What is the most common site of tumor involvement?	Lymph nodes, particularly periaortic
What is the working formulation?	The current standard of classification, with emphasis on clinical behavior. It is divided into low, intermediate, and high grades.
What histologic characteristics are associated with a good prognosis?	Nodular forms and small cell lymphomas. Conversely, large cell and follicular lymphomas have a poor prognosis.
Which lymphoma is characterized by destruction of the normal lymph node architecture?	Small lymphocytic
Which B-cell lymphomas commonly occur in elderly persons and usually follow an indolent course?	Follicular predominantly small cleaved cell and small lymphocytic
What cytogenetic abnormality is associated with follicular predominantly small cleaved cell lymphoma?	t(14;18) with expression of *bcl*-2, an oncogene
What is the most common form of non-Hodgkin lymphoma?	Follicular predominantly small cleaved cell
Which lymphoma is more commonly found in children?	Lymphoblastic lymphoma

| How does lymphoblastic lymphoma present? | As a mediastinal mass progressing rapidly to ALL |
| What is the cause of the mediastinal mass? | The neoplastic cells often arise from thymic lymphocytes. |

BURKITT LYMPHOMA

What is Burkitt lymphoma?	A high-grade T-cell lymphoma
What is the typical histologic appearance?	A "starry sky," caused by the uptake of excessive cellular debris by macrophages
Which virus is associated with the disease?	EBV
What cytogenetic abnormality is commonly present?	t(8;14); the c-*myc* oncogene on chromosome 8 is translocated to chromosome 14.

MYCOSIS FUNGOIDES

What is mycosis fungoides?	A cutaneous T-cell lymphoma
How does it present?	As an erythematous, eczematoid, or psoriasiform rash
Which cells characteristically infiltrate the dermis?	Mycosis cells: atypical CD4$^+$ T cells with cerebriform nuclei
What is found on skin biopsy?	Groups of intraepidermal mycosis cells (Pautrier abscesses)
What is the leukemic form of disease called?	Sézary syndrome

POWER REVIEW

What disease is characterized by lytic bone lesions?	Multiple myeloma
Which neoplasm has been linked to EBV?	Burkitt lymphoma
Which leukemia is characterized by low leukocyte alkaline phosphatase activity?	CML

What is the erythropoietin level in polycythemia vera?	Decreased
What leukemia is often associated with DIC?	APML
What leukemia commonly occurs in children?	ALL
What is another name for immunoglobulin light chains in the urine?	Bence-Jones protein
The Philadelphia chromosome is diagnostic of what disease?	CML
Which cells are present in acute leukemia, differentiating it from chronic leukemia?	Blasts
What disease arises from clonal proliferation of a malignant antibody-producing cell?	Multiple myeloma
What benign condition is characterized by an M spike on protein electrophoresis?	MGUS
The Reed-Sternberg cell is diagnostic of what disease?	Hodgkin disease

15

Hemorrhagic Disorders

DISORDERS OF PRIMARY HEMOSTASIS

What is the fundamental abnormality?

Defective platelet plug formation

How do disorders of primary hemostasis present?

Petechiae and mucocutaneous bleeding [oozing from nose, gums, and gastrointestinal (GI) tract]

Which vessels are involved?

Small vessels and capillaries

What lab abnormality is seen in these disorders?

Markedly prolonged bleeding time

Name some diseases that may cause vascular lesions resulting in defective primary hemostasis.

Scurvy, Henoch-Schönlein purpura (HSP), Osler-Weber-Rendu syndrome, amyloidosis, meningococcemia, and rickettsial diseases

What is Henoch-Schönlein purpura (HSP)?

A hypersensitivity vasculitis due to an immune reaction damaging the vascular endothelium

What are the clinical characteristics of HSP?

Fever, palpable purpura, arthralgias, and GI and renal involvement

Which disease often presents with gingival hemorrhage?

Scurvy (vitamin C deficiency)

What are some causes of thrombocytopenia?

Radiation exposure, drug side effects, disseminated intravascular coagulation (DIC), acute leukemia, splenic sequestration, dilutional effect from transfusion, AIDS

Describe idiopathic thrombocytopenic purpura (ITP).

Thrombocytopenia due to the production of antiplatelet antibodies that coat the platelets, leading to their destruction by splenic macrophages

How does ITP differ clinically in children and adults?	Adults tend to have a chronic form, whereas > 80% of children experience complete resolution in 6 months.
Name 5 clinical characteristics of thrombotic thrombocytopenic purpura (TTP).	1. Thrombocytopenia 2. Microangiopathic hemolytic anemia 3. Fever 4. Neurologic abnormalities 5. Renal insufficiency
What is the characteristic vascular lesion in TTP?	Hyaline microthrombi in small vessels
What is Bernard-Soulier disease?	An autosomal recessive disorder with defective platelet adhesion due to a lack of platelet glycoprotein Ib (GpIb)
What is Glanzmann thrombasthenia?	A defect in platelet aggregation due to lack of GpIIb and GpIIIa
What are some drugs that may cause bleeding by interfering with platelet function?	Aspirin, penicillin, cephalosporins, and antihistamines
How may aspirin cause a defect in platelet aggregation?	Inactivation of cyclooxygenase causes decreased production of thromboxane A_2 (a platelet aggregant).

DISORDERS OF SECONDARY HEMOSTASIS

What is the fundamental defect?	Lack of plasma clotting factors
Which vessels are affected?	Large vessels
Name 4 clinical characteristics of disorders of secondary hemostasis.	1. Hemarthrosis 2. Large hematomas 3. Ecchymoses —— bruising 4. Excessive bleeding with trauma
Which lab test results may be abnormal?	Prothrombin time (PT) and partial thromboplastin time (PTT)
How are bleeding time and platelet count affected?	They are not. They are usually normal.

What is thrombosis?	The intravascular coagulation of blood
What does the clotting cascade involve?	Two distinct, but connected, clotting pathways: intrinsic and extrinsic (Fig. 15–1)
Which clotting factors are tested in PT?	Factors II, V, VII, and X
What clotting factor is deficient in classic hemophilia (hemophilia A)?	Factor VIII
What defines severe hemophilia A?	< 1% factor VIII activity
How is hemophilia A inherited?	X-linked
Factor IX deficiency is also called?	Hemophilia B

Thrombosis and the Clotting Cascade

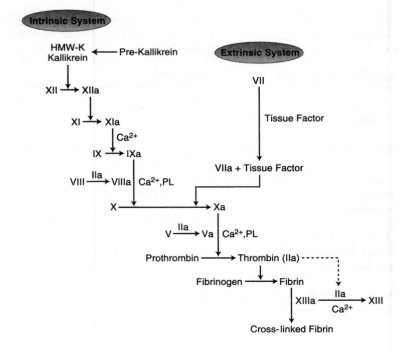

What is another name for hemophilia B?	Christmas disease
How is hemophilia B inherited?	X-linked
What type of hemophilia is most common?	Hemophilia A is 5 to 10 times more common than hemophilia B.
How does vitamin K deficiency cause clotting disorders?	Vitamin K is necessary for production of factors II, VII, IX, and X.
Why is vitamin K deficient in neonates?	Incomplete intestinal colonization by bacteria that produce vitamin K
What is the most common cause of vitamin K deficiency in adults?	Fat malabsorption

COMBINED PRIMARY AND SECONDARY HEMOSTATIC DEFECTS

What is the most common hereditary bleeding disorder?	von Willebrand disease
von Willebrand disease is a deficiency of what?	von Willebrand factor (vWF)
What is the function of vWF?	It is a multimeric protein that is a carrier molecule for factor VIII and a mediator of platelet adhesion at vascular injury sites.
What is DIC?	A condition in which both the intrinsic pathway of coagulation and the fibrinolytic system are activated, with consumption of clotting factors, platelets, and fibrinogen
What are the lab abnormalities in a patient with DIC?	Increased bleeding time, PT, PTT, thrombin time, and fibrinogen degradation products; thrombocytopenia
What conditions are associated with DIC?	Cancer, gram-negative sepsis, obstetric complications (e.g., toxemia, abruptio placentae), trauma, and immune-mediated illness (e.g., hemolytic transfusion reaction)

Why does liver disease cause bleeding disorders?	All coagulation factors, except vWF, are produced in the liver.

POWER REVIEW

Name the 4 vitamin K-dependent clotting factors.	Factors II, VII, IX, and X
How is hemophilia inherited?	X-linked
What platelet disorder is characterized by a lack of GpIIb-IIIa?	Glanzmann thrombasthenia
A healthy child presents with sudden onset of petechiae, but no other symptoms.	
What disease would you suspect?	ITP
What is the probable prognosis?	The condition likely will resolve spontaneously.
What lab value is routinely monitored for a patient on Coumadin?	PT
What lab value is routinely monitored for a patient on heparin?	PTT
Where are the majority of clotting factors produced?	In the liver
What condition is characterized by rapid consumption of clotting factors?	DIC
von Willebrand disease causes what 2 lab abnormalities?	Prolonged PTT and prolonged bleeding time
An abnormality in one of the clotting factors associated with the intrinsic pathway of coagulation leads to what lab abnormality?	Prolonged PTT

16

Hemodynamic Dysfunction

HEMORRHAGE

What is hemorrhage?	The escape of blood from the vasculature into the surrounding tissues, a hollow organ, a body cavity, or to the outside
What is the most common cause?	Trauma
List the 3 phases of response to vessel injury.	1. Vascular phase (vasoconstriction) 2. Platelet phase (primary homeostasis) 3. Coagulation (formation of fibrin clot)

HEMATOMA

Define hematoma.	A localized hemorrhage with resultant mass of blood (blood tumor)
What is the most common location?	Within a tissue or organ

PETECHIAE

What are petechiae?	Small punctate hemorrhages in the skin, mucous membranes, or serosal surfaces
Do they blanch with compression of the skin surface?	No. Accumulation of blood outside the vasculature will not blanch with compression.

ECCHYMOSIS

What is ecchymosis?	A diffuse hemorrhage, usually in the skin and subcutaneous tissue
What is a more common name?	Bruise

What color changes are seen with ecchymosis?	Initially purple, then green, and finally yellow
Explain the color changes.	They reflect the progressive oxidation of bilirubin released from degraded erythrocytes.

HYPEREMIA

What is hyperemia?	Localized increase in blood volume within capillaries and small vessels
Does hyperemia blanch with skin compression?	Yes
What are the 2 types of hyperemia?	Active and passive

ACTIVE HYPEREMIA

What is active hyperemia?	Localized arteriolar dilatation
Name 3 causes of active hyperemia.	Exercise, inflammation, and menopausal flush

PASSIVE HYPEREMIA

What is passive hyperemia?	Congestion of an organ with venous blood
What are the 2 phases of passive hyperemia?	Acute and chronic passive congestion
Name 3 causes of acute passive congestion.	Shock; acute inflammation; sudden right ventricular failure
In what organ systems does chronic passive hyperemia (CPH) usually occur?	Lung, liver, and lower extremities
Name 2 causes of CPH of the lung.	Left ventricular failure; mitral stenosis
What are "heart failure cells"?	Intra-alveolar hemosiderin-laden macrophages that engulf and degrade red blood cells (RBCs) released during alveolar capillary rupture associated with CPH of the lung

What causes CPH of the liver and lower extremities?	Right ventricular failure
What is a "nutmeg liver"?	Chronically congested liver exhibiting dark foci of centrilobular dilatation, surrounded by brownish yellow fatty liver cells
What complication is associated with prolonged liver congestion?	Cirrhosis from thickening of central veins and centrilobular fibrosis

INFARCTION

What is infarction?	Necrosis resulting from ischemia caused by obstruction of blood supply
Name the 2 types of infarctions.	Anemic and hemorrhagic infarcts

ANEMIC INFARCT

What is another name for anemic infarct?	Pale infarct
What causes it?	Arterial occlusion
Where does it typically occur?	In the heart, spleen, brain, and kidney

HEMORRHAGIC INFARCT

What is a hemorrhagic infarct?	Necrosis resulting from either arterial or venous occlusion. RBCs from adjacent vessels ooze into the necrotic area.
Where do they tend to occur?	At well-vascularized sites (e.g., lung) and sites with multiple anastomoses (e.g., gastrointestinal [GI] tract)
Is dry gangrene a hemorrhagic or anemic infarct?	Dry gangrene, often associated with diabetes, is a large anemic infarct.

THROMBOSIS

What is thrombosis?	An intravascular coagulation of blood adherent to the vascular endothelium. It often significantly interrupts blood flow.

How is a thrombus formed? By the interaction of platelets, damaged endothelial cells, and the coagulation cascade

PLATELETS

Where do platelets arise? Platelets are cytoplasmic fragments formed from megakaryocytes in bone marrow.

What are the 3 granular components of platelets?
1. α granules containing proteins such as fibrinogen, von Willebrand factor (vWF), factor V, and $α_2$-antiplasmin
2. Dense granules containing non-proteins such as calcium, serotonin, adenosine diphosphate (ADP), and adenosine triphosphate (ATP)
3. Lysozymes

What is the average life span of platelets? 10 days

What is the normal range of platelets in the blood? $150 \times 10^9 - 450 \times 10^9/L$

What are the 4 functions of platelets?
1. Maintain integrity of the vascular endothelium.
2. Release platelet-derived growth factor (PDGF) for endothelial repair.
3. Form platelet plugs.
4. Activate platelet factor 3 (PF3), which promotes the coagulation cascade.

What is the cell surface receptor, located on platelets, that is involved with adhesion of platelets to subendothelial collagen? Glycoprotein Ib (GpIb)

What cross-links platelets with subendothelial collagen? von Willebrand factor

What is the next step following the cross-linking of platelets to collagen? Platelets release their granule contents, mainly ADP, histamine, epinephrine, serotonin, calcium, and PDGF.

How do platelets activate the coagulation cascade? The conformational change that occurs in the platelet membrane from increased intracellular calcium makes PF3 available, thus activating the coagulation cascade.

How does arachidonic acid become available in the platelet?

By activation of platelet membrane phospholipases

What is the enzyme involved in the production of thromboxane A$_2$ (TXA$_2$) from arachidonic acid?

Cyclooxygenase

What is the function of TXA$_2$?

It is a potent vasoconstrictor and platelet aggregator.

What is the rationale for using low-dose aspirin as a prophylaxis of coronary artery disease?

Aspirin irreversibly inhibits cyclooxygenase, and therefore decreases the synthesis of TXA$_2$.

What agonists promote platelet aggregation?

ADP, thrombin, TXA$_2$, collagen, epinephrine, and platelet-activating factor (PAF). (Think PET CAT: **P**latelet, **E**pinephrine, **T**XA$_2$, **C**ollagen, **A**DP, **T**hrombin.)

What cells release PAF?

Basophils and mast cells

What receptor on platelets is involved with platelet aggregation?

Platelet glycoprotein IIb/IIIa complex (GpIIb-IIIa)

What mediates the cross-linking of platelets by binding to the receptor GpIIb-IIIa?

Fibrinogen and fibrin

What is prostacyclin (PGI$_2$)?

A product of cyclooxygenase pathway that antagonizes TXA$_2$ and limits further platelet aggregation

What cells produce PGI$_2$?

Endothelial cells

ENDOTHELIAL CELLS

What is the difference between endothelial cells and subendothelial cells with respect to hemostasis?

Subendothelial cells are thrombogenic, whereas endothelial cells are nonthrombogenic.

Describe 8 different ways endothelial cells resist thrombosis.

1. Release heparan sulfate, which activates antithrombin III, an inhibitor of factors II, IXa, Xa, XIa, and XIIa.
2. Secrete tissue plasminogen activator (TPA), which activates plasminogen and degrades fibrin.
3. Degrade ADP.
4. Take up, inactivate, and clear thrombin.
5. Synthesize thrombodulin, a cell surface protein that binds thrombin and converts it to an activator of protein C, which in turn inhibits factors Va and VIIIa.
6. Synthesize protein S, a cofactor for activated protein.
7. Synthesize and release PGI_2.
8. Synthesize and release nitrous oxide (NO), which has actions similar to PGI_2.

THE COAGULATION CASCADE

What are the 2 pathways of the coagulation cascade?

The intrinsic and extrinsic pathways

Intrinsic pathway of coagulation

How is the intrinsic pathway activated?

Exposure to collagen activates factor XII to form XIIa, and prekallikrein to form kallikrein with high-molecular-weight kininogen.

What is a different mechanism of activating the intrinsic pathway?

Conformational changes in the platelet membrane allow PF3 to become available, and activate the intrinsic pathway.

What is the laboratory test available to measure the intrinsic pathway?

Activated partial thromboplastin time (aPTT)

What is the normal range of aPTT?

22 to 35 seconds

What is the mechanism of heparin anticoagulation?

Heparin activates antithrombin III, which inhibits factors II and X and prolongs aPTT.

Extrinsic pathway of coagulation

How is the extrinsic pathway activated?	By tissue factor that activates factor VII
What is the laboratory test available for measuring the extrinsic pathway?	Prothrombin time (PT)
What are the vitamin K-dependent factors?	Factors II, VII, IX, and X
What is the mechanism of coumadin anticoagulation?	Coumadin blocks formation of the vitamin K-dependent factors, and therefore prolongs PT.
How does coumadin anticoagulation concurrently increase coagulability?	Coumadin inhibits protein C and protein S production. Protein C degrades factor Va and VIIIa, and protein S is a co-factor needed for protein C activation.

Fibrinolysis

What is the role of plasmin in thrombus dissolution?	Plasmin is a fibrinolytic enzyme that restores blood flow in vessels occluded by thrombus.
How is plasmin formed?	From activation of plasminogen
Where is plasminogen normally located?	Bound to fibrin within a blood clot
How is plasminogen activated to form plasmin?	Plasminogen activator is released by endothelial cells, binds to fibrin, and converts plasminogen to plasmin.
What is the site of action for plasmin?	Plasmin digests fibrin and lyses the thrombus.

CHARACTERISTICS OF THROMBI AND CLOTS

ARTERIAL THROMBI

In what areas of the arterial vasculature are thrombi formed?	In areas of active flow
What are the "lines of Zahn"?	Yellowish, alternating bands of platelets and fibrin that attach a thrombus to the vascular endothelium

What is the difference between an arterial thrombus, a blood clot, and a hematoma?

An arterial thrombus is coagulated blood adhering to vascular endothelium through the lines of Zahn. A blood clot is coagulated blood in the vasculature occurring without adhesion. A hematoma is coagulated blood outside vessels.

What is the most common cause of arterial thrombosis?

Atherosclerosis

What are 4 less common causes of arterial thrombi?

Trauma, arteritis, blood diseases, and aneurysms

VENOUS THROMBI

In what areas of the venous vasculature are thrombi formed?

Areas of less active blood flow (e.g., leg or pelvic veins)

What is the Homan's sign?

Pain in the calf with passive dorsiflexion of the toe. It is a sign of venous thrombosis in the deep veins of the calf.

What factors lead to thrombosis in the venous system (deep venous thrombosis)?

Stasis (postoperative immobilization), congestive heart failure, trauma, hypercoagulability (oral contraceptive use, pregnancy, cancer), advanced age, and sickle cell disease

Are lines of Zahn present in venous thrombi?

Lines of Zahn are less prominent and often absent in venous thrombi.

What is thrombophlebitis?

Venous thrombosis with concurrent inflammation of veins

Once formed, what are the 4 possible outcomes of arterial or venous thrombosis?

Lysis, propagation, organization, or canalization

MURAL THROMBI

What 4 conditions can lead to thrombus formation in the heart?

Myocardial infarction (MI), atrial fibrillation, cardiomyopathy, and bacterial endocarditis

What factors are associated with left atrial mural thrombogenesis?

Mitral stenosis and atrial fibrillation

What is commonly associ-ated with left ventricular thrombogenesis?	MI
What is the feared compli-cation of thrombi in any location of the heart?	Embolization and occlusion of arterial vessels (especially in the heart and the brain)

POSTMORTEM CLOTS

Do postmortem clots attach to vessel walls?	Unlike true thrombi, they do not attach to vessel walls.
Describe the two-layered appearance of postmortem clots.	Postmortem clots have a lower layer that is rich in red cells and has a currant-jelly appearance, and an upper layer that is cell poor and has a chicken-fat appearance.

EMBOLIZATION

What is embolization?	Passage through the venous or arterial circulations of any material capable of lodging in a blood vessel and thereby obstructing the lumen
What is the most common form of embolism?	Thromboembolism
What is a thrombo-embolism?	Embolism of thrombus fragments

PULMONARY EMBOLI

What 2 groups of patients are most likely to get pulmonary emboli?	Immobilized postoperative patients and those with congestive heart failure
What are "saddle emboli"?	Emboli that obstruct the bifurcation of the pulmonary artery. They can lead to sudden death.
What type of infarct occurs when the pulmonary arteries are obstructed by emboli?	Hemorrhagic pulmonary infarct. It is typically wedge shaped and located just below the pleura.

ARTERIAL EMBOLI

What is the most common origin for arterial emboli?	Mural thrombi

| What are 4 common sites of embolic arrest? | 1. Brain: especially in the middle cerebral artery, leading to cerebral infarction
2. GI tract: in branches of the mesenteric arteries, leading to bowel infarction
3. Kidney: in branches of the renal artery, producing characteristic wedge-shaped pale infarcts of the renal cortex
4. Heart: coronary artery embolism, resulting in MI |

PARADOXICAL EMBOLI

| What is a paradoxical embolus? | A venous thrombus that gains access to the arterial circulation through a right-to-left shunt, most often a patent foramen ovale or atrial septal defect |

FAT EMBOLI

What causes fat emboli?	Severe fractures that release particles of bone marrow and other fatty intraosseous tissue into the circulation
What are the 3 most common sites of arrest for fat emboli?	Lungs, brain, and kidneys
What are the clinical manifestations of fat emboli?	Pulmonary distress, cutaneous petechiae, and neurologic symptoms

GAS EMBOLI

How is air introduced into the circulation?	By means of penetrating chest wounds, thoracentesis, hemodialysis, and criminal abortions
What is caisson disease?	It occurs in deep-sea divers who ascend to the surface too rapidly. The inert gases (nitrogen and helium), which are dissolved in body fluids during descent, form gas bubbles in the circulation and other tissues with rapid ascent, obstructing blood flow and causing cell damage.
Why are obese persons at increased risk for caisson disease?	Nitrogen has a high affinity for adipose tissue.

AMNIOTIC FLUID EMBOLI

Who gets amniotic fluid emboli, the mother or the neonate?	Mother
How does it occur?	Amniotic fluid escapes into the maternal circulation.
What are the clinical manifestations?	Sudden onset of cyanosis and shock, followed by coma and death
What type of coagulation complication can result from amniotic fluid emboli?	Disseminated intravascular coagulation (DIC)

EDEMA

What is edema?	Abnormal accumulation of fluid in interstitial tissue spaces or body cavities
What is a transudative fluid?	A noninflammatory edema fluid with low protein content and specific gravity less than 1.012, usually resulting from increased hydrostatic pressure or decreased oncotic pressure
What is exudative fluid?	An inflammatory edema fluid with high protein content, large number of leukocytes, and specific gravity exceeding 1.020, associated with increased vascular permeability
Where is the edema fluid located in:	
Anasarca?	Generalized edema
Ascites?	Peritoneal cavity
Hydrothorax?	Pleural cavity
Hydropericardium?	Pericardial cavity
What are the 5 different causes of edema?	Increased hydrostatic pressure, increased capillary permeability, decreased oncotic pressure, increased sodium retention, and lymphatic obstruction

INCREASED HYDROSTATIC PRESSURE

What is the most common cause of increased hydrostatic pressure?

Congestive heart failure (CHF)

What type of heart failure causes pulmonary edema?

Right-sided failure

What type of heart failure causes systemic edema?

Left-sided failure

INCREASED CAPILLARY PERMEABILITY

What are the 3 typical causes of increased capillary permeability?

Inflammation, burns, and adult respiratory distress syndrome (ARDS)

DECREASED ONCOTIC PRESSURE

What disease processes increase the loss of protein?

Nephrotic syndrome and protein-losing gastroenteropathy

What disease processes decrease protein production?

Cirrhosis and malnutrition

INCREASED SODIUM RETENTION

How much extracellular volume expansion has occurred by the time peripheral edema is first clinically detectable?

At least 5 L

Typically, what is the cause when generalized edema and ascites are present?

Increased sodium retention

What are 3 common causes of increased sodium retention?

Congestive heart failure (CHF), cirrhosis, and renal disorders

How does CHF precipitate increased sodium retention?

With decreased cardiac output, renal blood flow is decreased, which stimulates the renin-angiotensin system and aldosterone production. This activates the renal system to retain sodium and water.

LYMPHATIC OBSTRUCTION

What are 3 causes of lymphatic channel obstruction?	1. Malignant tumors 2. Fibrosis secondary to inflammation or irradiation 3. Inflammatory response to parasitic infection

SHOCK

What is shock?	Hypoperfusion and decreased oxygenation of tissues
What are the 2 mechanisms of shock?	1. Decreased cardiac output 2. Widespread peripheral vasodilatation, resulting in decreased venous return
What are the 3 stages of shock?	Nonprogressive, progressive, and irreversible
What are the compensatory mechanisms involved in the early (nonprogressive) stage of shock?	Increased heart rate from sympathetic discharge, increased peripheral resistance, and shifting of blood flow away from the periphery and to the brain and heart
What is characteristic of the progressive stage of shock?	Compensatory mechanism is no longer adequate. Onset of circulatory and metabolic imbalance occurs, and increased production of lactic acid leads to metabolic acidosis.
What is the likelihood of survival at the irreversible stage of shock?	Impossible, due to severe organ damage and metabolic disturbances
What 6 organs are usually affected during shock, and what are the anatomic findings?	1. Kidney: acute tubular necrosis 2. Brain: areas of necrosis 3. Liver: centrilobular necrosis and fatty changes 4. Lung: pulmonary edema 5. Adrenal: depletion of lipid in the adrenal cortex 6. Colon: patchy mucosal hemorrhages in the colon
What are the 4 different types of shock?	Hypovolemic, cardiogenic, septic, and neurogenic

HYPOVOLEMIC SHOCK

What precipitates the circulatory collapse in hypovolemic shock?	A reduction in circulating blood volume caused by hemorrhage, massive loss of fluid from skin, and loss of fluid from the GI tract
What is the most common cause of massive fluid loss from the skin?	Burns

CARDIOGENIC SHOCK

What is the typical cardiac ejection fraction in cardiogenic shock?	Less than 20%
What are 3 common causes of cardiogenic shock (left ventricular failure)?	MI, myocarditis, and pericardial tamponade

SEPTIC SHOCK

What kind of bacterial infection is characteristically associated with septic shock?	Gram-negative infection
What bacterial products are usually implicated in septic shock?	Endotoxins
How do endotoxins impair perfusion?	Endotoxins release arachidonic acid derivatives and cytokines that activate the complement and kinin systems. This causes direct injury to vessels, leading to peripheral vasodilatation.
What is the possible coagulation complication associated with septic shock?	Endothelial injury can lead to DIC.

NEUROGENIC SHOCK

What causes neurogenic shock?	Severe neurologic injury, leading to reactive peripheral vasodilatation

POWER REVIEW

What is the difference between hemorrhage and hyperemia?

Hemorrhage is the escape of blood from the vasculature. Hyperemia is a localized increase in blood volume in capillaries and small vessels.

What are the 2 types of infarctions, and where do they typically occur?

1. Anemic infarct: heart, spleen, brain, and kidney
2. Hemorrhagic infarct: lung and GI tract

How is a thrombus formed?

From the interaction of platelets, damaged endothelial cells, and the coagulation cascade

What are the 4 functions of platelets?

1. Maintain the integrity of the vascular endothelium.
2. Release PDGF for endothelial repair.
3. Form platelet plugs.
4. Activate PF3, which promotes the coagulation cascade.

What is the difference between endothelial cells and subendothelial cells of the vascular wall, with respect to hemostasis?

Subendothelial cells are thrombogenic, whereas endothelial cells are nonthrombogenic.

What are the two pathways of the coagulation cascade?

The intrinsic and extrinsic pathways

How is the intrinsic pathway activated?

Exposure to collagen activates factor XII to form XIIa, and prekallikrein to form kallikrein with high-molecular-weight kininogen.

What are the vitamin K-dependent factors?

Factors II, VII, IX, and X (extrinsic factors)

What is the mechanism of heparin anticoagulation?

Heparin activates antithrombin III, which inhibits factor II and X and prolongs aPTT.

How does coumadin anticoagulation initially increase coagulability?

Coumadin inhibits protein C and protein S production.

What are the "lines of Zahn"?

Yellowish, alternating bands of platelets and fibrin that attach a thrombus to the vascular endothelium

Define embolization.

The passage through the venous or arterial circulations of any material capable of lodging in a blood vessel and thereby obstructing the lumen

What is caisson disease?

It occurs in deep-sea divers who ascend to the surface too rapidly. The inert gases (nitrogen and helium), which are dissolved in body fluids during descent, form gas bubbles in the circulation and other tissues with rapid ascent, obstructing blood flow and causing cell damage.

What are the 5 causes of edema?

Increased hydrostatic pressure, increased capillary permeability, decreased oncotic pressure, increased sodium retention, and lymphatic obstruction

List the 4 different types of shock.

Hypovolemic, cardiogenic, septic, and neurogenic

What 6 organs are usually affected during shock, and what are the anatomic findings?

1. Kidney: acute tubular necrosis
2. Brain: areas of necrosis
3. Liver: centrilobular necrosis and fatty changes
4. Lung: pulmonary edema
5. Adrenal: depletion of lipid in the adrenal cortex
6. Colon: patchy mucosal hemorrhages in the colon

17

Mediastinum

ANATOMY

Name the structures that make up the boundaries of the mediastinum.

1. Pleural cavities—lateral boundary
2. Thoracic inlet—superior boundary
3. Diaphragm—inferior boundary
4. Sternum—anterior boundary
5. Spine—posterior boundary

Name the 6 structures of the superior mediastinum that lie above the pericardium.

1. Aortic arch
2. Great vessels
3. Thymus
4. Trachea
5. Upper esophagus
6. Thoracic duct

What structures form the boundaries of the anterior mediastinum?

The pericardium and the sternum

What 3 structures does the anterior mediastinum contain?

1. Lymph nodes
2. Vessels
3. Fat

What structures form the boundaries of the posterior mediastinum?

The posterior mediastinum lies posterior to the trachea and pericardium, anterior to the vertebrae.

What 8 structures does the posterior mediastinum contain?

1. Descending aorta
2. Greater azygous vein
3. Lesser azygous vein
4. Intercostal veins
5. Vagus nerve
6. Greater splanchnic nerve
7. Esophagus
8. Thoracic duct

What 5 structures does the middle mediastinum contain?

1. Heart
2. Pericardium
3. Pulmonary arteries

4. Pulmonary veins
5. Tracheal bifurcation

CONGENITAL AND INFLAMMATORY DISORDERS

Name 3 different types of congenital mediastinal cysts.	1. Bronchogenic 2. Enteric 3. Pericardial
What complication is most commonly associated with congenital mediastinal cysts?	These cysts are usually asymptomatic, but abscess formation may occur.
Name 3 common causes of acute mediastinitis.	1. Descending infection 2. Esophageal perforation 3. Carcinomatous infiltration
What are 2 common causes of chronic mediastinitis?	1. Chronic granulomatous disease [e.g., tuberculosis (TB), histoplasmosis, sarcoidosis] 2. Idiopathic fibrosis
Chronic mediastinitis is most common in what compartment?	Anterior mediastinum

TUMORS AND MASSES

Name 4 tumors or masses common to the superior mediastinum.	1. Thymoma 2. Thyroid mass 3. Parathyroid mass 4. Metastatic tumor
Name 4 tumors or masses common to the anterior mediastinum.	1. **T**hymoma 2. **T**eratoma 3. (**T**errible) lymphoma 4. **T**hyroid mass "4 Ts"
Name 3 tumors or masses common to the posterior mediastinum.	1. Neurogenic tumors (e.g., schwannomas, neurofibromas) 2. Enteric cysts 3. Gastroenteric hernias
Name 2 tumors or masses common to the middle mediastinum.	1. Pericardial cysts 2. Bronchogenic cysts

Name 2 tumors or masses common to any mediastinal compartment.	1. Lymphomas 2. Mesenchymal tumors (lipomas, lymphangiomas, hemangiomas)
Which neoplasms of the mediastinum are most common?	Thymomas
Are thymomas benign or malignant?	Most thymomas are benign.
Thymomas are tumors composed of what type of cells?	Epithelial cells
Which other cell types are often seen in thymomas?	Lymphocytes
What is the most important factor that affects prognosis in patients with thymomas?	The pattern of growth and extent of the tumor. Its histologic composition does not affect prognosis in any way.
What is the 10-year survival rate after resection of well-encapsulated thymomas?	100%
What disease state is often associated with thymomas?	Myasthenia gravis
What lymphoma is most common in the mediastinum?	Hodgkin disease (60%)
What germ cell tumor is most common in the mediastinum?	Teratoma
Are teratomas more common in males or females?	Males
Are teratomas benign or malignant?	Benign
What malignant germ cell tumors of the mediastinum are most common?	Seminomas

What is the most common malignant neoplasm to involve the mediastinum secondarily?	Bronchogenic carcinoma
What other tumors commonly metastasize to the mediastinum?	Melanomas, as well as renal cell, breast, and germ cell tumors

POWER REVIEW

Name the most common anterior mediastinal masses.	Thymomas, teratomas, (terrible) lymphomas, thyroid masses ("4 Ts")
What neoplasms are most common in the mediastinum?	Thymomas
What disease state is associated with thymomas?	Myasthenia gravis
What malignant germ cell tumors are most common in the mediastinum?	Seminomas are seminomas usually found in the anterior mediastinum
What is the most common cause of chronic mediastinitis?	Chronic granulomatous diseases such as TB, histoplasmosis, or sarcoidosis
What structures form the boundaries of the posterior mediastinum?	The posterior mediastinum lies posterior to the trachea and pericardium, anterior to the vertebrae.
What is the most common complaint of patients with mediastinal cysts?	Patients rarely have problems, because these cysts are usually asymptomatic.

18   Heart

ANATOMY

What is the normal size of the heart?

Approximately the size of a fist
Males: 300–350 g
Females: 250–300 g

Name the 4 cardiac valves and the number of leaflets in each.

1. Tricuspid: 3
2. Pulmonic: 3
3. Mitral: 2
4. Aortic: 3

From where do the coronary arteries originate?

The extreme proximal aorta, just after the aortic valve, which is the region known as the sinus of Valsalva

What are the 2 major branches of the left coronary arterial system?

1. Left anterior descending coronary artery (LAD)
2. Left circumflex coronary artery (LCCA)

Normally, what areas of the heart do the left coronary arteries supply?

LAD: apex of the left ventricle, anterior surface of the left ventricle, anterior two-thirds of the septum, and adjacent part of the right ventricle
LCCA: anterolateral wall of the left ventricle, part of posterior wall of the left ventricle

What areas of the heart does the right coronary artery (RCA) supply?

Most of the right ventricle, posterior one-third of the septum, part of the posterior wall of the left ventricle, and occasionally the apex of the left ventricle

What determines "dominance" in the coronary system?

The artery supplying the posterior descending coronary

Which side of the coronary system is usually dominant?

The right side is dominant in 70%–80% of the population.

Describe the 3 layers of the heart.	1. Endocardium: single layer of endothelium with adjacent basement membrane 2. Myocardium: cardiac muscle, a unique form of striated muscle 3. Epicardium: thin layer of mesothelium overlying connective tissue merging with myocardium
What is the structure surrounding the heart?	The pericardial sac

ISCHEMIC HEART DISEASE

Describe ischemic heart disease.	Partial or complete interruption of blood flow to the myocardium, leading to inadequate oxygen delivery
What part of the body has the lowest oxygen content?	The coronary sinus; the heart extracts 70%–80% of the oxygen from the blood.
What is the incidence of ischemic heart disease in the United States?	> 500,000 deaths/year (about 25% of all deaths). Ischemic heart disease is the leading cause of death in industrialized nations.
What is the primary cause of ischemic heart disease?	Atherosclerosis (> 95% of all cases)
Name 5 other causes of ischemic heart disease.	1. Thromboemboli (valvular vegetations) 2. Coronary artery spasm (idiopathic etiology, cocaine) 3. Coronary arteritis (polyarteritis nodosa, Kawasaki disease, luetic aortitis) 4. Increased demand (increased heart rate or contractility, decreased compliance, hyperthyroidism, fever, pregnancy) 5. Decreased blood supply
What is the name for coronary artery spasm in an otherwise normal vessel?	Prinzmetal angina
What population is commonly affected by Prinzmetal angina?	Young women
What are the risk factors for ischemic heart disease?	Male gender, older age, and positive family history, hyperlipidemia [i.e.,

decreased high-density lipoprotein (HDL; < 35 mg/dl), increased lipoprotein A (> 30 mg/dl)], cigarette smoking, hypertension, diabetes mellitus, and obesity

When blood flow is compromised with exertion, how much is the cross-sectional area of vessels decreased?

50%–75%

When blood flow is compromised at rest, how much is the cross-sectional area of vessels decreased?

> 75%

What compensatory process accompanies chronic plaque formation in arteries?

Collateral blood flow

What are the 3 most common sites of severe vessel narrowing in the heart?

1. First 2 cm of the proximal LAD
2. Proximal one-third of the RCA
3. Proximal one-third of the LCCA

Name 3 clinical syndromes associated with ischemic heart disease.

1. Angina pectoris
2. Acute myocardial infarction (MI)
3. Chronic ischemic heart disease

ANGINA PECTORIS

Describe angina pectoris.

Episodic, paroxysmal, ischemic chest pain or shortness of breath caused by inadequate blood supply to the myocardium. It is not associated with measurable tissue damage.

Name and describe 3 distinct subsets of angina pectoris.

1. Stable angina: symptoms with exertion; limited duration (< 30 minutes); relieved by rest and/or nitroglycerin
2. Unstable angina: often occurs at rest; increase in frequency, duration, or severity of typical symptoms
3. Variant (Prinzmetal) angina: chest pain at rest; coronary artery spasm in relatively normal vessels

Which type of angina pectoris is most worrisome?	Unstable angina
What happens to the ST segment with ischemia?	ST-segment depression: if the ischemia is most severe in subendocardium ST-segment elevation: if the ischemia is transmural

ACUTE MYOCARDIAL INFARCTION (MI)

Define acute MI.	Irreversible cardiac injury resulting from prolonged ischemia
How does an acute MI present clinically?	Sudden onset of chest pain, unrelieved by nitroglycerin, with associated nausea, vomiting, and diaphoresis. Pain may radiate to the arms, neck, or jaw.
What individuals may have "silent" MIs?	Diabetics
Why does diabetes result in "silent" MIs?	Long-standing diabetes causes a peripheral neuropathy, usually manifested as a "stocking-glove" loss of sensation in the feet and hands. The neuropathy also involves fibers conducting visceral pain and autonomic nerves.
To diagnose an MI, 2 of what 3 criteria must be satisfied?	1. Clinical history of chest pain 2. Electrocardiographic (ECG) changes 3. Elevated cardiac enzymes

Tell what cardiac conditions are indicated by the following ECG changes:

T-wave inversion	Earliest ischemia
ST-segment depression	Worsening ischemia
ST-segment elevation	Myocardial injury
Q waves	Transmural infarction

Can there be an infarction in the absence of Q waves?

Yes, a non–Q-wave infarct can occur if the lesion remains subendocardial. New evidence suggests existence of a continuum between non–Q wave and Q wave findings, with the absence of Q waves indicating viable but jeopardized myocardium.

Tell what 4 cardiac enzymes are monitored and what should be remembered about these enzymes.

1. Creatine kinase (CK)-MB (isoenzyme): sensitive and specific marker that peaks 6–8 hours after infarction
2. Lactose dehydrogenase (LDH): ubiquitous, late-peaking enzyme (about 24 hours postinfarction)
3. LDH_1 (isoenzyme): produced by heart, kidney, and red blood cells (RBCs); "flipped" LDH_1/LDH_2 ratio (normally < 1) is a sensitive and specific marker
4. Troponin I: very specific and sensitive marker that peaks early and stays late

Name 5 changes that occur within the vasculature during an MI.

1. Chronic atherosclerosis
2. Acute change (ulceration, fissure)
3. Superimposed thrombosis
4. Platelet activation
5. Coronary vasospasm

List the 3 major coronary arteries in order of relative infarct involvement.

1. LAD ($\sim 50\%$)
2. RCA ($\sim 30\%$)
3. LCCA ($\sim 20\%$)

What type of infarct is usually associated with a globally hypoperfused state (shock)?

Subendocardial, usually circumferential

Name the macroscopic changes apparent at the following times postinfarction.

< 1 day post-MI

Pallor

2–3 days post-MI

Pallor, but with mottled, more circumscribed borders

3–7 days post-MI	Hyperemic border, with soft, yellow-brown center
1–3 weeks post-MI	Yellow center, red-brown margins, scar complete

Name the microscopic changes apparent at the following times postinfarction.

5–12 hours post-MI	Coagulation necrosis, "wavy" fibers
12–24 hours post-MI	First neutrophils, then contraction band necrosis
2–3 days post-MI	Increased neutrophils, necrosis
3–7 days post-MI	Macrophages, granulation tissue
1–3 weeks post-MI	Collagen deposition, scarring

At what time postinfarction is the myocardial muscle weakest? Days 3–7

Name 7 postinfarction complications and the incidence of each.
1. Arrhythmias (> 70%)
2–7. Mural thrombus/emboli (15%–40%), pericarditis (~ 30%), left ventricular failure (~ 10%), wall rupture (~ 5%), ventricular aneurysm (~ 5%), and infarct extension (< 5%)?

What is the most common cause of sudden cardiac death < 1 hour postinfarct? Ventricular tachycardia

What infarcts most commonly cause heart block? Posterior MIs (normally RCA lesions)

What infarcts most commonly cause complete heart block? Septal MIs (normally LAD lesions)

What size of infarct leads to cardiogenic shock? 40% of the left ventricle

During what time period post-MI is rupture of myocardium most common? 3–7 days

What does the occurrence of decreased heart sounds, hypotension, and jugular venous distention on day 5 post-MI suggest?	Cardiac tamponade from rupture into the pericardial sac
Describe the 2 postinfarct pericarditis syndromes.	1. Immediate (2–3 days) postinfarct pericarditis caused by irritation of infarcted area on pericardium 2. Delayed pericarditis (usually 2–4 weeks afterward), which is called Dressler syndrome and thought to be an autoimmune disorder
What is the overall prognosis for patients who have MIs?	For patients who reach the hospital, mortality is 3%–30%. For patients with cardiogenic shock, mortality exceeds 70%.

CHRONIC ISCHEMIC HEART DISEASE

Describe chronic ischemic heart disease.	Clinicopathologic changes invoked by long-standing perfusion that is inadequate to meet the metabolic needs of the myocardium and/or repeated small infarcts
Name 2 general physiologic categories that are used to classify chronic ischemic heart disease.	1. Systolic dysfunction 2. Diastolic dysfunction
What is systolic dysfunction?	An abnormality in the heart's ability to generate adequate contractility to maintain cardiac output, which may be manifested by decreased, abnormal, or absent movement of the ventricular walls. This irregularity can either involve a specific area of the myocardium or be a global deficit.
What causes systolic dysfunction?	Specific: infarct to a specific area of myocardium, leaving it unable to contract appropriately Global: dilated cardiomyopathy or a large enough ischemic "hit" that involves the majority of the ventricle
What is diastolic dysfunction?	An inability of the ventricle to adequately relax during diastole, which is manifested

by a persistently decreased filling of the ventricle. Hence, a decreased preload occurs, leading to a lower cardiac output via the Frank-Starling mechanism.

Name 3 causes of diastolic dysfunction.

1. Severe hypertrophy with relative stiffening, which is usually a manifestation of long-standing hypertension or aortic stenosis
2. Restrictive cardiomyopathy
3. Hypertrophic cardiomyopathy

CONGESTIVE HEART FAILURE

What is the most common clinical manifestation of systolic or diastolic dysfunction?

Congestive heart failure

What is congestive heart failure?

Inability of the heart to produce adequate cardiac output sufficient to meet the body's needs. Congestive heart failure is a complex of symptoms, not a disease entity.

Name 4 causes of left-sided heart failure.

1. Ischemic heart disease
2. Hypertension
3. Valvular disease (aortic or mitral)
4. Diseases of the myocardium (e.g., myocarditis, cardiomyopathy)

What are the signs and symptoms of left-sided failure?

Dyspnea, orthopnea, cerebral anoxia, relative hypotension, poor peripheral pulses, rales, S_3, and a large heart

Name 5 causes of right-sided failure.

1. Left-sided failure
2. Left-sided lesions without failure (e.g., mitral stenosis, mitral regurgitation)
3. Pulmonary hypertension
4. Valvular disease (tricuspid or pulmonic)
5. Diseases of the myocardium (e.g., myocarditis, cardiomyopathy)

What are the signs and symptoms of right-sided failure?

Fluid retention, congested liver and spleen, jugular venous distention, peripheral edema, ascites, fatigue, and anorexia

What is the most common cause of right-sided failure?	Left-sided failure
What is cor pulmonale?	Right-sided heart failure caused by a primary pulmonary disease, usually primary pulmonary hypertension
What 5 conditions should be considered when a patient becomes acutely decompensated (i.e., manifestations of heart failure are exacerbated)?	1. Ischemia 2. Infection 3. Indiscretion (noncompliance with medicines) 4. Anemia (Inemia) 5. Arrhythmia (Irrhythmia) "5 Is"
What is the classic appearance of the liver in congestive heart failure on gross examination?	"Nutmeg" liver

DISEASES OF THE MYOCARDIUM

What is the most common cause of acute myocarditis?	Viral, most commonly coxsackievirus (B > A) and other enteroviruses
Name several other causes of acute myocarditis.	Diseases: bacterial (e.g., Lyme disease); fungal; protozoan (e.g., Chagas disease); systemic (e.g., acute rheumatic fever, lupus); sarcoidosis; uremia Physical processes: chemotherapy, radiation
Describe the microscopic characteristics of myocarditis.	Nonspecific inflammatory infiltrate, sometimes with microabscess formation
Define cardiomyopathy.	A general term referring to a disorder of heart muscle not secondary to ischemic, hypertensive, congenital, valvular, or pericardial disease
Characterize the 3 major types of cardiomyopathy.	1. Dilated (congestive): hypocontractile muscle with poor systolic function 2. Hypertrophic [sometimes called idiopathic hypertrophic subaortic stenosis (IHSS)]: thick, noncompliant, hypercontractile muscle

3. Restrictive: normal-sized but stiff muscle

What is cor bovinum?

Literally, cow heart. This term refers to an extremely large heart (weight sometimes > 1000 g) caused by any cardiomyopathy, but usually reserved for one caused by syphilitic disease.

Overall, what is the most common type of cardiomyopathy?

Dilated idiopathic form

Name the 4 major causes of dilated cardiomyopathy.

1. Idiopathic mechanisms
2. Alcohol
3. Thiamine deficiency (beriberi)
4. Peripartum state

In hypertrophic cardiomyopathy, is the size of the ventricular chamber large, small, or unchanged?

Although the walls are thicker, the ventricular chamber is relatively unchanged.

What happens if the enlargement is asymmetric?

Significant outflow obstruction results if the septum is greatly involved.

If the heart is large and hypercontractile, what is seen microscopically?

Disoriented and tangled myocardial fibers

Name and describe 3 causes of restrictive cardiomyopathy.

1. Infiltrative: amyloid, sarcoid, hemochromatosis, and glycogen storage disease
2. Endocardial fibroelastosis: cartilage-like appearance of the heart; most common in infants
3. Loeffler eosinophilic endocarditis: peripheral blood and tissue eosinophilia

DISEASES OF THE PERICARDIUM

How much fluid is normally present within the pericardial space?

Approximately 30 ml

What is the purpose of the pericardial fluid?

To provide lubrication for the beating heart

What is a hydropericar-dium?

Excessive accumulation of serous, transudative fluid within the pericardial space

What causes a hydroperi-cardium?

Any condition that results in systemic edema, such as congestive heart failure or hypoproteinemia

What is a hemopericar-dium?

Accumulation of blood within the pericardial space.

What causes a hemoperi-cardium?

Usually, a rupture or perforation of the heart or aorta

✗ Define cardiac tamponade.

Compression of the heart caused by an accumulation of fluid (usually blood) within the sac such that the heart is hemodynamically compromised

Describe the 2 clinical fea-tures of acute pericarditis.

1. Chest pain
2. Pericardial friction rub

Name 4 different types of acute pericarditis and describe the character of the associated fluid.

1. Serous: clear, straw-colored, protein-rich exudate
2. Purulent/suppurative: cloudy, purulent, inflammatory exudate
3. Fibrinous ("bread and butter" pericarditis): fibrin-rich exudate
4. Hemorrhagic: bloody exudate

What is adhesive peri-carditis?

Postinflammatory fibrosis located outside of the pericardium, which causes adherence to adjacent structures

What is constrictive pericarditis? _oc HRonic pericarditis_

Residual fibrosis within the pericardium and calcification of the pericardial sac caused by chronic inflammation

What are causes of constrictive pericarditis?

Tuberculosis (TB), pyogenic bacteria, metastatic invasion, radiation treatment, or connective tissue disease

What conditions may result from constrictive peri-carditis?

Decreased diastolic filling, decreased cardiac output, and untreated heart failure

Hemodynamically, what is the difference between cardiac tamponade and constrictive pericarditis?	Cardiac tamponade involves a pressure-limited system. Constrictive pericarditis involves a volume-limited system.

VALVULAR HEART DISEASE

RHEUMATIC HEART DISEASE

Define rheumatic fever.	A systemic inflammatory disorder that most often affects children 5–15 years of age. Cardiac manifestations are among the most prominent sequelae.
What usually triggers the systemic manifestations of rheumatic fever?	Pharyngitis caused by group A β-hemolytic streptococci (*Streptococcus pyogenes*). The disease develops 1–4 weeks later.
How does "strep throat" cause the various sequelae of rheumatic fever?	Rheumatic fever is thought to involve an autoimmune reaction. It is not a direct bacterial infection.
What is the chance of developing acute rheumatic fever if streptococcal pharyngitis is left untreated?	< 1%
How are the modified Jones criteria used to diagnose acute rheumatic fever?	In the presence of supportive evidence of a previous streptococcal pharyngitis, at least 2 major criteria or 1 major and 2 minor criteria are required for diagnosis.
Name the 6 major Jones criteria.	1. Carditis 2. Polyarthritis (usually migratory, involving larger joints) 3. Chorea (e.g., Sydenham) 4. Erythema marginatum 5. Subcutaneous nodules 6. History of previous acute rheumatic fever (new addition)
Name the 4 minor Jones criteria.	1. Fever 2. Arthralgia 3. Elevated erythrocyte sedimentation rate (ESR) 4. Prolonged PR interval on ECG

What type of carditis is found in acute rheumatic fever?	Pancarditis (involving all 3 layers)
Involvement of what heart layer accounts for the majority of deaths in the early stages of rheumatic fever?	The myocardium, because it can lead to cardiac failure
What intracardiac lesion is a classic pathologic finding in rheumatic fever?	Aschoff body
What is the characteristic microscopic appearance of rheumatic fever?	Areas of focal myocardial inflammation, with collagen and fibrin deposition, and Anitschkow and Aschoff cells
What are Anitschkow cells?	Large mesenchymal cells
What are Aschoff cells?	Multinucleated giant cells
Are Aschoff bodies found in places other than the heart?	Yes; these structures may be identified in joints, tendons, and other connective tissue.
During an acute episode of rheumatic fever, what happens to the heart valves?	They are grossly inflamed with tiny, wart-like, rubbery vegetations (verrucae) that form along the lines of closure.
Are the vegetations usually a source of emboli?	No, because they are not overtly friable at this stage.
What are the late sequelae of rheumatic heart disease?	Thickened, fibrotic, and calcified heart valves.
In what 2 ways are the heart valves affected by these late changes?	1. Stenosis 2. Insufficiency
What 2 valves are most commonly involved in rheumatic heart disease?	1. Mitral valve 2. Aortic valve
How often does trivalvular involvement (i.e., mitral, aortic, and tricuspid valves) occur in rheumatic heart disease?	Approximately 5% of the time

Which heart valve is least often involved in rheumatic heart disease?	Pulmonic
Why are the mitral and aortic valves most often affected in rheumatic heart disease?	The vegetations occur most prominently at points of stress, and left-sided pressures are greater than right-sided.

NONRHEUMATIC ENDOCARDITIS

Define infective endocarditis.	Bacterial or fungal infection of the endocardium, most prominently involving the heart valves
What types of heart valves are prone to infection in endocarditis?	Previously damaged or abnormal valves Prosthetic valves
Name the species of bacteria that is most commonly implicated in the following conditions:	
Acute endocarditis	*Staphylococcus aureus*
Subacute endocarditis	*Streptococcus viridans*
Prosthetic heart valve use	*Staphylococcus aureus* or *S. epidermidis*
Intravenous drug abuse (IVDA)	*Staphylococcus aureus*
Which heart valve is the most frequently involved in endocarditis?	Mitral
Which heart valve is the second most frequently involved in endocarditis?	Aortic
Which heart valve is most frequently involved in IVDA and endocarditis?	Tricuspid
Describe the complications associated with endocarditis.	1. Sepsis

2. Valve destruction, which may lead to congestive heart failure/regurgitation
3. Distal embolization of vegetations, which may lead to infarcts (stroke, bowel ischemia, MI) or abscesses

Define nonbacterial thrombotic endocarditis.
(NBTC)

Marantic endocarditis, characterized by small, sterile vegetations along the valve commissures

With what disorders is thrombotic endocarditis often associated?

Metastatic cancers and other debilitating disorders

What causes thrombotic endocarditis?

Increased blood coagulopathy or immune complex deposition

What is the valve plaque formation called when seen in association with systemic lupus erythematosus (SLE)?

Libman-Sacks endocarditis

On which side of the valve surface are the vegetations located in Libman-Sacks endocarditis?

On either side. In all other conditions, they are located on the outflow side of the valve.

What specific tumor type may result in thickened endocardial plaques?

Carcinoid tumor

In carcinoid endocarditis, which side of the heart is involved and why?

Right-sided endocardium and valves, because the carcinoid secretory products are filtered by the lung

OTHER VALVULAR DISEASE

What are the 3 major causes of valvular heart disease?

1. Rheumatic fever
2. Inflammatory processes
3. Congenital conditions

What valvular lesion occurs most frequently?

Mitral valve prolapse

What is the incidence of mitral valve prolapse?

5%–10% (normal population)

In what population is mitral valve prolapse commonly seen?

Young women

What is the classic patho-logic finding in mitral valve prolapse?

An excess of mucopolysaccharide in valve spongiosa (myxoid degeneration)

What physical finding is characteristic of mitral valve prolapse? = phub closing

A midsystolic click

What causes a midsystolic click?

A "floppy" cusp of at least one of the leaflets prolapsing into the atrium during systolic contraction

To what condition are individuals with mitral valve prolapse predisposed?

Infective endocarditis, because bacteria can more easily proliferate within the cusp

What condition is the most common cause of mitral valve stenosis and insufficiency? phub opening

Rheumatic heart disease

What are other causes of mitral valve insufficiency?

Mitral valve prolapse, infective endocarditis, post-MI papillary muscle rupture, and widely dilated left ventricle (leaflets are unable to reach each other)

What 2 long-term problems are caused by chronic mitral valve disease?

1. Left atrial dilatation from chronic increased pressures
2. Cor pulmonale from subsequent pulmonary hypertension

Individuals with left atrial dilatation are predisposed to what condition?

Arrhythmias, notably atrial fibrillation

Individuals with atrial fibrillation are predisposed to what condition?

Formation of a mural thrombus, which can lead to emboli (stroke, infarcted bowel)

Name 3 common causes of aortic valve stenosis.

1. Rheumatic heart disease
2. Congenital bicuspid valve
3. Age-related degenerative valvular changes

Aortic valve stenosis can lead to what problem?

Concentric left ventricular hypertrophy and eventual dilatation with failure caused by chronic resistance to outflow

Name 3 symptoms associated with aortic stenosis.	1. Angina 2. Syncope 3. Dyspnea
Name 4 common causes of aortic insufficiency.	1. Rheumatic heart disease 2. Luetic (syphilis) aortitis 3. Nondissecting aortic aneurysm 4. Worsening aortic sclerosis and/or calcification
Name 4 causes of tricuspid valve failure.	1. Rheumatic heart disease 2. Carcinoid syndrome 3. Right ventricle dilatation 4. Age-related changes
Name 4 causes of pulmonic valve failure.	1. Congenital malformations 2. Carcinoid syndrome 3. Rheumatic heart disease 4. Age-related changes

CONGENITAL HEART DISEASE

What is the most common cause of congestive heart disease?	Idiopathic mechanisms
What are 3 other frequently occurring causes of congestive heart disease?	1. Down syndrome 2. Turner syndrome 3. Intrauterine rubella infection
What is the most frequent type of congestive heart disease?	Ventral septal defect (VSD) [25%–30%]
What is the natural history of VSD?	If a VSD is small enough, it may close on its own. If not, or if it is unstable, surgery is indicated.
What causes an atrial septal defect (ASD)?	Patent foramen ovale
Describe the 3 different types of ASDs?	1. Septum primum: lower part of septum 2. Septum secundum: defect in fossa ovalis 3. Sinus venosus: upper part of septum, near coronary sinus

What is a paradoxical embolus?

An embolus that forms in the venous circulation and passes to the systemic circulation, bypassing the lungs. It may be seen with ASDs or VSDs.

What is Lutembacher syndrome?

An ASD with mitral stenosis

What causes patent ductus arteriosus (PDA)?

Failure of the fetal ductus arteriosus to close

What type of shunt is usually associated with cyanosis?

Right-to-left

Why is a right-to-left shunt compatible with cyanosis?

Cyanosis occurs when a certain percentage of hemoglobin is deoxygenated. Blood must bypass the lungs or the ventilated portions of the lungs to allow development of clinical cyanosis. Therefore, in the absence of severe lung disease, a cardiovascular right-to-left shunt must exist.

Can a left-to-right shunt cause cyanosis?

Not initially. However, a left-to-right shunt may reverse to a right-to-left shunt secondary to increased pulmonary arterial pressure.

What is the eponym for the conversion of a left-to-right shunt to a right-to-left shunt?

Eisenmenger complex

What are the 5 cyanotic congenital lesions?

"5 Ts"
1. **T**etralogy of Fallot
2. **T**ransposition of the great vessels
3. **T**ricuspid atresia
4. **T**otal anomalous pulmonary venous return
5. **T**runcus arteriosus

Name the abnormalities that constitute tetralogy of Fallot.

VSD, pulmonary stenosis, overriding aorta, right ventricular hypertrophy

What compensatory mechanism is often necessary for survival in some types of congestive heart disease?

A PDA is often the only way oxygenated blood can pass to the systemic circulation.

What is coarctation of the aorta?	A discrete narrowing of the aortic arch
What is the most common location of coarctation of the aorta?	Postductal, or after the subclavian "takeoff"

Name the classic signs of coarctation of the aorta:

If it occurs after the subclavian "takeoff"?	Blood pressure in arms > legs
If it occurs before the subclavian "takeoff"?	Blood pressure in right arm > left arm
What anomaly is commonly associated with coarctation of the aorta?	Bicuspid aortic valve (50% of patients)
What is Ebstein anomaly?	Displacement of the tricuspid valve into the right ventricle, resulting in a small functional right ventricle

TUMORS OF THE HEART

What are the most common cardiac neoplasms?	Metastatic tumors
What are the most common primary cardiac tumors and where are they located?	Myxomas are found in the left atrium.
Are left atrial myxomas benign or malignant?	Benign
What are the most common primary malignant tumors?	Angiosarcomas
What are the most common primary cardiac tumors in infants and children?	Rhabdomyomas
What condition is associated with hamartomas?	Tuberous sclerosis (approximately one-third of patients)

POWER REVIEW

What patients develop "silent" MIs?	Diabetics
At how many days post-MI is a soft, yellow-brown center with a hyperemic border visible macroscopically?	3–7
What is the most common cause of death post-MI?	Arrhythmias, specifically ventricular tachycardia
What are the classic ECG changes associated with the following:	
Ischemia	ST-segment depression
Ongoing myocardial injury	ST-segment elevation
Infarction (if transmural)	Presence of Q waves
If an individual has shortness of breath, poor peripheral pulses, an S$_3$, and rales, which side of the heart has failed?	Left side
What is cor pulmonale?	Right-sided heart failure caused by a primary pulmonary disease
If an individual has a large liver or spleen, pedal edema, and jugular venous distention, which side of the heart has failed?	Right side
What is the classic appearance of a congested liver on gross examination?	"Nutmeg" liver
What is the most common cause of acute myocarditis?	Coxsackievirus B
Overall, what is the most common form of cardiomyopathy?	Dilated, idiopathic type

Name 4 major causes of dilated cardiomyopathy.

1. Idiopathic etiology
2. Alcohol
3. Thiamine deficiency (beriberi)
4. Peripartum

What is cardiac tamponade?

Compression of the heart caused by an accumulation of fluid (usually blood) within the pericardial sac

What is the initial causative agent in rheumatic heart disease?

Pharyngeal infection with *Streptococcus pyogenes*

What intracardiac lesion is the classic pathologic finding in acute rheumatic fever?

Aschoff body

Which valve is most commonly involved in rheumatic heart disease?

Mitral

Which valve is least often involved in rheumatic heart disease?

Pulmonic

Which heart valves are prone to infection?

Any abnormal valve

What are the most common cause of acute and subacute endocarditis?

Staphylococcus aureus and *Streptococcus viridans,* respectively

What is the name of the valve plaque formation that is seen in association with SLE?

Libman-Sacks endocarditis

In newborns with Down syndrome, what should you look for on physical examination?

Cyanosis, tachypnea, murmurs, and other abnormal heart sounds. One-third of these infants have a congenital heart defect.

Left atrial dilatation predisposes to what condition?

Arrhythmia

What abnormalities are associated with tetralogy of Fallot.

VSD, pulmonary stenosis, overriding aorta, and right ventricular hypertrophy

What is the most frequent form of congestive heart disease?

VSD (25%–30%)

A child is seen in the emergency department. Blood pressure in her legs is difficult to elicit. Arm pressures measure about 105/65 mm Hg, while pressures taken over her thigh measure 80/50 mm Hg. What condition should you consider?

Coarctation of the aorta

What are the most common primary cardiac tumors?

Myxomas, which are usually found in the left atrium

19

The Respiratory System

ANATOMY

Name the 7 descending anatomic portions of the bronchial tree, starting with primary bronchi.

1. Lobar/secondary bronchi
2. Segmental/tertiary bronchi
3. Bronchioles
4. Terminal/lobular bronchioles
5. Respiratory/alveolar bronchioles
6. Alveolar ducts
7. Alveoli

What is the conducting portion of the respiratory system?

Trachea to terminal bronchioles

What is the respiratory portion?

Respiratory bronchioles, alveolar ducts, and alveoli

What is the vascular supply to the conducting airways?

Bronchial arteries

What is the vascular supply to the respiratory portion of the lung?

Branches of the pulmonary artery

What is the acinus?

The basic unit of lung function. It includes respiratory bronchioles, alveolar ducts, alveoli, and a capillary bed derived from the pulmonary artery.

What cells make up the alveolar septa?

Type I alveolar cells, endothelium, and interstitial cells

HISTOLOGY

Which cells secrete pulmonary surfactant?

Type II alveolar cells

What are the minute openings in the alveolar septae through which alveolar macrophages pass from one alveolar space to another?	Pores of Kohn
What 2 cell types line the bronchi?	1. Pseudostratified ciliated columnar epithelial cells 2. Mucus-secreting goblet cells
What 2 cell types line the bronchioles?	1. Columnar cells 2. Secretory Clara cells

CONGENITAL PULMONARY ABNORMALITIES

What defect causes congenital lobar emphysema?	Congenital absence or hypoplasia of bronchial cartilage
What is pulmonary sequestration?	A mass of isolated, nonfunctioning lung tissue with an aberrant blood supply
What congenital pulmonary abnormality is frequently associated with hydrops fetalis and polyhydramnios?	Congenital adenomatoid malformation
What is bronchopulmonary dysplasia?	Diffuse alveolar damage occurring in neonates following respiratory failure, particularly in premature infants who have received oxygen and mechanical ventilation. It causes chronic pulmonary disease characterized by bronchospasm and interstitial edema.
What are bronchogenic cysts?	Cysts arising from accessory lung buds and lined by bronchial epithelium
With what other cysts may they be associated?	Cysts of the pancreas, liver, and kidney

COMMON INFECTIOUS DISORDERS OF THE UPPER RESPIRATORY TRACT

What are the most common clinical manifestations of the common cold?	Coryza, sneezing, nasal congestion, and mild sore throat

What is the most common virus causing the common cold?	Adenovirus
What type of immune reaction mediates allergic rhinitis?	IgE type I immune reaction. It is characterized by increased eosinophils in the peripheral blood.
What usually precedes bacterial rhinitis?	Acute viral or allergic rhinitis that causes injury to mucosal cilia
Name the 3 most common bacteria that cause bacterial rhinitis.	1. Streptococci 2. Staphylococci 3. *Haemophilus influenzae*
What is the agent responsible for acute epiglottitis in children?	*H. influenzae*
What is laryngotracheobronchitis?	Inflammation of the larynx, trachea, and epiglottis most often caused by a virus
What is croup?	The harsh cough and inspiratory stridor characterizing laryngotracheobronchitis
Name the agents responsible for acute bronchitis.	Common cold viruses, influenza viruses, bacteria (staphylococci, streptococci, and *H. influenzae*), and irritant dusts and gases

PNEUMONIAS

INFECTIOUS PNEUMONIAS

What are the clinical manifestations of pneumonia?	Cough, chills, fever, sputum production, pleuritic pain, dyspnea, hypoxia, and cyanosis
Identify and describe the 4 different morphologic types of pneumonia.	1. Segmental pneumonia—affects only a segment of a lobe 2. Lobar pneumonia—affects an entire lobe 3. Bronchopneumonia—affects both alveoli and bronchi 4. Interstitial pneumonia—occurs in the interstitial areas of alveolar walls
What is the most common cause of community-acquired bacterial pneumonia?	*Streptococcus pneumoniae*

What type of pneumonia results from *Mycoplasma pneumoniae* infection?

Interstitial pneumonia

What 3 organisms cause hospital-acquired Gram-negative pneumonia?

1. *Klebsiella*
2. *Pseudomonas aeruginosa*
3. *E. coli*

What frequent cause of pneumonia in children and young adults may occur in epidemics, has a relatively insidious onset, and is characterized by intra-alveolar hyaline membrane formation?

Mycoplasma pneumoniae

What bacterial pneumonia often complicates influenza or viral pneumonia?

S. aureus

What 4 viruses most commonly cause pneumonia?

1. Influenza
2. Parainfluenza
3. Adenovirus
4. Respiratory syncytial virus

What type of pneumonia is produced by the measles virus?

Giant cell pneumonia

What agents can cause bronchopneumonia?

Staphylococcus, Pseudomonas, Klebsiella, Proteus, and other Gram-negative coliform bacteria

Name 4 important causes of interstitial pneumonia or pneumonitis in immuno-suppressed patients.

1. Cytomegalovirus
2. Herpes virus
3. Measles virus
4. Respiratory syncytial virus (RSV)

What is the most common opportunistic infection in AIDS patients?

Pneumocystis carinii pneumonia

What is Q fever and how is it caused?

The most common rickettsial pneumonia. It is caused by *Coxiella burnetii.* People may become infected by working with infected cattle or sheep, inhaling dust particles containing the organism, or

drinking unpasteurized milk from
infected animals.

What is the agent respon-
sible for ornithosis and how
is it transmitted?

An organism of the genus *Chlamydia*. It
is transmitted by inhalation of dried
excreta of infected birds.

What 3 organisms cause
atypical pneumonia?

1. *Mycoplasma*
2. *Legionella*
3. *Chlamydia*

Name 4 frequent complica-
tions of infection with
Staphylococcus pneumoniae.

1. Abscess formation
2. Empyema
3. Bronchopleural fistula
4. Bacterial endocarditis

NONINFECTIOUS PNEUMONIAS

What are the pathologic
changes that occur in
aspiration/chemical
pneumonitis?

Acute tracheobronchitis with edema and
hyperemia of the airways; eventual
necrosis of the bronchial mucosa with
consequent peribronchiolar hemorrhages;
pulmonary edema; and acute infiltration
of inflammatory cells

List 4 complications of
aspiration pneumonia.

1. Bacterial pneumonia
2. Abscesses
3. Bronchiectasis
4. Extensive necrosis

What causes lipid
pneumonia?

Aspiration of small oil droplets (e.g.,
mineral oil)

What are 4 possible causes
of eosinophilic pneumonia?

1. Löffler syndrome: necrotizing arteritis,
   granuloma formation, and lymphoid
   interstitial inflammation
2. *Ascaris* infestation
3. Polyarteritis nodosa
4. Hypersensitivity states

LUNG ABSCESS

What events or conditions
precede the formation of a
lung abscess?

Bronchial obstruction (often caused by
cancer), aspiration, bacterial pneumonia,
bronchiectasis, septic emboli, pulmonary
embolism, cavernous sinus thrombosis, or
postpartum endometriosis

Who is predisposed to developing a lung abscess?	Patients who aspirate following loss of consciousness from alcohol or drug abuse, neurologic disorders, or general anesthesia
What organisms are typically involved?	*Staphylococci, Pseudomonas, Klebsiella,* or *Proteus*

BRONCHIECTASIS

Define bronchiectasis.	Permanent bronchial dilatation associated with suppuration
What 2 genetic disorders are associated with bronchiectasis?	1. Cystic fibrosis 2. Kartagener syndrome
What 2 states may predispose one to developing bronchiectasis?	1. Bronchial obstruction, most often by a tumor 2. Chronic sinusitis accompanied by postnasal drip
What are the clinical signs and symptoms of bronchiectasis?	Copious purulent sputum, hemoptysis, and recurrent pulmonary infection, which may lead to abscess formation

TUBERCULOSIS

How is the pulmonary form of tuberculosis (TB) spread?	By inhalation of droplets containing the organism *Mycobacterium tuberculosis*
How is the nonpulmonary form of TB most often spread?	By ingestion of infected milk
What is primary tuberculosis?	The initial infection, characterized by the primary, or Ghon complex. Primary TB is most often asymptomatic and usually does not progress to clinically evident disease.
What is the difference between the Ghon focus and the Ghon complex?	Ghon focus: initial tuberculous lesion Ghon complex: initial primary lesion plus involved lymph nodes
Where does the Ghon lesion usually occur?	It is usually subpleural, in the inferior portion of the upper lobe or in the superior segments of the lower lobe.
What type of inflammation characterizes these lesions?	Granulomatous

What is the name of the granuloma of tuberculosis?

Tubercle

What are the characteristics of a tubercle?

Central caseous necrosis surrounded by multinucleated giant cells (Langhans giant cells)

What is secondary tuberculosis?

A prior Ghon complex is reactivated with blood-borne spread to a new pulmonary site—usually the apical or posterior segments of the upper lobes

List 5 clinical manifestations of secondary TB.

Fever, hemoptysis, pleural effusion, generalized wasting, and progressive disability

What are the pathologic changes associated with the lesions of secondary TB?

Tubercles form, then coalesce and rupture into the bronchi. The caseous contents may liquefy and be expelled, resulting in cavitary lesions. This is followed by scarring and calcification.

How does TB spread to distant organs?

Via the lymphatics or bloodstream

What is miliary TB?

Hematogenous spread resulting in seeding of distal organs with innumerable small millet seed-like lesions

Name 4 examples of extrapulmonary TB.

1. Tuberculous meningitis
2. Pott disease (TB in the spine)
3. Paravertebral abscess
4. Psoas abscess

A positive tuberculin skin test represents what type of immune reaction?

Delayed hypersensitivity

When is a tuberculin skin test positive?

In cases of either primary or secondary TB. Once infected, a person will usually test positive throughout life.

OTHER INFECTIOUS CONDITIONS OF THE LUNGS

ATYPICAL MYCOBACTERIA

Which nontuberculous mycobacterium most commonly causes infection in patients with AIDS and other states of immunodeficiency?

Mycobacterium avium-intracellulare

FUNGAL INFECTIONS OF THE LUNG

What type of inflammation is seen with fungal infections?

Granulomatous inflammation

In what 2 geographic areas is *Histoplasmosis capsulatum* endemic?

Ohio and Mississippi River valleys
Southern Appalachian Mountain area

Describe the pathologic changes of a pulmonary infection with *Histoplasmosis*.

The commonly asymptomatic primary lesion is characterized by a mass of phagocytes containing the engulfed organisms. This usually results in scarred calcified granulomas, but may occasionally progress to chronic cavitary disease and/or hematogenous dissemination.

Name another fungus endemic to the Mississippi and Ohio River valleys and the Great Lakes which causes pulmonary infection and often disseminates to the skin and bones.

Blastomyces dermatitidis

In what geographic areas might one become infected with coccidioidomycosis?

In the San Joaquin Valley and in arid desert regions of the southwestern United States

What is an aspergilloma?

A fungus ball occurring in pulmonary cavities or areas of bronchiectasis caused by inhalation of *Aspergillus* spores

What is allergic bronchopulmonary aspergillosis?

Inhalation of *Aspergillus* spores initiates an allergic response in asthmatics

Who is especially predisposed to invasive aspergillosis?

Neutropenic patients

What is seen microscopically with aspergillosis?

Branching hyphae

How is cryptococcosis diagnosed?

The characteristic encapsulated appearance of *Cryptococcus neoformans* is seen with India ink stains.

MISCELLANEOUS LUNG INFECTIONS

What is a Gram-positive anaerobic filamentous bacteria that causes abscess and sinus tracts?

Actinomyces

What is the Gram-positive aerobic, weakly acid-fast bacterium closely related to *Actinomyces*, which is typically an opportunistic infection and may disseminate to the brain and meninges?

Nocardia

OBSTRUCTIVE LUNG DISEASE

ASTHMA

Define asthma.

Inflammatory disease of the lungs, characterized by reversible airflow obstruction

Differentiate between extrinsic and intrinsic asthma.

Extrinsic (allergic) asthma

Mediated by a type I (IgE) hypersensitivity response to inhaled allergens (e.g., bacterial proteins, aspirin, organic and inorganic industrial and occupational materials). Usually begins in childhood, in patients with a family history of allergy.

Intrinsic (nonallergic) asthma

Usually begins in adult life and is not associated with a history of allergy. Inhaled irritants or infection precipitates symptoms.

What are the 2 classic symptoms of asthma?

Dyspnea and expiratory wheezing

What are 4 pathologic findings in asthma?

1. Bronchial smooth muscle hypertrophy
2. Hyperplasia of bronchial submucosal glands and goblet cells
3. Edema of the bronchial wall
4. Airways plugged by viscid mucus

containing Curschmann spirals, eosinophils, and Charcot-Leyden crystals

Name 4 complications of asthma.

1. Superimposed infection
2. Chronic bronchitis
3. Pulmonary emphysema
4. Status asthmaticus

CHRONIC OBSTRUCTIVE PULMONARY DISEASE (COPD)

What is the main risk factor for COPD (both chronic bronchitis and emphysema)?

Cigarette smoking

How is chronic bronchitis clinically defined?

Productive cough for 3 consecutive months over 2 consecutive years

What are 2 pathologic findings in chronic bronchitis?

1. Hyperplasia of bronchial submucosal glands with increased Reid index (ratio of the thickness of the gland layer to that of the bronchial wall)
2. Hypersecretion of mucus

EMPHYSEMA

What is emphysema?

Dilatation of the acinar airspaces due to destruction of the interalveolar septae and reduced lung elasticity

What is the probable etiology of emphysema?

Septal destruction is thought to be caused by proteolytic enzymes (e.g., elastase) that are released from leukocytes during inflammation. Elastase can induce destruction of elastin unless neutralized by the antiproteinase/antielastase activities of α-1-antitrypsin.

What are 3 pieces of evidence that support this theory?

1. Emphysema is strongly correlated with cigarette smoking and air pollution, both of which cause a low-grade pulmonary inflammation.
2. Patients with α-1-antitrypsin deficiency develop early, severe emphysema.
3. Cigarette smoking inactivates α-1-antitrypsin.

What are the clinical features of emphysema?

Progressive dyspnea and hypoxemia

Identify and differentiate the 3 major subtypes of emphysema.

1. **Centrilobular emphysema.** The most common type, it begins in the upper lobes and primarily involves the respiratory bronchioles and spares the alveoli. It predominantly affects men and is associated with cigarette smoking.
2. **Pan-lobular and pan-acinar emphysema.** Involves dilatation of the alveoli, respiratory bronchioles, and terminal bronchioles; most often distributed uniformly throughout the lung. Associated with α-1-antitrypsin deficiency.
3. **Paraseptal emphysema.** Involves mainly the distal acinus and localizes subjacent to the pleura and interlobar septae. Occasionally associated with large subpleural bullae, which may rupture and cause a pneumothorax.

What is the genetic basis for hereditary α-1-antitrypsin deficiency?

Variants in the *pi* (protease inhibitor) gene on chromosome 14

pi ZZ = homozygous state ↓ anti trypsin act.

What are 2 serious consequences of long-standing emphysema and/or chronic bronchitis?

Pulmonary hypertension and cor pulmonale

RESTRICTIVE OR INFILTRATIVE LUNG DISEASES

What is markedly decreased in infiltrative lung diseases?

Lung compliance

What produces the characteristic honeycomb appearance?

Diffuse interstitial fibrosis of the alveolar wall

What is eosinophilic granuloma?

An interstitial lung disease characterized by proliferation of histiocytic cells

What are the cytoplasmic inclusions in the histiocytes called?

Birbeck granules

What is idiopathic pulmonary fibrosis?	Immune complex disease with progressive fibrosis of the alveolar wall with alveolar spaces remaining patent
And what is the prognosis?	Often results in death within 5 years
What is the desquamative interstitial pneumonitis?	Marked proliferation and desquamation of the alveolar lining cells
What syndrome may be associated with lymphoid interstitial pneumonitis?	Sjögren syndrome
What is Goodpasture syndrome?	Hemorrhagic pneumonitis and glomerulonephritis caused by antibodies directed against glomerular basement membranes
What interstitial lung disease resembles the pulmonary component of Goodpasture syndrome but lacks the renal component?	Idiopathic pulmonary hemosiderosis
What is hypersensitivity pneumonitis?	Interstitial pneumonia caused by inhalation of antigenic substances
What causes farmer's lung?	Antigens of the molds *Micromonospora vulgaris, Micropolyspora faeni,* and *Thermopolyspora polyspora,* which grow on improperly stored hay, corn, tobacco, and barley.

SARCOIDOSIS

What is the pathologic finding in sarcoidosis?	Noncaseating granulomas
What population gets sarcoidosis more frequently?	African Americans
What is the usual age of onset of sarcoidosis?	Teenage years
Name 5 common pathologic changes of sarcoidosis.	1. Interstitial lung disease 2. Bilateral hilar lymphadenopathy 3. Anterior uveitis 4. Erythema nodosum of the skin 5. Polyarthritis

What are the 2 immuno-logic findings of sarcoidosis?	Reduced sensitivity and often anergy to skin test antigens (negative tuberculin test) Polyclonal hyperglobulinemia
What are 3 laboratory findings in sarcoidosis?	1. Hypercalcemia and hypercalciuria 2. Hypergammaglobulinemia 3. Increased activity of serum angiotensin-converting enzyme
What is required for definitive diagnosis?	Biopsy demonstrating noncaseating granulomas

PNEUMOCONIOSES

What are pneumoconioses?	Environmental lung diseases caused by inhalation of inorganic dust particles
What is the pneumoconiosis caused by carbon dust inhalation?	Anthracosis
What are the medical implications for a patient with anthracosis?	Anthracosis causes no harm; carbon-carrying macrophages result in irregular black patches visible on gross inspection of the lung.
What causes coal worker's pneumoconiosis?	Inhalation of coal dust (a combination of carbon and silica)
Differentiate simple coal worker's pneumoconiosis from progressive massive fibrosis.	The former is marked by coal macules around the bronchioles and usually produces no disability. The latter is marked by fibrotic nodules filled with necrotic black fluid and may result in bronchiectasis, pulmonary hypertension, or death from respiratory failure or cor pulmonale.
What occupations are predisposed to silicosis?	Miners, glass manufacturers, and stonecutters
Describe the pathophysiology of silicosis.	Alveolar macrophages ingest silica dust, which initiates an inflammatory response. Silicotic nodules enlarge and eventually obstruct the airways and blood vessels.
Describe the pathophysiology of asbestosis.	The uptake of asbestos fibers by alveolar macrophages results in release of

fibroblast-stimulating growth factors, which leads to diffuse interstitial fibrosis, principally in the lower lobes.

What are 2 distinctive pathologic findings of asbestosis?

1. Ferruginous bodies. Yellow-brown, rod-shaped bodies with clubbed ends that stain positively with Prussian blue, they arise from iron and protein coating on fibers.
2. Hyalinized fibrocalcific plaques of the parietal pleura

Patients with asbestosis are predisposed to what form of cancer?

Malignant mesothelioma

PULMONARY VASCULAR DISORDERS

What is the origin of most pulmonary embolisms (PEs)?

Venous thrombosis in the lower extremities or pelvis

Give 4 examples of non-thrombotic particulate material that could cause a PE.

Fat, amniotic fluid, clumps of tumor cells or bone marrow, or foreign matter such as bullet fragments

What are 5 examples of clinical settings that could predispose one to developing a PE?

1. Venous stasis: Primary venous disease, CHF, states of vascular insufficiency (shock), prolonged bed rest or immobilization, and prolonged sitting while traveling
2. Cancer
3. Multiple fractures
4. Oral contraceptives
5. Septicemia

A PE results in what type of pulmonary infarct?

Hemorrhagic (or red) infarct

What is the name of a PE occurring in the pulmonary artery near its origin from the right ventricle?

Saddle embolus

What factors increase the risk for saddle embolism?

Advanced age and morbid obesity

Pulmonary veno-occlusive disease occurs primarily in what age group?	Children younger than 15 years of age
What are clinical signs of pulmonary veno-occlusive disease?	1. Severe pulmonary hypertension, accompanied by right ventricular hypertrophy and enlarged central pulmonary arteries 2. Pulmonary congestion, edema, interstitial fibrosis, hemosiderosis, and arterial hypertensive changes with lymphatic dilatation
Name 3 morphologic changes of pulmonary hypertension.	1. Intimal proliferation 2. Medial hypertrophy 3. Arterial sclerosis
What is primary pulmonary hypertension?	A disorder of unknown etiology and poor prognosis that arises despite the absence of heart or lung disease. It occurs most frequently in young women and is rapidly fatal.
What is the major cause of secondary pulmonary hypertension?	COPD
List 3 other causes of COPD.	1. Increased pulmonary blood flow as in congenital heart disease (ASD, VSD) 2. Increased resistance within the pulmonary circulation, from embolism, hypoxic vasoconstriction, left ventricular heart failure, restrictive lung diseases, vasculitis, and aortic or mitral stenosis. 3. Increased blood viscosity from polycythemia
What impact does pulmonary hypertension have on the heart?	Right ventricular hypertrophy and eventual cor pulmonale
Define pulmonary edema.	Intra-alveolar accumulation of fluid
List 2 causes of pulmonary edema.	1. Increased hydrostatic pressure: LV failure, mitral stenosis, and massive intravenous saline infusion 2. Increased alveolar permeability:

	pneumonia, irritant gases, shock, sepsis, pancreatitis, uremia, and drug overdose
What cells fill the alveolar lumen in chronic pulmonary congestion, as in mitral stenosis?	Hemosiderin-laden macrophages
Name the 3 pulmonary vasculitides.	Wegener granulomatosis, polyarteritis nodosa, and Churg-Strauss syndrome

ADULT RESPIRATORY DISTRESS SYNDROME

Define adult respiratory distress syndrome (ARDS).	Diffuse alveolar damage with resultant increase in alveolar capillary permeability, causing leakage of protein-rich fluid into alveoli and formation of intra-alveolar hyaline membranes composed of fibrin and cellular debris
List several causes of ARDS.	Postoperative state, septicemia, shock, uremia, pancreatitis, severe thermal burns, severe pulmonary infections, oxygen toxicity, inhalation of chemical irritants, drug overdose, hypersensitivity reactions, and major tissue trauma
How does the administration of high concentrations of oxygen result in ARDS?	Oxygen-derived free radicals may cause necrosis of alveolar epithelium by affecting the cell membrane lipids. Focal atelectasis and alveolar collapse occur because of altered surface tension.
How does hypoperfusion of the distal pulmonary microvasculature contribute to the pathogenesis of ARDS?	Direct pulmonary vascular endothelial damage occurs, often accompanied by platelet microthrombi, sludging of capillary red blood cells, and sequestration of neutrophils. Pulmonary microvascular constriction from platelet-derived serotonin causes shunting of blood away from atelectatic areas and local tissue acidosis.

NEOPLASIA

TUMORS OF THE UPPER RESPIRATORY TRACT

What is the most frequently occurring malignant nasal tumor?	Squamous cell carcinoma

Define:

Neoplasia

Uncontrolled, autonomous proliferation of cells

Invasion

Infiltration of neoplastic cells into adjacent tissue

Grade

Pathologic classification of a tumor based on histology and cytology of a sample of cells, examining specifically for the degree of differentiation. Scale ranges from grade I through IV where I = well-differentiated, and IV = highly anaplastic.

Stage

Clinical classification of a patient's disease based on the size of the primary tumor and extent of invasion or metastasis. Scale ranges from stage I through IV where I = local disease, and IV = metastatic

What cell types cannot regenerate?

Permanent cells: neurons, lens cells, myocardial cells

What cell types are in a constant state of renewal?

Labile cells: GI mucosa, bone marrow cells

Name the appropriate antibody for each description.

Specific for Sle?

DsDNA, smith Ag (Sm)

Associated with CREST syndrome?

Anti-centromere

Specific for scleroderma?

Scl-70

Sensitive general marker of autoimmunity?

Anti-nuclear antibodies

Associated with mixed connective tissue disease?

Anti-smooth muscle

Associated with poly/dermatomyositis?

Anti JO-1 and PM1

Specific for Sjogren syndrome?

SS-B

Visit medrevu.com on the internet

The Science of Review™

PATHOLOGY

RECALL

BOOKMARK

PATHOLOGY RECALL is organized in a self-study/quiz format.
By covering the right side of the page with this bookmark, you can
attempt to answer the questions on the left side of the page to
assess your understanding of the information.

Name the 5 common techniques used to analyze tissues.
**Cytology, immunohistochemistry, flow cytometry for DNA
analysis, hybridization procedures for DNA analysis, electron
microscopy**

What are the cardinal signs of inflammation?
Rubor, calor, tumor, dolor

What are the nuclear changes in necrosis?
**Pyknosis (chromatin clumps); karyorrhexis (nucleus
fragments); karyolysis (chromatin dissolves and fades);
nuclear loss**

Name 4 adaptive responses to stress.
Hyperplasia, hypertrophy, atrophy, metaplasia

What are the 5 components of the extracellular matrix (ECM)?
**Collagen, elastic fibers, structural glycoproteins, basement
membrane, proteoglycans**

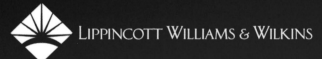
LIPPINCOTT WILLIAMS & WILKINS

What is the infectious agent associated with nasopharyngeal carcinoma?

Epstein-Barr virus

In what 2 geographic areas is nasopharyngeal carcinoma most common?

Southeast Asia and East Africa

Name 2 other malignant tumors of the nose and nasal sinuses.

Adenocarcinoma, plasmacytoma

What is the name of a small, benign laryngeal polyp usually localized to the true vocal cords and induced by chronic irritation, such as excessive use of the voice or heavy cigarette smoking?

Singer's nodule

What is a laryngeal papilloma?

A benign neoplasm usually located on the true vocal cords

How are laryngeal papillomas in children different from those in adults?

Children often have multiple lesions caused by human papillomavirus. Adults have a single lesion that sometimes undergoes malignant change.

What is the most common malignant tumor of the larynx?

Squamous cell carcinoma

Name the 2 biggest risk factors for cancer of the head and neck.

Tobacco use, alcohol use

Where is the most common site of laryngeal carcinoma—supraglottic, glottic, or subglottic?

Glottic

Which of these has the best prognosis?

Glottic

CANCER OF THE LUNG

What is the most common tumor of the lung?

Metastatic carcinoma

What is the leading cause of death from cancer in both men and women?

Bronchogenic carcinoma

What histologic change is seen in cigarette smokers and precedes bronchogenic carcinoma?

Squamous metaplasia of the respiratory epithelium

How is the incidence of bronchogenic carcinoma related to cigarette smoking?

The incidence is directly proportional to the number of cigarettes smoked daily and to the number of years of smoking.

How much greater is the risk of developing lung cancer in heavy cigarette smokers?

20 times higher

Name 4 other etiopathogenic factors for lung cancer.

1. Air pollution
2. Radiation: increased incidence in radium and uranium workers
3. Asbestos: greater increase with combination of cigarette smoking and asbestos
4. Industrial exposure to nickel and chromates

What is the overall 5-year survival rate?

Less than 10%

What are the symptoms?

Cough, hemoptysis, and recurrent pneumonia

What type of bronchogenic carcinoma is unrelated to smoking?

Bronchoalveolar

What types of lung cancer are central in location?

Squamous cell, small cell/oat cell, and carcinoid

What types of lung cancer are peripheral in location?

Adenocarcinoma, large cell carcinoma

Which type of lung cancer has a low malignancy, spreads by direct extension into adjacent tissues, and

Carcinoid

may rarely result in a syndrome characterized by bronchospasm, facial flushing, and diarrhea?

Which type of tumor is undifferentiated, most aggressive, and usually already metastatic at diagnosis?

Small cell

Which tumor develops on site of prior pulmonary inflammation or injury and is less clearly linked to smoking?

Bronchial-derived adenocarcinoma

What 2 types of bronchogenic carcinoma are often associated with ectopic hormone secretion?

Small cell, squamous cell

What tumor appears as a hilar mass, frequently results in cavitation, and is clearly linked to smoking?

Squamous cell

Name 3 paraneoplastic conditions that occur with small cell carcinoma.

1. ACTH-like activity
2. Antidiuretic hormone-like activity
3. Carcinoid syndrome

What paraneoplastic condition most commonly occurs in squamous cell carcinoma?

Hypercalcemia secondary to parathyroid hormone-like activity

Name 3 peripheral clinical signs found in all types of lung cancer.

Digital clubbing, Horner syndrome, and pulmonary osteoarthropathy

Which type of bronchogenic carcinoma has the best prognosis?

Adenocarcinoma

Which tumor may produce myasthenic (Eaton-Lambert) syndrome?

Small cell

What is the 5-year survival rate of bronchial carcinoid tumors?	80%
Bronchial carcinoid tumors occur primarily in what age group?	Patients under 45 years of age
Which 2 primary lung cancers have secretory granules like the amine precursor uptake and decarboxylation (APUD) system?	Carcinoid, small cell
Name 2 bronchial gland neoplasms thought to arise from the subbronchial seromucous glands.	Mucoepidermoid carcinoma, adenoid cystic carcinoma
Which type of carcinoma produces uniformly tall and columnar cells that line the alveolar spaces and appear to reproduce terminal bronchial architecture?	Bronchoalveolar carcinoma
Which tumor cells may have a lymphocyte-like character?	Small cell carcinoma
Which type of lung cancer consists of nests of uniform circular to polygonal cells arranged in tubular glands and ribbons, next to blood vessels, and usually involves the large bronchi?	Carcinoid
Describe the 2 variant forms of bronchial carcinoid.	1. Spindle-cell variant: more mitoses and spindle cells; more aggressive course 2. Tumorlet variant: small round or spindle-shaped cells; small in diameter; very low malignancy
What is the superior vena cava (SVC) syndrome?	Obstruction of the superior vena cava, resulting in dilatation of the veins of the head and neck with facial swelling and flushing

What is the name of the tumor that involves the apex of the lung and produces Horner syndrome?	Pancoast tumor
What clinical feature would suggest recurrent laryngeal nerve paralysis?	Hoarseness

DISORDERS OF THE PLEURA

List 4 causes of pleuritis.

1. Infection (bacterial, viral, or fungal)
2. Rheumatologic disorders (SLE, rheumatoid arthritis)
3. Uremia
4. Pulmonary infarction

What is a hydrothorax?

Accumulation of clear serous fluid (transudate) in the pleural cavity due to an increase in extravascular fluid

What are the 5 common causes of a transudate?

1. Congestive heart failure
2. Renal failure
3. Cirrhosis
4. Hypoalbuminemia (starvation)
5. Abdominal fluid collection (ascites, peritoneal dialysis)

What is the differential diagnosis for the cause of an exudate?

Lung problems—pneumonia, primary or metastatic lung cancer, pulmonary infarction, pulmonary embolism, tuberculosis
Environmental causes—asbestos
Gastrointestinal problems—pancreatitis, intraabdominal abscess, esophageal perforation, post-abdominal surgery
Other systemic conditions—rheumatoid arthritis, SLE, dressler syndrome (pleuropericarditis after MI, trauma, or surgery to pericardium), uremia, drug sensitivity, myxedema, lymphedema

What is an empyema?

Suppurative exudate

On what side does a chylothorax usually occur?

On the left side

What is a pneumothorax?	Air in the pleural cavity
What are 12 possible causes of a pneumothorax?	1. Idiopathic 2. Mechanical ventilation 3. Emphysema 4. Trauma 5. Thoracentesis 6. Interstitial lung disease 7. Lung biopsy 8. Eosinophilic granuloma 9. Cystic fibrosis 10. Asthma 11. Malignancy 12. Esophageal perforation
What is a hemothorax?	Hemorrhage into the pleural space resulting from damage to any vessel, but especially from a ruptured aortic aneurysm or trauma to the ascending aorta

MISCELLANEOUS DISORDERS OF THE LUNG

What is atelectasis?	Alveolar collapse caused by bronchial obstruction or external compression of lung parenchyma by tumors or by pleural accumulation of fluid
What is atelectasis neonatorum?	Failure of alveolar spaces to expand adequately at birth
Differentiate primary from secondary atelectasis.	1. Primary atelectasis: failure of initial aeration of the lungs at birth associated with prematurity and fetal anoxia 2. Secondary atelectasis: collapse of previously aerated bronchi
What is the most common cause of respiratory failure in the newborn and the most common cause of death in premature infants?	Neonatal respiratory distress syndrome (hyaline membrane disease)
How does a newborn manifest respiratory distress syndrome (RDS)?	Dyspnea, cyanosis, and tachypnea
What are the 3 predisposing factors to RDS?	1. Prematurity 2. Maternal diabetes 3. Birth by caesarean section

Why are premature infants predisposed to RDS?

Premature infants have a deficiency of surfactant.

What is the role of surfactant?

It reduces surface tension within the lung, facilitating expansion during inspiration and preventing atelectasis during expiration.

How can fetal pulmonary maturity be assessed?

By measuring the ratio of surfactant lecithin to sphingomyelin in the amniotic fluid. Lecithin increases starting at approximately the 33rd week of pregnancy, while sphingomyelin remains stable. A ratio of 2:1 or greater indicates pulmonary maturity.

What are the pathologic findings in RDS?

Areas of atelectasis alternating with occasional dilated alveoli or alveolar ducts

Small pulmonary blood vessels are engorged, with leakage of blood products into the alveoli and formation of intra-alveolar hyaline membranes.

What are 4 conditions associated with RDS?

1. Bronchopulmonary dysplasia, which is precipitated by treatment with high-concentration oxygen and mechanical ventilation
2. Patent ductus arteriosus secondary to immaturity and hypoxia
3. Intraventricular brain hemorrhage
4. Necrotizing enterocolitis

What is pulmonary alveolar proteinosis?

A chronic lung disease of unknown cause characterized by accumulation of amorphous, PAS-positive material in the alveolar air spaces

What are the symptoms of pulmonary alveolar proteinosis?

Progressive dyspnea, chest pain, marked fatigue, and thick yellow sputum production

What abnormality is thought to cause alveolar microlithiasis?

The carbonic anhydrase system. An increase in pH causes calcium salts to precipitate within the alveolar spaces.

POWER REVIEW

Which organism causes acute epiglottitis?	*H. influenzae*
What tumor of the upper respiratory tract is associated with Epstein-Barr virus?	Nasopharyngeal carcinoma
What is a singer's nodule?	A benign laryngeal polyp induced by chronic irritation and associated most commonly with heavy cigarette smoking
Which type of asthma is mediated by a type I hypersensitivity response involving IgE?	Extrinsic asthma
What are the 4 pathologic findings in asthma?	1. Bronchial smooth muscle hypertrophy 2. Hyperplasia of bronchial submucosal glands and goblet cells 3. Charcot-Leyden crystals 4. Curschmann spirals
What is the pathologic finding in chronic bronchitis?	Hyperplasia of the bronchial submucosal glands
What is emphysema?	Abnormal dilatation of the air spaces with destruction of alveolar walls
Which type of emphysema is caused by α-1-antitrypsin deficiency?	Panacinar emphysema
What is bronchiectasis?	Permanent abnormal bronchial dilatation
What is anthracosis?	Pneumoconiosis caused by inhalation of carbon dust
What disease is characterized by ferruginous bodies?	Asbestosis
What type of cancer is associated with asbestosis?	Malignant mesothelioma
What interstitial lung disease is caused by anti-	Goodpasture syndrome

bodies directed against
glomerular basement
membrane?

What is sarcoidosis?   Granulomatous disorder of unknown
                                            etiology

What are the 5 clinical man-   1. Interstitial lung disease
ifestations of sarcoidosis?   2. Bilateral hilar lymphadenopathy
                                            3. Anterior uveitis
                                            4. Erythema nodosum
                                            5. Polyarthritis

What are 2 names for inter-   Hypersensitivity pneumonitis, or extrinsic
stitial pneumonia caused   allergic alveolitis
by inhalation of various
antigenic substances?

Name the characteristic   Birbeck granules
cytoplasmic inclusions of
histiocytes in eosinophilic
granuloma?

Define idiopathic   Immune complex disease with
pulmonary fibrosis.   progressive fibrosis of the alveolar wall

What is the most common   Venous thrombosis in the lower
origin of a pulmonary   extremities or pelvis
embolism?

What is the most common   COPD
cause of secondary pul-
monary hypertension?

What is most likely cause of   *Streptococcus pneumoniae*
a community-acquired
pneumonia?

What morphologic variant   Lobar pneumonia
of pneumonia is caused by
pneumococcus?

What are 3 organisms   1. *Mycoplasma pneumoniae*
responsible for atypical   2. *Legionella*
pneumonia?   3. *Chlamydia*

What main Gram-negative   1. *Klebsiella*
organisms cause hospital-   2. *Pseudomonas aeruginosa*
acquired pneumonia?   3. *E. coli*

What is the pathologic lesion seen in primary tuberculosis?

Ghon focus

What is a Ghon complex?

Ghon focus plus involved lymph nodes

Where does secondary TB usually occur?

Apical or posterior segments of upper lobes

Which fungus is diagnosed based on the characteristic appearance on India ink preparations?

Cryptococcus neoformans

Which fungal infection has pulmonary manifestations similar to tuberculosis and occurs in primary and secondary forms?

Histoplasmosis

What results from a deficiency of surfactant?

Neonatal respiratory distress syndrome

What lung disorder is produced by diffuse alveolar damage and results in intra-alveolar hyaline membrane formation?

Adult respiratory distress syndrome (ARDS)

How is fetal pulmonary maturity assessed?

By measuring the lecithin-sphingomyelin ratio. (If >2:1, indicates pulmonary maturity.)

What is the most common lung tumor?

Metastatic

What 3 types of bronchogenic carcinoma are central in location?

Squamous cell, small cell, carcinoid

Which type of bronchogenic cancer is unrelated to smoking?

Bronchoalveolar

Which type of bronchogenic cancer is associated with myasthenic (Eaton-Lambert) syndrome?

Small cell

What 3 paraneoplastic syndromes occur in small cell carcinoma?

1. Cushing syndrome
2. Diabetes insipidus
3. Carcinoid syndrome

What is the most common paraneoplastic syndrome in squamous cell carcinoma?

Hypercalcemia

What is superior vena cava (SVC) syndrome?

Obstruction of the SVC causing facial plethora and erythema as well as dilatation of the head and neck veins

What tumor involves the apex of the lung and may cause Horner syndrome?

Pancoast tumor

20

Male Reproductive System

THE PENIS

ANOMALIES OF THE PENIS

What are the 3 most common congenital anomalies of the penis?

1. Hypospadias
2. Epispadias
3. Phimosis

Define hypospadias.

The urethral meatus opens on the ventral surface of the penis.

Define epispadias.

The urethral meatus opens on the dorsal surface of the penis.

Define phimosis.

An abnormally tight foreskin. It is caused by inflammation, trauma, or congenital defects.

What are the 2 possible consequences of phimoses that are of most concern?

Secondary infections, carcinoma

Define priapism.

An intractable, painful erection. It is often associated with thrombosis of the corpora cavernosa.

INFLAMMATORY DISORDERS OF THE PENIS

What are the most common inflammatory disorders of the penis? (Name 7)

Balanitis, syphilis (lues), gonorrhea, chlamydia, lymphopathia venereum, genital herpes, and granuloma inguinale

How does primary syphilis manifest itself?

Painless chancre (see Ch 21)

What are 3 microscopic interstitial changes associated with syphilis?

Edema, lymphoplasmacytic inflammatory cells, and obliterative endarteritis

What is the most common presentation of gonorrhea?	Acute purulent urethritis
What does *Neisseria gonorrhoeae* look like under the microscope?	Intracellular Gram-negative diplococci
What is the most common cause of nongonococcal urethritis?	Chlamydial infection
How frequently is orchitis seen as a complication of mumps infection in children?	Rarely
How frequently is orchitis seen as a complication in post-pubertal males?	20%–30% of cases

NEOPLASMS OF THE PENIS

Name the 3 major types of carcinoma in situ of the penis.	1. Bowen disease 2. Erythroplasia of Queyrat 3. Bowenoid papulosis
Which type is associated with visceral malignancies?	Bowen disease
Which type is associated with a viral infection?	Bowenoid papulosis is associated with human papilloma virus (HPV) type 16 infection.
What are the microscopic features associated with Bowen disease?	Marked epithelial atypia with no invasion of underlying stroma.
How does Bowen disease usually present?	A gray-white plaque over the shaft of the penis
How does erythroplasia of Queyrat usually present?	Single or multiple shiny red or velvety plaques on the glans and prepuce
How does Bowenoid papulosis usually present?	Multiple pigmented papular lesions on external genitalia

Carcinoma of the penis is usually which histologic type?	Squamous cell
In which parts of the world is there an increased risk of carcinoma of the penis?	The Far East, Africa, and Central America
Which virus is carcinoma of the penis associated with?	HPV types 16 and 18
Is there any association between circumcision and hygiene and the risk of carcinoma?	Yes. Penile carcinoma is rare in circumcised men and is predisposed by poor personal hygiene and venereal disease.
In what age range are most of these cancers seen?	40–70 years of age
Describe the clinical course of squamous cell carcinoma of the penis.	The cancer is slow-growing, with metastases to regional lymph nodes. Distant metastases are uncommon.

THE TESTES

DISEASES OF THE TESTES

What is cryptorchidism?	Developmental failure of a testis to descend into the scrotum
What are 3 causes of cryptorchidism?	Idiopathic (most common), genetic abnormalities, and hormonal abnormalities
What is the clinical significance of cryptorchidism?	There is an increased prevalence of inguinal hernias, sterility, testicular atrophy, and an increased incidence of germ cell tumors.
What 2 germ cell tumors are most common with cryptorchidism?	Seminoma and embryonal carcinoma
Is there any way to prevent the possible complications of cryptorchidism?	Yes, orchiopexy (surgical correction) can be performed; however, this does not decrease the risk of neoplasia.
What is spermatic cord torsion?	Compromise of the blood supply, resulting in testicular gangrene

Define the following terms.

Hydrocele

A serous fluid filling and distending the tunica vaginalis. It may be secondary to infection or to lymphatic blockage by tumor.

Hematocele

An accumulation of blood that distends the tunica vaginalis. Most often it occurs due to trauma but can also be due to tumor.

Varicocele

Varicose dilation of the veins of the spermatic cord

Spermatocele

A sperm-containing cyst

Which of the above "cele"'s is sometimes congenital in origin? What causes it?

Hydrocele. It occurs due to the persistence of continuity (failure to close) of the tunica vaginalis with the peritoneal cavity.

What conditions are associated with testicular atrophy?

Orchitis, trauma, hormonal excess or deficiency, cryptorchidism, Klinefelter syndrome, chronic debilitating disease, old age (risk factor)

Which organisms are most commonly associated with epididymitis?

Chlamydia trachomatis and *Neisseria gonorrhoeae* (in sexually active men < 35 years of age); *E. coli* and *Pseudomonas species* (in men > 35 years of age); *Mycobacterium tuberculosis* (in men of any age)

Which organisms are most commonly associated with orchitis?

Viral orchitis—mumps virus; bacterial orchitis—same organisms as for epididymitis. Syphilis infection is also associated with orchitis.

Which is more commonly seen—orchitis or epididymitis?

Epididymitis

What is the worst consequence of orchitis?

Sterility

TESTICULAR TUMORS

Into which 2 major categories are testicular tumors divided?

1. Germ cell tumors (90%)
2. Sex cord-stromal tumors (10%)

Name 6 common types of germ cell tumors.

1. Seminoma (40%)
2. Embryonal carcinoma
3. Endodermal sinus (yolk sac) tumor
4. Teratoma
5. Choriocarcinoma
6. Mixed germ cell tumors

Name 2 common types of stromal tumors.

1. Leydig cell (interstitial) tumor
2. Sertoli cell (androblastoma) tumor

Are testicular tumors usually benign or malignant?

Malignant

To which tumor of the ovary is the seminoma analogous?

Dysgerminoma (see Ch 21)

Which tumor is derived from more than one embryonic layer?

Teratoma (components: cartilage islands, ciliated epithelium, liver cells, neuroglia, embryonic gut, or striated muscle)

What tumor of the ovary is analogous to the mature teratoma?

Dermoid cyst (see Ch 21)

Which testicular tumors are associated with an elevation in a tumor marker? Identify the tumor and name the marker.

Endodermal sinus tumor: serum α-fetoprotein (AFP)
Choriocarcinoma: serum human chorionic gonadotropin (hCG)

How is the choriocarcinoma characterized histologically?

Cells resembling syncytiotrophoblasts and cytotrophoblasts

What are the 3 most common combinations of mixed germ cell tumors?

1. Teratocarcinoma (teratoma and embryonal carcinoma)
2. Teratoma, embryonal carcinoma, and seminoma
3. Embryonal carcinoma and seminoma

What determines the prognosis of mixed germ cell tumors?

The least mature element

What type of cells are Leydig cell tumors derived from?

Testicular stroma

What type of cells are Sertoli cell tumors derived from?	Sex-cord stroma
What histologic structure is characteristic of Leydig cell tumors?	Intracytoplasmic Reinke crystals
Which of the stromal sex-cord tumors is known for its endocrine manifestations?	Leydig cell tumor. It is characteristically androgen producing, but may produce both androgens and estrogens (sometimes corticosteroids). It may be associated with precocious puberty in children and with gynecomastia in adults.
Are stromal sex-cord tumors usually benign or malignant?	Benign

THE PROSTATE

What are the 3 major disorders of the prostate?	Inflammation (prostatitis), nodular hyperplasia, and carcinoma
Prostatitis is diagnosed by what 3 modalities?	1. Microscopic examination 2. Urine culture (>15 WBC/hpf) 3. Prostatic secretions by prostatic massage
Name 3 organisms associated with bacterial prostatitis.	The same organisms that are associated with UTIs: 1. *Escherichia coli* (and other Gram-negative rods) 2. *Enterococcus* 3. *Staphylococcus aureus*
How does acute bacterial prostatitis present?	Fevers, chills, and dysuria, with a boggy, markedly tender prostate
How does chronic bacterial prostatitis present?	Suprapubic and perineal discomfort, low back pain, dysuria, and a history of multiple recurrent urinary tract infections
What is the most common form of prostatitis?	Chronic abacterial prostatitis
What population is predisposed to chronic abacterial prostatitis?	Sexually active males

What percentage of males are affected by benign prostatic hypertrophy (BPH)

by 40 years of age?	20%
by 60 years of age?	70%
by 70 years of age?	90%

What is the etiology of BPH?

Uncertain. It is likely related to androgens by dihydrotestosterone (DHT), which is derived from testosterone via 5-α-reductase activity.

Which part of the prostate gland is enlarged in BPH?

The inner (periurethral) portion

How are the prostate glands affected microscopically in BPH?

Nodules are composed of mixtures of proliferating glands and fibromuscular stroma.

What percentage of men experience symptoms of BPH?

50% by 60 years of age

Name 4 clinical symptoms associated with BPH.

1. Symptoms related to urinary tract obstruction
2. Urinary frequency
3. Nocturia
4. Difficulty starting and stopping stream

What is the most common form of cancer in men?

Prostate cancer. It is currently the third leading cause of cancer death. 20% of cases prove fatal.

Prostate cancer is predominantly seen in what population?

Men over 50 years of age

Is there any racial predilection for prostate cancer?

Yes, high prevalence in African Americans; low prevalence in Asians.

What is the cause of prostate cancer?

Unknown. Its development may be related to advancing age, race, endocrine influences, viral infection, or environmental influences (cadmium exposure).

Where in the prostate gland does carcinoma usually arise?

It can arise anywhere, but most commonly in the posterior lobe, near the outer margins.

How is prostate cancer diagnosed clinically?

By an indurated area in the gland palpated on rectal exam. Patients are usually asymptomatic.

What are pain and urinary symptoms suggestive of in prostate cancer?

Tumor extension. Pain may reflect involvement of capsular perineural spaces.

Which tumor marker is associated with prostate cancer?

Prostate specific antigen (PSA). It cannot be used to diagnose prostate cancer, but rather to detect recurrences and metastases.

What laboratory finding is consistent with prostatic carcinoma?

Serum acid phosphatase (specifically of prostate origin)

Is there any role for radiologic diagnosis in prostate cancer?

Yes. Bone scan and radiograph show osteoblast metastatic lesions in the pelvis, ribs, skull, and spine when the disease has spread outside the prostate gland.

How does prostatic carcinoma appear upon gross examination?

Nodular, ill-defined areas of stone-hard consistency, ranging from gray-white to yellow in color

What is the histologic type of most prostate cancers?

Adenocarcinoma

What are 3 microscopic findings seen in a cancerous prostate gland?

1. Two cell types: clear cells or dark spindle cells
2. Malignant acini
3. Perineural invasion

What classification system is used to grade prostate carcinoma?

Gleason classification is based on degree of glandular differentiation and pattern of growth in relation to the stroma.

Name 3 treatment modalities for prostate cancer.

Antiandrogenic therapy, radiotherapy, and chemotherapy

POWER REVIEW

What is the most common congenital anomaly of the penis?

Hypospadias

Which secondary infection is most commonly associated with phimosis?	Balanitis
What is the characteristic lesion of primary syphilis?	Painless chancre
What disorder would be suspected in a patient who presents with acute purulent urethritis?	Infection with *Neisseria gonorrhoeae*
What is a major concern in a patient diagnosed with Bowen disease?	The association with visceral malignancies
Which type of carcinoma of the penis is associated with viral infection?	Bowenoid papulosis
Which virus is most commonly seen in the above question?	HPV type 16
Are circumcised men more or less likely to develop penile carcinoma?	Less likely
Why is cryptorchidism clinically significant?	There is an increased incidence of hernias, sterility, and germ cell tumors.
Which testicular tumor often has endocrine activity?	Leydig cell tumors
AFP is elevated in which two tumors?	Endodermal sinus tumor, hepatocellular carcinoma
HCG is elevated in which tumor?	Choriocarcinoma
In general, which testicular tumors are usually considered benign and which are considered malignant?	Benign: sex-cord tumors Malignant: germ cell tumors
Which bacterial organisms are most often seen in prostatitis?	*E. coli, Enterococcus,* and *Staphylococcus aureus*

How does BPH usually present clinically?	Urinary frequency, nocturia, and difficulty starting and stopping the stream
How is prostate cancer diagnosed clinically?	Digital rectal exam
In a patient who has been diagnosed with prostate cancer, what does pain often suggest?	Tumor extension

21

Female Reproductive System

THE VULVA AND VAGINA

INFECTIOUS DISORDERS OF THE VULVA AND VAGINA

Bacterial Vaginosis

What is the claim to fame of bacterial vaginosis?

It is the most common infectious vaginitis in the United States.

What organism is most commonly associated with bacterial vaginosis?

Gardnerella vaginalis

Name 3 clinical findings.

1. Vaginal odor (particularly after coitus)
2. Vaginal discharge is frequently but not always present
3. Vulvar irritation is mild or absent

Describe the pH of the discharge.

Elevated

What is a positive "whiff" test?

A pungent, amine-like odor is elicited upon addition of potassium hydroxide to the vaginal discharge.

What other cause of vaginitis is associated with a positive "whiff" test?

Trichomoniasis

Why does coitus exacerbate the odor in a patient with bacterial vaginosis?

Semen has an elevated pH and will alkalinize the vaginal contents in vivo, having the same effect as potassium hydroxide in eliciting a pungent, amine-like odor.

What is the characteristic finding on cytologic smears?

Clue cells and few polymorphonuclear neutrophils (PMNs)

What are "clue cells"?

Desquamated epithelial cells with many adherent tiny coccobacilli, giving the cell a freckled appearance and obscuring the edges of the cell.

What if there are large numbers of PMNs in the discharge?

Suggests a coincident vaginal process, such as trichomoniasis or the presence of coincident cervicitis, prompting further evaluation.

Trichomoniasis

What is the second-most common organism of vaginitis?

Trichomoniasis, caused by the protozoan *Trichomonas vaginalis*

Who is most commonly infected?

Sexually active women of reproductive age

What are some clinical features associated with trichomoniasis?

Copious, malodorous, greenish-yellow or gray, frothy vaginal discharge sometimes associated with pruritus. Asymptomatic infection is common, however, particularly in men.

What is seen under the microscope?

Motile, flagellated, ovoid protozoan and many PMNs

Describe the pH of the discharge.

Elevated

Candidiasis

What organism is the usual cause of candidiasis?

Candida albicans, a normal inhabitant of the vaginal flora

What are 6 conditions that predispose an individual to candidiasis?

1. Diabetes mellitus
2. Cancer
3. Pregnancy
4. Use of broad-spectrum antibiotics
5. Oral contraceptive use
6. Immunosuppression

What are 3 clinical features associated with candidiasis?

1. Reddened vulvar and vaginal mucosa with characteristic white patches
2. Thick white discharge
3. Vulvovaginal pruritus

What are the microscopic findings?

Yeast and branching hyphae

What is the pH of the discharge?

Normal pH (4.5)

How is the diagnosis made?

Clinical exam with confirmation by cytologic smears that demonstrate the causative fungus

Pelvic Inflammatory Disease

What is pelvic inflammatory disease (PID)?

An inflammatory (predominantly infectious) condition of the fallopian tubes and paratubal tissues that can lead to fibrosis, scarring, and obstruction

What is the most common cause of PID?

Gonorrhea (50%–65% of cases)

What are some other causes?

Chlamydial infection, coliform organisms such as *Escherichia coli,* and tubal tuberculosis (more common in third world countries).

What form of contraception is associated with a higher rate of PID?

Intrauterine devices (IUDs), which are found to increase rate of salpingitis by coliform organisms

What are some clinical features of PID?

Fever, abdominal pain, and other signs of infection

What are the major complications of PID?

1. Pyosalpinx (tube filled with pus)
2. Hydrosalpinx (tube filled with watery fluid)
3. Tubo-ovarian abscess
4. Sterility (when bilateral)
5. Increased risk of ectopic pregnancy

How does the acutely inflamed fallopian tube appear macroscopically?

Red and swollen

How does the acutely inflamed fallopian tube appear microscopically?

Capillaries are congested and pus is present in the lumen, wall, and mucosa.

Gonorrhea

What organism causes gonorrhea?

Neisseria gonorrhoeae, a Gram-negative diplococcus

What characteristics of this organism facilitate its ability to lead to infection?

Surface pili that preferentially attach to endocervical and fallopian tube epithelium, allowing the organism access to host cells

What are some clinical features of gonorrhea?

Vaginal discharge, dysuria

What percentage are asymptomatic?

50%

What do constitutional symptoms such as fever, abdominal pain, and vomiting suggest in a woman with gonorrhea?

Acute salpingitis with pelvic peritonitis

How is gonorrhea diagnosed?

Identification of the Gram-negative diplococcus either by Gram-stained direct smears of infected material or appropriate bacteriologic cultures

Chlamydia

To what group of bacteria does *Chlamydia trachomatis* belong?

Rickettsia

What subtypes cause lymphogranuloma venereum?

Chlamydia trachomatis L1,L2,L3 serotypes

What is lymphogranuloma venereum (LGV)?

A sexually transmitted disease characterized initially by a small, painless papule or ulcer, followed by superficial ulcers and enlargement of regional lymph nodes, which then become matted together

What does the ulcer look like histologically?

Non-necrotizing granulomatous inflammation

In what geographic region is LGV most frequently found?

In the Tropics

What complications can follow LGV?	Lymph node involvement is associated with abscess and fistula formation, often involving the rectum, vagina, and inguinal area, and may ultimately lead to scarring and strictures.
How is LGV diagnosed?	Usually by serologic testing (e.g., micro-immunofluorescent antibody testing or complement fixation)
Name 3 other chlamydial genital infections.	Urethritis, cervicitis, and salpingitis
Are these infections caused by the same subtypes?	No
What are the clinical features?	Most often these infections are asymptomatic and are discovered only when brought to clinical attention by a concomitant venereal disease.
Why is it important to recognize these chlamydial infections?	To prevent possible transmission to neonates at delivery, which can result in neonatal conjunctivitis and pneumonia
How is the definitive diagnosis made?	Finding characteristic intracytoplasmic inclusion bodies in cervicovaginal cytologic smears

Herpes Simplex Virus Infections

What subtype of herpes simplex virus causes genital herpes?	HSV type 2 (90% of cases); HSV type 1 (10%)
How is genital herpes contracted?	Sexual contact
Where does the virus remain in the latent phase of genital herpes?	Sacral ganglia
What are some clinical features of symptomatic genital herpes infection?	Small, painful 1-mm vesicles and shallow ulcers involving the cervix, vagina, clitoris, vulva, urethra, and perianal skin
What are the pathologic features seen under the microscope?	Multinucleated giant cells with viral inclusions found in Tzanck smear

What is a Tzanck smear?

Cytologic smear from the lesions

How sensitive is the Tzanck smear?

Only about 30% sensitive on herpetic ulcers

What are 2 complications of HSV infection?

1. Possible association with cervical cancer
2. Active infection in a pregnant woman usually demands cesarean section to avoid systemic, and possibly fatal, infection in the newborn

Syphilis

What organism is involved in syphilis?

A spirochete called *Treponema pallidum*

Describe a typical spirochetal organism.

Thin, motile, spiral-shaped bacterium

Name 2 ways in which syphilis is transmitted.

1. Sexual contact with an infected person
2. Transplacental syphilis (congenital syphilis)

What are the clinical features of primary syphilis?

Usually it is asymptomatic, but a shallow, indurated, and painless ulcer (chancre) may be found. It is usually in the genital area at the point of inoculation.

What is the histology of the chancre?

Ulceration, chronic inflammation with plasma cells, and evidence of endarteritis

What characteristic features are found in secondary syphilis?

Diffuse skin rash and generalized lymphadenopathy accompanied by fever and malaise

What other characteristic skin lesion develops in secondary syphilis?

Condyloma lata, which are highly contagious, gray, flattened wartlike lesions

What characteristic features are found in tertiary syphilis?

1. Cardiovascular involvement (syphilitic aortitis)
2. Central nervous system involvement (tabes dorsalis, dementia)
3. Gummas, which may involve the liver, bones, and joints

Describe the pathologic features found in a gumma.

Fibrogranulomatous wall with a central area of coagulative necrosis

How is a diagnosis of syphilis made?	Darkfield examination of material from the primary chancre (if present) or by serologic tests (i.e., RPR, VDRL, MHA-TP).

Chancroid

What are chancroid ulcers?	Soft, painful ulcers caused by *Haemophilus ducreyi,* a gram-negative coccobacillus
How are chancroid ulcers transmitted?	Via sexual contact
In what geographic areas are chancroid ulcers most prevalent?	In tropical areas; rare in the U.S.
What is the clinical appearance?	The lesions are ragged, painful ulcers often accompanied by tender inguinal lymphadenopathy.
What are some pathologic features of the chancroid ulcer?	Superficial necrosis with underlying granulation tissue and fibrosis
What clinical features develop as the disease progresses?	Early, rapid enlargement of regional lymph nodes, which may manifest as fluctuant abscesses in the inguinal nodes (bubo) followed by acute, tender, suppurative lymphadenitis and eventual scarring of affected lymph nodes and ulcer sites
How is chancroid diagnosed?	Isolation of *H. ducreyi* from an ulcer or bubo

Granuloma inguinale

What organism causes granuloma inguinale?	*Calymmatobacterium (Donovania) granulomatis,* a Gram-negative intracellular rod
How is the disease thought to be contracted?	Sexual transmission
What are the clinical features?	Initially, a papule at the site of inoculation. This develops into a large painless ulcer with multiple surrounding satellite lesions, which can become secondarily infected.

What are Donovan bodies?	Characteristic intracellular bacteria which, on Wright stain, are seen filling vacuolated macrophages

Molluscum contagiosum

What type of organism is the molluscum contagiosum?	Double-stranded DNA virus in the poxvirus group
What is its clinical appearance?	Multiple small, smooth papules with central umbilication
What is the histology of the papules?	Characteristic large, intracytoplasmic inclusions called "molluscum bodies"

NON-INFECTIOUS DISORDERS OF THE VULVA AND VAGINA

What is hidradenitis suppurativa?	Apocrine gland disorder
What is its clinical appearance?	Subcutaneous, painful nodules in the vulva, which progress to form a confluent mass that eventually ulcerates the epidermis
What causes a Bartholin cyst to form?	Obstruction of Bartholin ducts, which are located in the vestibule
What type of epithelium lines the cyst?	Transitional epithelium
What are the complications?	Secondary infection and abscess formation
Name 3 other common cysts of the vulva and vagina.	Mesonephric duct cysts, mucinous cysts, and keratinous cysts

DYSTROPHIES OF THE VULVA

What are vulvar dystrophies?	Disorders of epithelial growth often including leukoplakia
What does leukoplakia look like?	White, patch-like lesion on the mucous membrane
What are the 3 histological forms of vulvar dystrophy?	1. Lichen sclerosus 2. Squamous hyperplasia

3. Mixed dystrophy (combination of these two forms)

Which is the only form with malignant potential?

Squamous hyperplasia

What are the clinical findings?

Pruritus and leukoplakia. Skin is often atrophic with parchment-like appearance.

How can one use the patient's age to help distinguish squamous hyperplasia from lichen sclerosus?

Women younger than 50 years of age develop squamous hyperplasia more frequently; women older than 50 more frequently develop lichen sclerosus.

What are the histologic features of squamous hyperplasia?

Hyperkeratosis and acanthosis with or without dysplasia and atypical cells

What percentage of women with squamous hyperplasia have dysplastic cells?

10% have dysplastic cells, which is a low risk factor for development of squamous cell carcinoma (1%–5% with dysplastic cells will develop squamous cell carcinoma).

What are the histologic features of lichen sclerosus?

Hyperkeratosis, epidermal and dermal atrophy, hyalinization of dermal collagen, and chronic inflammation

How is the diagnosis of lichen sclerosus confirmed?

Biopsy

NEOPLASTIC DISORDERS OF THE VULVA

What is the normal histology of the vulva?

Keratinized, stratified squamous epithelium; labia majora with skin and its appendages (hair follicles, sebaceous glands, sweat glands, apocrine glands); Bartholin glands with lobules of mucus-secreting cells, normally not palpable glands

What are the most common neoplastic disorders of the vulva?

Papillary hidradenoma (most common benign tumor), condyloma acuminatum, squamous cell carcinoma (most common malignant tumor), Paget disease of the vulva, and malignant melanoma

Papillary hidradenoma

Where do papillary hidradenomas originate?

Apocrine sweat glands of the vulva

What race is most commonly affected?

Seen virtually only in Caucasian women

What is the clinical presentation?

Small labial nodule, which may ulcerate and bleed

What are the histologic findings?

Numerous tubules and acini with apocrine differentiation

Condyloma acuminatum

What is a condyloma acuminatum?

Benign squamous cell papilloma

What is the etiologic agent causing condyloma acuminatum?

Human papillomavirus (HPV); most frequently types 6 and 11

What is the mode of transmission?

Sexual contact

What are the clinical manifestations?

Multiple wart-like lesions in the vulvo-vaginal and perianal regions and sometimes on the cervix

What are the histologic findings?

Acanthosis, papillomatosis; characterized by koilocytes

What do koilocytes look like?

Expanded epithelial cells with peri-nuclear clearing

Vulvar Dysplasia [Vulvar Intraepithelial Neoplasia (VIN)]

What organism is associated with vulvar dysplasia?

HPV infection

What ages are affected?

All ages, but most commonly older women

How many women with vulvar dysplasia have concomitant dysplasia or squamous cell carcinoma of the cervix or vagina?

25%

What are the histologic findings?	Dysplastic cells that are basaloid and undifferentiated, reflecting loss of epithelial maturation
What is the grading system?	1. Vulvar Intraepithelial Neoplasia (VIN 1): one third of epithelium replaced by dysplastic cells 2. VIN 2: two thirds of epithelium replaced by dysplastic cells 3. VIN 3 (carcinoma in situ): entire epithelium layer replaced by dysplastic cells
What is the natural history?	Recurrences are common, but VIN may or may not progress to squamous cell carcinoma.

Squamous cell carcinoma

What is the age group of peak occurrence of squamous cell carcinoma?	Older women; however, it is beginning to occur with increasing frequency in younger women
What percentage of vulvar malignancies are squamous cell carcinoma?	90%
What etiologic agent is often responsible?	HPV infection, usually types 16 and 18
What is commonly the first symptom?	Pruritus
What is the clinical appearance?	An exophytic mass or endophytic ulcer
What are the histologic findings?	Usually well differentiated and keratinizing
What clinical feature determines prognosis?	Regional lymph node status and degree of invasiveness of tumor

Paget Disease of the Vulva

In what age group of women does Paget disease of the vulva occur?	Older women
What are the common presenting symptoms?	Pruritus and burning sensation of long duration

What is the clinical appearance?	Sharply demarcated, red velvety skin similar to (and often mistaken for) dermatitis
What is the histology?	Large cells (Paget cells) with pale, vacuolated cytoplasm containing mucin
With what other neoplastic disorder is Paget disease associated?	Rarely associated with adenocarcinoma of apocrine sweat glands

NEOPLASTIC DISORDERS OF THE VAGINA

What is the normal histology of the vagina?	Squamous epithelial cells

Squamous cell carcinoma

How common is dysplasia and squamous cell carcinoma (SCC) of the vagina?	Much less common than in the vulva or cervix
What age group is most commonly affected?	Older women with peak incidence between 60 and 70 years of age
What is the usual cause of SCC of the vagina?	Extension of SCC of the cervix. Only rarely is the vagina the primary site.
What is the most common site of invasive SCC of the vagina?	Posterior upper third of the vagina
What is the clinical appearance?	Exophytic mass

Clear cell adenocarcinoma

In what age group is the peak incidence of clear cell adenocarcinoma?	Teenagers and young women
What therapy is associated with clear cell adenocarcinoma?	Diethylstilbestrol (DES) during pregnancy, markedly increasing the incidence in daughters of women who received it.
What other lesions have been associated with exposure to DES?	1. Vaginal adenosis and cervical ectropion 2. Gross structural changes in the vagina and cervix

3. Structural and functional abnormalities of the upper genital tract

What is the most common site of clear cell carcinoma?

Upper anterior vagina

What are the histologic findings?

Glands, nests, or sheets of hobnail cells

What do hobnail cells look like?

Cells with clear or eosinophilic cytoplasm

What is the prognosis?

80% 5-year survival

Vaginal adenosis

What is vaginal adenosis?

Benign condition characterized by mucosal columnar epithelial-lined crypts in areas normally lined by stratified squamous epithelium

Sarcoma botryoides

What is sarcoma botryoides?

A rare variant of rhabdomyosarcoma

At what age is it diagnosed?

90% of cases are in children younger than 2 years of age

What is the clinical presentation?

Multiple polypoid masses resembling "bunches of grapes" protrude into the vagina and often from the vulva.

What is the prognosis?

Poor. Death is more often caused by direct extension of the tumor than by distant metastases.

THE CERVIX

NON-NEOPLASTIC DISORDERS OF THE CERVIX

What is the normal anatomy of the cervix?

Exocervix: portion of cervix that protrudes into the upper vagina
Endocervix: portion of cervix that leads to the endometrial cavity
External os: junction between the exocervix and endocervix

What is the normal histology of the cervix?

Exocervix: nonkeratinizing stratified squamous epithelium

Endocervix: longitudinal mucosal ridges lined by a single layer of mucinous columnar cells

Where is the squamo-columnar junction?

Junction of the stratified squamous epithelium of the exocervix and the columnar epithelium of the endocervix

Where is the location of this junction in relation to the anatomic external os?

The epithelium remodels continuously throughout life so that the exact location varies depending on a number of factors, including age, hormonal status, and parity.

What is endocervical ectropion?

Areas where the columnar endocervical epithelium extends onto the exocervix, appearing as reddish discoloration on colposcopy

What is the transformation zone?

Area between the original squamo-columnar junction and the new squamo-columnar junction

Cervicitis

What is the cause of cervicitis?

Constant exposure to the bacterial flora of the vagina

What are the organisms most commonly responsible?

Endogenous vaginal aerobes and anaerobes, streptococci, staphylococci, enterococci, *Gardnerella vaginalis*, *Trichomonas vaginalis*, *Candida albicans*, and *Chlamydia trachomatis*

What is the clinical presentation?

Acute cervicitis: cervix is red, swollen, and edematous with pus seen at the external os
Chronic cervicitis: hyperemic cervical mucosa with epithelial erosions

DYSPLASIA AND CARCINOMA IN SITU OF THE CERVIX

What site is most frequently involved?

Transformation zone

What organism is most closely associated?

HPV infection, particularly types 16 and 18

What is the histology of dysplasia?

Disordered epithelial growth manifest by loss of polarity, increased mitotic figures, and nuclear hyperchromasia, beginning at the basal layer and extending outward

What is the definition of carcinoma in situ?

Atypical changes extending through the entire thickness of the epithelium but not invading to the underlying stroma

What percentage of carcinoma in situ of the cervix progress to invasive carcinoma?

70% after 12 years

NEOPLASIA OF THE CERVIX

In what age group is the peak occurrence of carcinoma of the cervix?

Middle-aged women (30–50 years of age)

What type of cervical carcinoma is most common?

Squamous cell carcinoma is most common (95%); adenocarcinoma may also occur (5%).

Why has mortality due to cervical carcinoma taken such a dramatic reduction?

The Papanicolaou cytologic screening (Pap smear)

Name 5 epidemiologic factors related to invasive cervical carcinoma.

1. Early sexual contact
2. Multiple sexual partners
3. History of prostitution
4. Low socioeconomic status
5. HSV-2 infection, which may act as a cocarcinogen with HPV infection

What are the gross pathologic features?

Exophytic, ulcerating, or infiltrating lesions

What is koilocytosis?

Similar to HPV-induced condyloma acuminatum, this process is frequently exhibited in dysplastic cells, where expanded epithelial cells with perinuclear clearing are seen.

THE UTERUS

NON-NEOPLASTIC DISORDERS OF THE UTERUS

What is the normal histology of the uterus?

Endometrium composed of glands with simple columnar epithelium and specialized endometrial stroma; myometrium composed of smooth muscle

What is the histology of the endometrium in a post-menopausal female?

Thin endometrial mucosa, scant and atrophic glands, and dense stroma

What is the histology of endometrium in women on oral contraceptives?

Small inactive glands and predecidualized stroma due to progesterone effect

What is the histology of women with dysfunctional uterine bleeding due to estrogen stimulation without subsequent progesterone stimulation?

Proliferative glands; breakdown and collapse of stroma

Acute endometritis

What are the most common causes of acute endometritis?

Intrauterine trauma secondary to instrumentation, IUDs, or complications of pregnancy (postpartum retention of placental fragments)

What organisms are most commonly involved?

Staphylococcus aureus, streptococci, and *Neisseria gonorrhoeae*

Endometriosis

What is endometriosis?

The presence and proliferation of ectopic, non-neoplastic endometrial tissue

What are the common locations of ectopic tissue?

1. Ovary
2. Uterine ligaments
3. Rectovaginal septum
4. Pelvic peritoneum

Name 3 theories of pathogenesis.

1. Retrograde dissemination of endometrial fragments through the fallopian tubes during menstruation (Sampson theory)
2. Metaplasia of the specialized surface epithelium of any part of the müllerian system to endometrial tissue (Novak theory)
3. Blood-borne or lymphatic-borne dissemination and emboli of fragments

What are the clinical manifestations of endometriosis?	Severe menstrual-related pain
What are pelvic exam findings?	Menstrual-type bleeding into the ectopic endometrium, resulting in blood-filled or "chocolate" cysts
What important complication may result?	Infertility

Adenomyosis

What is uterine adenomyosis?	Islands of endometrium within myometrium
What is endometrial hyperplasia?	Abnormal proliferation of endometrial glands
What are the causes of adenomyosis?	Excess estrogen stimulation secondary to one or more of the following: 1. Anovulatory cycles 2. Estrogen-secreting ovarian tumors 3. Estrogen medication
What are the clinical manifestations of adenomyosis?	Vaginal bleeding

Leiomyomas (Fibroids)

What is the incidence of leiomyomas?	Most common uterine tumor and most common of all tumors in women; there is increased incidence in African-American women.
What is their pattern of growth?	They are estrogen-sensitive; therefore, they increase in size during pregnancy and decrease in size following menopause
Name the 3 most common locations of leiomyomas.	1. Within the myometrium (intramural) 2. Subendometrial (submucous) 3. Subperitoneal (subserous)
What are the clinical manifestations?	Vaginal bleeding, especially in the subendometrial leiomyomas
What is the pathogenesis of leiomyosarcoma.	Almost always arises de novo, rarely due to malignant transformation of a leiomyoma

NEOPLASIA OF THE UTERUS

Describe the incidence of endometrial carcinoma.	The most common gynecologic malignancy, now increasing in incidence
In what age group is the peak occurrence?	Older women
What are the associated risk factors of endometrial carcinoma?	Related to prolonged unopposed estrogen stimulation, including exogenous estrogen therapy, estrogen-producing tumors, nulliparity, and obesity; also diabetes, hypertension, and high socioeconomic status.
What is the most significant clinical manifestation?	Vaginal bleeding
What are the histologic findings of endometrial carcinoma?	Most commonly endometrioid tumor, but also clear cell, adenosquamous, and papillary serous tumor
What is the prognosis?	90% 5-year survival rate with 75% of patients presenting with stage I disease

THE OVARY

CYSTIC DISORDERS OF THE OVARY

What is the normal histology of the ovary?	Each ovary is composed of a fibrous tissue layer, called the tunica albuginea, a mesenchymal stroma containing steroid-producing cells, and numerous follicles containing gametes.
What are the 5 most common types of ovarian cysts?	1. Follicular cyst 2. Corpus luteum cyst 3. Theca-lutein cyst 4. Chocolate cyst 5. Polycystic ovary (Stein-Leventhal) syndrome
What causes a follicular cyst?	Distention of the unruptured graafian follicle
What is the clinical presentation of a follicular cyst?	The cyst is usually small and clinically insignificant, but may cause abdominal

pain or, rarely, abnormal uterine bleeding.

Why may women with follicular cysts develop abnormal uterine bleeding?

The lining granulosa cells of the follicular cyst may produce enough excess estrogen to stimulate endometrial hyperplasia and, consequently, uterine bleeding.

What is the cause of a corpus luteum cyst?

Hemorrhage into a persistent mature corpus luteum

What are other factors associated with a corpus luteum cyst?

Menstrual irregularity, sometimes with intraperitoneal hemorrhage

What is the cause of theca-lutein cyst?

Gonadotropin stimulation

Polycystic Ovarian Syndrome (PCOS)

At what age does PCOS usually present?

It occurs in women in their 20s and 30s.

Name 4 clinical manifestations of PCOS.

1. Amenorrhea with abnormal uterine bleeding
2. Infertility
3. Obesity
4. Hirsutism

What is the pathogenesis of PCOS?

Due to excess androgen production and inhibition of follicle stimulating hormone (FSH), luteinizing hormone (LH) is elevated, which results in anovulation with follicle cyst formation.

Name 4 pathologic features of the ovary in PCOS.

1. Markedly enlarged ovary
2. Thickened ovarian capsule consisting of dense fibrous tissue
3. Multiple small follicular cysts containing a granulosa cell layer and a luteinized theca interna
4. Cortical stromal fibrosis with islands of focal luteinization

Is a corpora luteum present in PCOS?

No, because there is no ovulation

Do the lesions of PCOS regress once ovulation is achieved?

Yes

NEOPLASIA OF THE OVARY

What is the incidence of ovarian neoplasms?	It is the 5th most common form of cancer in women
How are ovarian tumors classified? Give 4 classes.	Based on the site of tumor origin: 1. Epithelial origin 2. Germ cell origin 3. Sex cord-stromal origin 4. Tumors metastatic to ovary

Ovarian tumors of epithelial origin

What is the incidence of ovarian tumors of epithelial origin?	Almost 75% of all ovarian tumors
What is the age of presentation for ovarian tumors of epithelial origin?	Women older than 20 years of age
What are the 5 types of ovarian tumors of epithelial origin?	1. Serous (most common) 2. Mucinous 3. Endometrioid 4. Clear cell 5. Brenner (rare)
What is the incidence of malignant serous tumors?	About 50% of ovarian carcinomas
What is the histology of benign serous tumors?	Benign cystic tumor lined with cells similar to fallopian tube epithelium; often cystic and filled with clear serous fluid or mucinous fluid
What is the histology of borderline and malignant serous tumors?	More complex configuration with frond-like masses protruding into the cystic space lined by more atypical-appearing cells, and abundant calcified psammoma bodies
How are borderline serous tumors differentiated from malignant serous tumors?	Invasion of the ovarian stroma
Name 3 characteristics of mucinous tumors that differentiate them from serous tumors.	1. Less common than serous tumors 2. Less often bilateral 3. More frequently multilocular

What is the histology of malignant mucinous tumors?	Increase in glandular complexity, atypical cells, and presence of ovarian stromal invasion
Name a complication of mucinous tumors.	Pseudomyxoma peritonei ("jelly belly") in 5% of cases
What is pseudomyxoma peritonei?	Presence of large quantities of mucinous material in the abdomen
What are the complications of pseudomyxoma peritonei?	Development of fibrous adhesions and intestinal obstruction
What is the histology of malignant endometrioid tumors?	Presence of tubular glands resembling uterine endometrial adenocarcinoma
What percentage of ovarian endometrioid carcinomas are associated with endometrial carcinoma of the uterus?	15%–30%, because of the field effect
What type of clear cell tumor is most common?	Malignant type. Benign and borderline types are extremely rare.
What is the most common type of Brenner tumor?	It is almost always benign and is discovered only incidentally. Borderline and malignant forms are extremely rare.

Ovarian tumors of germ cell origin

What is the incidence of ovarian cancer of germ cell origin?	About 15%–20% of ovarian tumors
What is the age at presentation?	Tumors of germ cell origin account for most ovarian tumors in women younger than 20 years of age.
Name 4 types of germ cell tumors.	1. Teratoma 2. Dysgerminoma, or ovarian seminoma 3. Endodermal sinus (yolk sac) tumor 4. Ovarian choriocarcinoma
Most common type of germ cell tumor?	95% of germ cell tumors are benign cystic teratomas (also called dermoid cysts).

What are the three forms of teratomas?	1. Immature teratoma 2. Mature teratoma (dermoid cyst) 3. Monodermal teratoma
Histology of the immature teratoma?	Immature (fetal) cellular elements
What is the most common immature element found in immature teratomas?	Neuroepithelium (brain tissue)
What may develop in association with rupture of an immature teratoma?	Gliomatosis peritonei, which develops as a result of peritoneal tumor implants of neural tissue that may either mature or remain immature.
Which is a better prognostic sign in a patient with gliomatosis peritonei: immature neural tissue or mature neural tissue?	Gliomatosis peritonei with mature neural tissue implants is a benign condition, but if the implants remain immature, there is a high mortality rate.
What are the gross pathological findings of mature teratoma?	Tumors are lined by skin, including hair follicles and other skin appendages; other elements often include bone, tooth, cartilage, and GI, neurologic, respiratory, thyroid gland tissues.
What is unique about monodermal teratomas?	They contain only a single tissue element.
What is the most common tissue element in monodermal teratomas?	Thyroid tissue, called struma ovarii
Is struma ovarii functional?	Yes, it may be hyperfunctional and result in hyperthyroidism.
What is the incidence of dysgerminomas?	2% of all malignant ovarian neoplasms and 50% of all malignant germ cell tumors are dysgerminomas.
What is the histology of dysgerminomas?	They are homologous to testicular seminoma, consisting of uniform sheets of undifferentiated germ cells surrounded by an intense lymphoid infiltrate.

In what population do endodermal sinus tumors usually develop?

Young girls and women

What is the histology of endodermal sinus tumors?

Resemble extraembryonic yolk sac structures

What serum tumor marker is produced?

α-fetoprotein

What are the characteristic features of endodermal sinus tumors?

Rapidly growing, clinically aggressive tumors

What is the most common location at which choriocarcinoma arises?

Within the uterus and, much less commonly, in the ovary

What is the serum tumor marker for choriocarcinoma?

Human chorionic gonadotropin (HCG)

Which cells show production of HCG by immunohistochemical staining?

Syncytiotrophoblasts, but not in cytotrophoblastic cells

What are potential complications of choriocarcinoma?

Intracranial, intrapulmonary, or intrahepatic hemorrhage due to widespread hematogenous metastasis of this very aggressive tumor

Ovarian tumors of sex cord-stromal origin

What are the 3 types of sex cord-stromal ovarian tumors?

1. Fibromas
2. Granulosa-theca cell tumors
3. Sertoli-Leydig cell tumors

What is the incidence of sex cord-stromal ovarian tumors?

They comprise only a small percentage of ovarian neoplasms.

What is the age of presentation?

Any age group may be affected.

What is the histology of a fibroma?

A solid tumor consisting of bundles of well-differentiated spindle-shaped fibroblasts

Name a condition associated with fibroma.

Meigs syndrome

What is the triad of Meigs syndrome?	1. Ovarian fibroma 2. Ascites 3. Hydrothorax
What percentage of granulosa-theca cell tumors are hormonally active?	Almost all tumors with a prominent theca cell component are hormonally active and 75% of pure granulosa cell tumors are associated with hormone production.
What is the characteristic histological feature of granulosa-theca cell tumors?	Call-Exner bodies, which are small follicles filled with eosinophilic secretion
What hormone is secreted by these tumors?	Estrogen
What are some conditions associated with granulosa-theca cell tumors?	1. Precocious puberty in children 2. Endometrial hyperplasia 3. Endometrial cancer
What are the 2 types of Sertoli-Leydig tumors?	Androblastoma and arrhenoblastoma
What is the hormone secreted by these tumors?	Androgen
What is the clinical presentation associated with Sertoli-Leydig tumors?	Variable—either virilizing, feminizing, or inactive
What is the histology of Sertoli-Leydig tumors?	Well-differentiated tumors containing tubules composed of Sertoli cells and surrounded by a stroma filled with Leydig cells, which mimics the histology of the testis

Tumors Metastatic to the Ovary

What is the incidence of tumors metastatic to the ovary?	5% of all ovarian tumors
What is the most common site of origin of metastatic ovarian tumors?	1. GI tract 2. Breast 3. Uterus
What are Krukenberg tumors?	Tumors that replace the ovaries bilaterally by mucin-secreting signet ring cells

| Which primary site is most often associated with Krukenberg tumors? | Stomach |

DISORDERS OF PREGNANCY

PLACENTAL ABRUPTION

| What is it? | Premature separation of the placenta from the uterine wall |

| Name 6 possible clinical findings. | 1. Antepartum bleeding
2. Uterine rigidity
3. Severe abdominal pain
4. Shock
5. Disseminated intravascular coagulation (DIC)
6. Fetal distress or fetal death |

| How often is placental abruption associated with maternal hypertension? | 25%–50% |

PLACENTA ACCRETA

| What is it? | Attachment of placenta directly to myometrium as a result of defective decidual layer |

| Name 2 types of placenta accreta. | 1. Placenta increta
2. Placenta percreta |

| What is the difference between these 2 types? | In placenta increta, chorionic villi penetrate the uterine muscle, and in placenta percreta it penetrates the entire myometrial wall to extend into the uterine serosa. |

| What are some predisposing factors for placenta accreta? | Events that result in defective decidual layer such as endometrial inflammation, and old scars caused by previous infection, trauma, or prior cesarean sections and other surgery |

| What are some clinical manifestations? | Impaired placental separation after delivery; massive hemorrhage sometimes follows. |

PLACENTA PREVIA

What is it?	The attachment of placenta to lower uterine segment, sometimes covering the internal cervical os
What is the most common symptom?	Painless vaginal bleeding

ECTOPIC PREGNANCY

What are the most common sites of ectopic pregnancy?	Fallopian tubes (95%), ovary, abdominal cavity, cervix
What are some predisposing risk factors?	History of chronic salpingitis (PID), endometriosis, postoperative adhesions
Do all cases have an obvious cause?	No
Name some complications of ectopic pregnancy.	Hematosalpinx, tubal rupture
How far do most tubal pregnancies progress before rupturing?	6–12 weeks

GESTATIONAL TROPHOBLASTIC DISEASE (GTD)

Name 2 types of gestational trophoblastic disease (GTD).	1. Hydatidiform mole 2. Gestational choriocarcinoma

Hydatidiform mole

What is the incidence of hydatidiform mole?	1 in 2000 pregnancies in the U.S.; in Asian countries, 1 in 125—250 pregnancies
Name 2 variants of hydatidiform moles.	1. Complete hydatidiform mole 2. Partial hydatidiform mole
What are the distinguishing characteristics of these two variants?	1. Complete hydatidiform moles contain no embryo, and the karyotype is 46,XX, with exclusively paternal derivation (androgenesis) 2. Partial hydatidiform moles contain an

embryo, triploidy and tetraploidy often occur, due to fertilization of ovum by two or more spermatozoa

What are some predisposing risk factors to hydatidiform mole?

Poor nutrition, consanguinity, very young or very old maternal age

What is the gross pathology?

Large mass of edematous tissue with grapelike bulbs of hydropic villi.

What is the histology of hydatidiform mole?

Hydropic villi are sparsely cellular and avascular with a syncytiotrophoblast covering them and, on occasion, highly proliferative trophoblastic lesions.

What hormone is most significantly elevated and used as a marker?

HCG

In which trimester does it usually present?

The first trimester

What are the clinical manifestations of hydatidiform mole?

Vaginal bleeding, rapid increase in uterine size, may be associated with toxemia

What is the incidence of transformation of hydatidiform mole to choriocarcinoma?

2%–3%

Choriocarcinoma

What is the histology of choriocarcinomas?

Soft, sometimes necrotic, hemorrhagic nodules consisting of mixed syncytiotrophoblastic and cytotrophoblastic cells and vascular invasion.

What are the characteristics of choriocarcinomas?

Aggressive, malignant

Name 4 preceding conditions of choriocarcinomas.

1. Hydatidiform mole (50%)
2. Abortion of pregnancy (20%–25%)
3. Ectopic pregnancy (3%)
4. Full-term normal pregnancy (20%–30%)

What serum tumor marker is produced and followed to determine response to therapy and prognosis?	HCG
Where is metastases from choriocarcinoma most commonly found and by what route?	In the lungs via hematogenous spread

POWER REVIEW

Name a group at high-risk for clear cell adenocarcinoma.	Mothers treated with diethylstilbestrol therapy during pregnancy
What is the etiologic agent of chancroid?	*Haemophilus ducreyi*
What condition is caused by Donovan bodies?	Granuloma inguinale
What are the risk factors associated with endometrial cancer?	Nulliparity, obesity, diabetes, and hypertension leading to increased estrogen stimulation
What is the most common organism responsible for PID?	Gonorrhea (50%–65% of cases)
What characteristic of *Neisseria gonorrheae* facilitates its ability to cause infection?	The presence of surface pili that preferentially attach to endocervical and fallopian tube epithelium
What are the major complications of PID?	Pyosalpinx, hydrosalpinx, tubo-ovarian abscess, sterility, and increased risk for ectopic pregnancy
What are the HPV types most often associated with cervical dysplasia and invasive carcinoma?	Types 16, 18
Name a form of teratoma containing hyperfunctional thyroid tissue.	Struma ovarii

Identify the triad of Meigs syndrome?

Ovarian fibroma, hydroperitoneum, hydrothorax

What site is most frequently involved in dysplasia and carcinoma of the cervix?

Transformation zone

Why do leiomyomas (fibroids) increase in size during pregnancy and decrease following menopause?

They are estrogen-sensitive

What microscopic evidence indicates a diagnosis of chlamydial infection?

Intracytoplasmic inclusion bodies in the cervicovaginal cytologic smears

What is the term for a gastric cancer metastatic to the ovary?

Krukenberg tumor

What are the complications of granulosa cell tumors and what causes them?

Precocious puberty, endometrial hyperplasia, and cancer. These complications are more likely because the granulosa cell tumors secrete estrogen.

Which type of ovarian cancer consists of psammoma bodies?

Malignant serous tumors

What is the most common benign germ cell tumor of the ovary in premenopausal women?

Dermoid cyst

Name the condition in which the placenta partially or completely covers the internal os.

Placenta previa

For what infectious disease would a Tzanck smear be useful?

HSV infections, where you may see multinucleated giant cells containing viral inclusions

In what phase of syphilis might you find condyloma lata on physical examination?

Secondary syphilis

What age group more commonly develops lichen sclerosus?

Women over 50 years of age (women under 50 years of age more commonly develop squamous hyperplasia)

What is the pathogenesis of PCOS?

Excess LH and androgen production with inhibition of FSH, resulting in anovulatory state with follicle cyst formation

Name 4 clinical manifestations of PCOS.

1. Amenorrhea
2. Infertility
3. Obesity
4. Hirsutism

What are "clue cells" and in what condition are they found?

Clue cells are desquamated epithelial cells with many tiny adherent coccobacilli; they are pathognomonic of bacterial vaginosis.

What etiologic agent is responsible for koilocytosis?

HPV

How do koilocytes appear?

Expanded epithelial cells with perinuclear clearing

When does sarcoma botryoides appear and what is the prognosis?

It usually presents before 2 years of age and carries a poor prognosis.

What tumor marker is produced by

Endodermal sinus tumors?

α-fetoprotein (AFP)

Choriocarcinomas?

HCG

Hydatiform moles?

HCG

22   The Breast

**What is the normal histol-
ogy of the female breast?**

Normal microscopic anatomy includes
epithelial and myoepithelial cells. Lobules
containing many small ductules and acini
when lactating lead to terminal ducts,
which join with segmental ducts and then
large lactiferous ducts that finally open on
the nipple.

**What causes the majority
of palpable breast masses?**

Proliferation of ductal epithelium usually
accompanied by increase in fibrous stroma

**Into what 4 categories do
most breast lesions fall?**

1. Inflammatory disorders
2. Fibrocystic disease
3. Benign tumors
4. Carcinoma

INFLAMMATORY DISORDERS OF THE BREAST

**Name 4 common inflamma-
tory disorders of the breast.**

1. Acute mastitis
2. Chronic mastitis
3. Duct ectasia
4. Fat necrosis

**When does acute mastitis
most commonly affect
women?**

During lactation

**What are the most common
causative agents?**

Staphylococci and streptococci

**What are the clinical
manifestations?**

The breast (mastitis is usually unilateral)
is swollen, erythematous, and painful.

**What diseases most
commonly lead to chronic
mastitis?**

Systemic granulomatous diseases such as
tuberculosis and sarcoidosis

**When does duct ectasia
most commonly occur?**

Postmenopause

What is the histology of duct ectasia?

Dilatation of collecting ducts with periductal fibrosis and amorphous material in the lumen of the ducts

What history is usually given in women with fat necrosis?

Preceding injury or traumatic event to the breast

What is the clinical presentation of fat necrosis?

May produce a mass that can simulate carcinoma

What are the histologic features of fat necrosis?

Inflamed, necrotic adipose tissue with areas of calcification. Chronic inflammatory cells and lipid-filled macrophages also are seen.

FIBROCYSTIC DISEASE

What is the incidence of fibrocystic disease?

It is the most common disorder of the breast and most common cause of a palpable breast mass in women 25–50 years of age.

What are the clinical manifestations of fibrocystic disease?

Lumpy breasts with midcycle tenderness

What is the pathogenesis of fibrocystic disease?

The cause is most likely increased activity of, or sensitivity to, estrogen or decreased progesterone activity.

Is fibrocystic disease usually unilateral or bilateral?

Usually bilateral

What are some conditions associated with fibrocystic disease?

Slightly increased incidence of cancer when epithelial hyperplasia is marked and clearly higher risk of cancer when hyperplastic epithelium demonstrates atypia. However, there is no risk of cancer in nonproliferative fibrocystic disease.

What is the morphology?

A variety of histologic changes are seen, including:
1. Fibrosis of variable degree
2. Cystic dilation of ducts

3. Epithelial hyperplasia (papillomatosis)
4. Apocrine metaplasia
5. Sclerosing adenosis

What is adenosis?

Proliferation of small ducts and myo-epithelial cells

BENIGN TUMORS OF THE BREAST

FIBROADENOMA

What is the incidence of fibroadenoma?

Most common breast tumor in women younger than 18–36 years of age but commonly seen in women 20–35 years of age.

Is fibroadenoma benign or malignant?

Benign

What are the clinical manifestations of a fibroadenoma?

Freely movable, firm, rubbery, painless lesion that is well demarcated from adjacent breast tissue

What percentage of fibroadenomas are multiple?

Approximately 10%, either in same breast or bilateral

What is the histology of fibroadenoma?

Proliferation of fibrous stroma and lobular epithelium with multiplication of ducts and acini

What are the classifications and distinguishing features of fibroadenoma?

1. Intracanalicular fibroadenoma: stroma compresses and distorts glands into slitlike spaces
2. Pericanalicular fibroadenoma: glands retain round shape

INTRADUCTAL PAPILLOMA

What tissue is involved in intraductal papilloma?

Major lactiferous ducts

What age group is most commonly affected?

Women 30–50 years of age, but usually at or shortly before menopause

What is the clinical presentation of intraductal papilloma?

Small masses located near the nipple; however, serous and bloody nipple discharge without a palpable mass is also commonly seen.

Are intraductal papillomas benign or malignant?

They are benign tumors.

What is different about the site of origin for intraductal papilloma as compared with fibroadenoma and fibrocystic disease?

Intraductal papilloma arises from the large ducts, whereas all fibroadenomas and fibrocystic changes originate from lobules.

CARCINOMA OF THE BREAST

What is the incidence of breast carcinoma?

It is the second most common malignancy in women (after lung cancer), and the leading cause of death in women over 40 years of age.

What is the most common cause of breast mass in the postmenopausal patient?

Carcinoma of the breast

What is the most common site of mass?

Upper outer quadrant of the breast

What are the most common sites of breast cancer metastases?

Lung, liver, bone, and brain

What are the risk factors for breast cancer?

1. Increasing age, particularly over 40 years of age
2. Positive family history, particularly in first-degree female relatives
3. Prior history of breast cancer
4. Early menarche
5. Late menopause
6. Nulliparity
7. First pregnancy after 30 years of age

What are the clinical features of breast cancer?

1. Palpable, fixed lump or mass
2. Pain
3. Edema, erythema, and dimpling of overlying skin
4. Nipple retraction
5. Lymphadenopathy

What are the histologic types of breast cancer?

1. Intraductal carcinoma in situ
2. Lobular carcinoma in situ
3. Infiltrating ductal carcinoma
4. Infiltrating lobular carcinoma

5. Medullary carcinoma
6. Mucinous (colloid) carcinoma
7. Tubular carcinoma
8. Invasive cribriform
9. Paget disease of the breast
10. Inflammatory carcinoma

Which histologic types of breast cancer are non-invasive?

Intraductal carcinoma in situ and lobular carcinoma in situ

What characteristics make a breast cancer invasive?

Invasion beyond the basement membrane, therefore allowing access to lymphatics and blood vessels and creating potential for distant metastases

Which of the invasive histologic types of breast cancer are potentially lethal?

Infiltrating ductal, infiltrating lobular, medullary, mucinous

What are 3 important prognostic factors for invasive carcinomas?

1. Histologic type/grade
2. Size of the tumor
3. Presence or absence of lymph node metastases

How many breast carcinomas contain estrogen-receptor proteins?

About 50%

Why are estrogen-receptor proteins important?

Patients with estrogen-receptor proteins are more likely to respond to endocrine therapy (e.g., tamoxifen), which can lead to objective remissions and a better prognosis.

What age group is more likely to have tumors with estrogen-receptor status?

Postmenopausal women (Premenopausal women have high levels of endogenous estrogen, which blocks the receptor sites.)

INTRADUCTAL CARCINOMA IN SITU

What is the incidence of intraductal carcinoma in situ of the breast?

5%–10% of all breast cancers

What are the 2 subtypes of intraductal carcinoma in situ of the breast?

1. Comedocarcinoma
2. Cribriform or micropapillary carcinoma in situ

What is the subsequent risk of developing invasive carcinoma of the breast for each of these subtypes?

Comedocarcinoma is thought to have a 100% chance of becoming invasive if untreated, while cribriform or micro-papillary carcinoma in situ has only about a 30% chance.

What are the histological differences between comedocarcinoma and cribriform or micropapillary carcinoma in situ?

Comedocarcinoma contains large pleomorphic tumor cells with a central area of necrosis (comedone), whereas cribriform or micropapillary carcinoma in situ has small, uniform cells that lack an area of necrosis.

What other characteristic features have been seen in comedocarcinoma?

High S phase and aneuploidy

What percentage of non-invasive carcinomas progress to invasive cancer?

Only about 30% of most subtypes; the exception is comedocarcinoma, in which almost 100% will progress to invasive cancer if left untreated.

LOBULAR CARCINOMA IN SITU

In what percentage of breast biopsy specimens taken for a suspicious mass will lobular carcinoma in situ be found?

About 3%

Why is lobular carcinoma in situ so often an incidental, unsuspected finding on biopsy?

Because it cannot be palpated on physical examination or felt at operation

What percentage of women with lobular carcinoma in situ go on to develop invasive carcinoma?

About 33%

Of the women with lobular carcinoma in situ who go on to develop invasive carcinoma, what is the chance that it will develop in the breast contralateral to the one that had the lobular neoplasia?

50%

What is the histology of lobular carcinoma in situ?	Clusters of neoplastic cells fill intralobular ductules and acini

INFILTRATING DUCTAL CARCINOMA AND INFILTRATING LOBULAR CARCINOMA OF THE BREAST

What percentage of invasive carcinoma is infiltrating ductal carcinoma?	80% of the invasive carcinomas
What is the histology of infiltrating ductal carcinoma?	Tumor cells larger than normal epithelium and arranged in cords, islands, and glands embedded in a dense fibrous stroma with abundant fibrous tissue giving it a firm consistency
What is the incidence of infiltrating lobular carcinoma?	10% of the invasive carcinomas
What is the histology of infiltrating lobular carcinoma?	Small, uniform cells about the same size as normal epithelium and usually arranged in single-file rows of cells
What features are used in determining the grading system for infiltrating ductal and lobular carcinomas of the breast?	1. Tubule formation 2. Nuclear pleomorphism 3. Mitotic counts
What is the single most important prognostic factor for infiltrating ductal carcinoma and infiltrating lobular carcinoma?	Status of the lymph nodes

MEDULLARY CARCINOMA AND MUCINOUS CARCINOMA

What is the incidence of medullary carcinoma?	2% of the invasive carcinomas
What is the histology of medullary cancer?	Mixture of malignant epithelial cells and many plasma cells and lymphocytes
What is the incidence of mucinous carcinoma?	2% of the invasive carcinomas
What is the histology of mucinous cancer?	Pools of extracellular mucus surrounding clusters of tumor cells

What features are characteristic on palpation of a medullary or mucinous carcinoma mass?	Sharply circumscribed, soft and gelatinous consistency due to lack of fibrous tissue in both types
Is the prognosis for both medullary and mucinous carcinoma worse or better than that of invasive ductal carcinoma?	Better

TUBULAR CARCINOMA AND INVASIVE CRIBRIFORM CARCINOMA

What is the incidence of tubular carcinoma?	2% of the invasive carcinomas
What are the histology findings?	Well-formed glands
What is the incidence of invasive cribriform carcinoma?	2% of the invasive carcinomas
What are the histology findings?	Well-formed lumens surrounded by broader nests of cells
What percentage of tubular carcinomas and invasive cribriform carcinomas have lymph node metastases?	5%–10%
Why are these types usually only locally invasive and thus non-lethal?	Neither type is able to metastasize hematogenously.

PAGET DISEASE OF THE BREAST

What is the incidence?	1%–2% of all breast cancers
What are the clinical features?	Eczematous, excoriated lesion involving the nipple and adjacent skin
What do Paget cells look like histologically?	Large cells with prominent nuclei and abundant eosinophilic cytoplasm
Name an associated underlying condition.	Infiltrating intraductal carcinoma is almost always present.

INFLAMMATORY CARCINOMA

What is the histology?	Lymphatic involvement of skin by underlying carcinoma
What are the clinical manifestations?	Red, swollen, hot skin resembling an inflammatory process or lymphatic edema resembling an orange peel

CYSTOSARCOMA PHYLLOIDES

What are the clinical manifestations?	Rapidly growing large, bulky mass with ulceration of overlying skin
Is cystosarcoma phylloides benign or malignant?	Variable malignancy
What are the histologic features?	Very cellular stroma composed of atypical spindle cells, abundant mitotic figures, and cystic spaces containing leaf-like projections from the cyst walls

POWER REVIEW

What is the most common breast mass in

A woman less than 18–36 years of age?	Fibroadenoma
A woman 25–50 years of age?	Fibrocystic disease
A woman over 50 years of age?	Carcinoma of the breast
Name some risk factors for breast cancer.	Increasing age, history of breast cancer in first-degree relative, prior history of breast cancer, early menarche, late menopause, nulliparity, first pregnancy after 30 years of age
What is the histology of fibroadenoma?	Pattern of compressed glands and young fibrous stroma
Which histologic feature is the hallmark of invasive lobular carcinoma of the breast?	Small, uniform cells arranged in single-file rows

What is the most likely diagnosis for a woman who presents with bloody discharge from one nipple?

Intraductal papilloma

Which breast disorder occurs most commonly during lactation and breast-feeding?

Acute mastitis

What is the most common type of invasive carcinoma of the breast?

Infiltrating ductal carcinoma

Which type of breast carcinoma is associated with involvement of the contralateral breast in 50% of cases?

Lobular carcinoma in situ

What type of breast carcinoma is associated with distant metastases consisting of malignant stromal cells?

Cystosarcoma phylloides

What is the single most important prognostic factor for infiltrating carcinomas?

Status of the lymph nodes

What type of carcinoma in situ of the breast progresses to invasive cancer in almost 100% of cases?

Comedocarcinoma

23

Kidney and Urinary Tract

CONGENITAL ANOMALIES OF THE KIDNEY AND URINARY TRACT

KIDNEY

Name 4 anomalies of kidney formation.	1. Renal agenesis: complete or unilateral 2. Renal ectopia 3. Horseshoe kidney 4. Renal hypoplasia
What finding in the prenatal period suggests renal agenesis?	Oligohydramnios (decrease in amniotic fluid—fetus normally swallows and excretes it continuously)
What is the most common ectopic site for the kidney?	Pelvis
What is a horseshoe kidney?	Connection (usually of the lower poles) secondary to failure of separation; may impinge on ureters and lead to obstruction
Is renal function impaired with a horseshoe kidney?	Usually not
What is Potter syndrome?	Bilateral (complete) renal agenesis. It is incompatible with life.

CONGENITAL ANOMALIES OF THE URINARY TRACT

Name 4 congenital anomalies of the urinary tract.	1. Bladder diverticula 2. Persistent urachus 3. Exstrophy of the bladder 4. Double ureters
What are diverticula?	Pouchlike eversions of the bladder wall. They may be congenital due to failure of

development of normal musculature, or acquired due to obstruction in the urethra or bladder neck.

Are diverticula most commonly found in men or women?

Men

What is a persistent urachus?

A patent connection between the apex of the bladder and the umbilicus

What is exstrophy of the bladder?

Absence of the anterior musculature of the bladder

With what other developmental defects is exstrophy associated?

Anterior abdominal wall defects

RENAL CYSTIC DISEASES

What is the etiology of simple renal cysts?

Inflammation and scarring creates cystic dilatation of the proximal nephron. The incidence increases with age and is usually asymptomatic.

What is medullary sponge kidney?

An incidental condition seen in adults, not a true cystic disease. Renal function is normal. Papillary ducts of the medulla are dilated to form small cysts lined by cuboidal or transitional epithelium.

What is cystic renal dysplasia?

A condition in which the kidney is distorted by cysts. It is often associated with obstructive abnormalities of the lower urinary tract.

Name the 3 most common renal cystic diseases.

1. Adult polycystic kidney disease
2. Autosomal-recessive polycystic kidney disease
3. Medullary cystic disease

ADULT POLYCYSTIC KIDNEY DISEASE

What is the mode of inheritance?

Autosomal-dominant with high penetrance

What are 3 signs of polycystic kidney disease (PKD)?	1. Enlarging flank and abdominal mass 2. Flank and back pain 3. Hematuria
What is the typical age of presentation?	15–40 years of age
What is the prognosis?	Two-thirds of patients with adult PKD die of renal failure and vascular complications
Name the intracranial lesion associated with adult PKD.	Berry aneurysms (usually in Circle of Willis)
Name the hematologic complication of APKD.	Secondary polycythemia ($\uparrow$ erythropoietin)
What is the pathology of polycystic kidneys?	Massively enlarged kidneys with numerous cysts replacing parenchyma and compressing nephrons

AUTOSOMAL-RECESSIVE POLYCYSTIC KIDNEY DISEASE

What is the typical presentation of autosomal-recessive PKD?	Renal failure in a newborn or infant; it can be delayed until later childhood
What is the pathology of autosomal-recessive PKD?	Bilaterally enlarged kidneys, massive dilatation of collecting tubules
With what extrarenal diseases is it associated?	Congenital hepatic fibrosis, liver cysts
What is the prognosis of autosomal-recessive PKD?	Death shortly after birth

MEDULLARY CYSTIC DISEASE

Name 4 pathologic features of medullary cystic disease.	1. Progressive tubular atrophy 2. Interstitial fibrosis 3. Medullary cysts 4. Small kidneys
What is the pattern of inheritance of medullary cystic disease?	Autosomal dominant

What is the age of presentation of medullary cystic disease?	20–40 years of age
What are the signs and symptoms of medullary cystic disease?	Polyuria, polydipsia, sodium wasting, and tubular acidosis
What is the prognosis of medullary cystic disease?	Progression to renal failure over several years
What is familial juvenile nephronophthisis?	Medullary cystic disease with autosomal-recessive inheritance. Severe growth retardation is common.

GLOMERULAR DISEASES

Name 2 mechanisms of immune-mediated glomerular disease.	1. Antibodies to glomerular basement membrane 2. Immune complex deposition
What are the signs of glomerular damage?	Increased glomerular filtration rate (GFR), salt and water retention, hypertension, edema, oliguria, proteinuria, and urinary RBCs
In what situation does effacement of podocytes occur?	Loss of glomerular polyanion resulting in heavy proteinuria when visceral epithelial cells show swelling of cell bodies
What is the significance of glomerular polyanion?	It creates a charge-selective barrier, which is essential to glomerular ultrafiltration. Loss of polyanion results in heavy proteinuria.
What antibodies are responsible for Goodpasture disease?	Anti-collagen type IV antibodies (also called anti-glomerular basement membrane antibodies)
Name and describe 4 general classifications of glomerulonephritis.	1. Focal—some glomeruli affected 2. Diffuse—all glomeruli affected 3. Segmental—part of one glomerulus affected 4. Global—entirety of one glomerulus affected
List 3 causes of thickened glomerular capillary loops.	1. Deposition of immune complexes 2. Increase in glomerular basement membrane material (diabetes)

	3. Infiltrate of abnormal material (amyloid)
What is hyalinosis?	Accumulation of homogenous, eosinophilic, amorphous material that probably represents precipitated plasma protein
With what is hyalinosis associated?	Increased mesangial matrix and collagenosis
Name 3 techniques used to evaluate biopsy tissue.	Light microscopy, immunofluorescence, and electron microscopy
What is the major histology of nephritic syndrome?	Inflammation and proliferation
What is a crescent?	Circumferential proliferation of epithelial cells in Bowman capsule
List some patterns of glomerular injury.	1. Cellular proliferation (endothelial, mesangial, epithelial)
	2. Leukocyte infiltration (PMNs, monocytes, lymphocytes)
	3. Thickening of glomerular capillary loops
	4. Basement membrane reaction: epimembranous projections ("spikes"), splitting of basement membrane (double contour)
	5. Hyalinosis
	6. Fibrosis (collagenous scarring)
	7. Epithelial cell change

IMMUNE COMPLEX DEPOSITION

Describe immune complex-associated injury of the glomerulus.	Antigen-antibody aggregates precipitate in the glomerulus. They are either preformed in the circulation or arise in situ with antibodies versus endogenous glomerular antigens.
Name the site of immune complex deposition for each condition.	
Post-infectious glomerulonephritis	Sub-epithelial

IgA nephropathy	Mesangium
SLE	Sub-endothelial
What happens to complement levels in glomerulonephritis?	Complement deposits in glomeruli and systemic levels decrease.
How does immunofluorescence work?	Antibodies tagged with a fluorochrome are used to localize immunoreactants in the glomerulus.
With which technique can you most accurately detect the position of immune complexes (ICs)?	Electron microscopy

MISCELLANEOUS RELATING TO GLOMERULAR DISEASE

Name the disease for each serologic test:

Anti-streptolysin Ab (ASLO)	Post-streptococcal glomerulonephritis (PSGN)
Anti-neutrophil cytoplasmic Ab (ANCA)	Vasculitis
Anti-GBM	Goodpasture disease
Anti-DNA	SLE
Anti-HepB and Anti-HepC	Membranoproliferative glomerulonephritis (MPGN)
Blood cultures	Post-infectious glomerulonephritis
Cryoglobulins	MPGN
Name forms of glomerulonephritis associated with low serum complement levels.	SLE, subacute bacterial endocarditis, "shunt" nephritis, cryoglobulinemia, acute PSGN, and MPGN.
Name forms of glomerulonephritis associated with normal serum complement levels.	PAN, Wegener, Henoch-Schönlein purpura, Goodpasture disease, hypersensitivity vasculitis, IgG-IgA nephropathy, and idiopathic RPGN.

What pattern of glomerulo-nephritis accompanies vasculitic syndromes?	Focal and segmental glomerulonephritis.
What is the best diagnostic test for glomerulonephritis?	Renal biopsy
Who should be considered for biopsy?	All patients with new onset of acute glomerulonephritis without signs or symptoms of PSGN
List the three major staining procedures for adequate diagnosis of biopsy specimen.	1. Routine staining (H&E, Trichrome for collagen, PAS for glycoproteins in GBM and mesangium) 2. Immunofluorescence (for presence of Ig's, complement and fibrin) 3. Electron microscopy (to detect immune deposits)

NEPHROTIC SYNDROME

What is nephrotic syndrome?	Kidney disease characterized by greater than 3.5 g per day of proteinuria
What is the major histologic finding of nephrotic syndrome?	Sclerosis
What allows urinary loss of proteins?	Increased permeability of the basement membrane
Name 4 key features of nephrotic syndrome.	1. Proteinuria 2. Hypoalbuminemia (often < 3 g/100 mL) 3. Generalized edema (from decreased oncotic pressure in plasma) 4. Hyperlipidemia/hypercholesterolemia (increased hepatic lipoprotein synthesis)
What stimulates hepatic lipoprotein synthesis?	Hypoalbuminemia
Describe a common thrombotic complication.	Renal vein thrombosis and pulmonary embolus may occur, secondary to loss of anticoagulant factor antithrombin III in the urine.

Name 5 disorders manifested by nephrotic syndrome.	1. Minimal change disease (lipoid nephrosis) 2. Focal and segmental glomerulosclerosis 3. Membranous glomerulonephritis 4. Diabetic nephropathy 5. Renal amyloidosis

MINIMAL CHANGE DISEASE

In what age group does it most frequently present?	Young children—age 2–3 years of age is peak incidence
What is the etiology of minimal change disease?	Unknown, possible immune etiology. It sometimes follows respiratory tract infection or immunization.
Describe 3 characteristic features of minimal change disease.	1. Normal glomeruli by light microscopy 2. Lipid-laden renal cortices 3. Effacement of epithelial foot processes (seen on EM)
To what does "lipoid" nephrosis refer?	The presence of numerous lipid droplets in tubules and fat bodies in the urine
What therapy is used for lipoid nephrosis?	Steroids; relapses more common in adults.

FOCAL AND SEGMENTAL GLOMERULOSCLEROSIS

In what age group does it most frequently present?	Older patients
What is the etiology?	Unknown
What is the pathology?	Hyalinosis and increased mesangial cellularity and matrix are found, along with interstitial fibrosis and tubular atrophy.
What is the distribution of pathology?	Some, but not all, glomeruli are involved. Only part of each glomerulus is diseased.
What is the treatment?	Most patients do not respond to steroids. 20% have a rapid downhill course with renal failure within 2 years. Others have slowly progressive renal failure.

MEMBRANOUS GLOMERULONEPHRITIS

What population is most affected?	Teenagers and young adults have the highest incidence.
What are the clinical features?	Severe proteinuria with excretion of albumin and globulins
What is the pathology?	Thickened capillary walls. Immune complexes are present in intra-membranous and epimembranous (subepithelial) locations within the basement membrane.
What is the characteristic staining pattern?	Spike and dome appearance (spikes are basement membranes, domes are intra-cellular deposits).
What is the immunofluores-cence pattern?	Granular immunofluorescence (granular deposits of IgG or C3)
Name several associated diseases.	HBV, syphilis, malaria, schistosomiasis, malignancy (colon, lung), and auto-immune diseases
What 2 drugs cause mem-branous glomerulonephritis as a potential side effect?	1. Gold salts 2. Penicillamine
What is the prognosis?	Most patients show slow progression to renal failure over several years (20% have more benign course).

DIABETIC NEPHROPATHY

What are the effects of diabetes mellitus on the kidney?	Diabetic glomerulosclerosis, arterio-sclerosis, and increased susceptibility to pyelonephritis and papillary necrosis
How long before the disease affects the kidneys?	Usually after 10–20 years, accompanied by retinopathy, coronary artery disease, and peripheral vascular disease
What are the predominant symptoms of diabetic nephropathy?	Early symptoms are proteinuria, glucosuria, and declining renal function. Later symptoms are dependent edema and hypertension.

Describe the earliest form of diabetic microangiopathy.	Capillary thickening in basement membrane
What part of the nephron is typically affected by diabetic glomerulosclerosis?	The mesangial matrix is increased.
Name 2 patterns of diabetic glomerulosclerosis.	1. Diffuse glomerulosclerosis 2. Nodular glomerulosclerosis
What are Kimmelstiel-Wilson nodules?	Nodular accumulations of mesangial matrix material seen in diabetic nephropathy

AMYLOIDOSIS

How does amyloidosis present?	Proteinuria and a variable degree of renal failure
What is the macroscopic appearance of kidneys?	Normal or enlarged in size; waxy appearance
What is the microscopic appearance of kidneys?	Amyloid deposits are brightly eosinophilic and homogeneous on H&E stain, in mesangium, and capillary loops.
Where are amyloid deposits predominately found?	Subendothelium and mesangium
How are amyloid deposits identified?	Congo red stain gives birefringence under polarized light.
What is the treatment?	None
What is the prognosis?	Poor

NEPHRITIC SYNDROME

Name 4 clinical findings indicative of a nephrotic syndrome.	1. Hematuria ("smoky brown urine") 2. Hypertension 3. Azotemia (increased BUN and Cr) 4. Oliguria
What causes the leakage of RBCs into urine?	Inflammatory rupture of glomerular capillaries with escape of RBCs into Bowman space

What is the cause of fluid retention in nephritic syndrome?	Decreased renal excretion of salt and H_2O (rather than hypoalbuminemia)
What is the degree of edema in the nephritides?	Minimal, often limited to periorbital edema
Name 4 disorders manifested by nephritic syndrome.	1. Postinfectious glomerulonephritis (PIGN) 2. Rapidly progressive glomerulonephritis (crescentic) (RPGN) 3. Goodpasture syndrome 4. Alport syndrome

POSTINFECTIOUS GLOMERULONEPHRITIS

What is the typical infection associated with PIGN?	Group A β-hemolytic streptococci (nephritogenic strains), which cause tonsillitis, impetigo
Describe the gross pathology of PIGN.	Many punctuate hemorrhages on surface of both kidneys
Describe 3 features of the microscopic pathology.	1. Enlarged, hypercellular, swollen, bloodless glomeruli with proliferation of mesangial and endothelial cells 2. Subepithelial "humps" (immune complex deposition) 3. "Lumpy-bumpy" immunofluorescence (IgG or C3)
What is the immunofluorescence finding in PIGN?	Complement in the basement membrane
What is the prognosis?	Complete recovery in almost all children and many adults
What are the typical lab abnormalities in PIGN?	Azotemia, decreased serum C3, increased ASO titer (antistreptolysin O), urinary RBCs and RBC casts
What is the worst-case scenario?	Progression to rapidly progressive glomerulonephritis

RAPIDLY PROGRESSIVE GLOMERULONEPHRITIS

What predisposes a patient to rapidly progressive glomerulonephritis (RPGN)?	Streptococcal infection, lupus, vasculitis, and cryoglobulinemia

What is the most common clinical presentation?	Severe oliguria or anuria
What is the characteristic pathology of RPGN?	Crescents between Bowman capsule and glomerular tuft (deposition of fibrin in Bowman space)
What are crescents?	Circumferential proliferation of epithelial cells and monocytes in Bowman space. This occurs in response to fibrin leaked from damaged capillary loops.
What is the prognosis of RPGN?	Progression to renal failure in weeks to months
Approximately what percentage is of poststreptococcal etiology?	50%
Approximately what percentage is characterized by anti-GBM antibodies?	10%

GOODPASTURE DISEASE

List the 3 characteristic findings.	1. Alveolar hemorrhage 2. Glomerulonephritis 3. Antibody deposition along alveolar and GBM
What are the common presenting features of Goodpasture disease?	Hemoptysis, anemia, pulmonary infiltrate, and hematuria
What is the immunofluorescence pattern?	Linear (IgG)
What is the pathology of Goodpasture disease?	Initially, focal and segmental proliferation; later crescentic glomerulonephritis
What is the treatment?	Elimination of antibodies by plasma exchange and immunosuppression
What is the sex and age group most commonly affected?	Men in their mid-20s

ALPORT SYNDROME

What is it?	Hereditary nephritis associated with cranial nerve VIII deafness
What is the electron microscopy finding?	GBM splitting

GLOMERULAR DISEASES ASSOCIATED WITH NEPHROSIS AND NEPHRITIS

Name 4 glomerular diseases associated with nephrosis and nephritis.	1. Lupus nephritis 2. Membranoproliferative glomerulonephritis (MPGN) 3. IgA nephropathy (Berger disease) 4. Henoch-Schönlein purpura

LUPUS NEPHROPATHY

What percentage of SLE cases have renal involvement?	50%–80% of cases
What are the common clinical features?	Proteinuria, hematuria, cylindruria
Describe the 5 patterns of lupus nephropathy characterized by the World Health Organization (WHO).	
Type 1	No observable renal involvement
Type 2	Mesangial proliferative form (focal and segmental increase in matrix)
Type 3	Focal proliferative form (endocapillary and epithelial proliferation and necrosis)
Type 4	Diffuse proliferative form (prototype and most severe form)
Type 5	Membranous form (similar to idiopathic membranous glomerulonephritis)
Describe 3 features of Type 4 lupus nephritis.	1. Wire-loop abnormality (results from immune complex deposition and thickening of GBM)

2. Endothelial cell proliferation
3. Subendothelial immune complex deposition

What are the immunofluo-
rescence findings?

Granular deposits of IgG, IgM, IgA, C3, and fibrin. In Type 2 lupus nephritis, they are confined to mesangial space. In Types 3, 4, and 5, deposits are also seen along capillary loops.

What is the prognosis?

Variable. Prognosis corresponds with the chronicity of damage.

MEMBRANOPROLIFERATIVE GLOMERULONEPHRITIS

What is the characteristic
microscopic finding of
MPGN?

Tram-track appearance, which results from reduplication of GBM into 2 layers due to expansion of mesangial matrix into glomerular capillary loops

Describe the histology of
MPGN.

Irregular thickening of GBM and cellular proliferation

What is the most prominent
clinicopathologic change?

Serum hypocomplementemia and glomerular deposition of complement components

Describe the 2 types of
MPGN.

1. Complement activation proceeds via the classic pathway.
2. Activation of complement by alternative pathway. C3 nephritic factor acts as antibody versus C3 convertase and stabilizes the enzyme leading to unopposed complement activation.

What is the clinical
presentation?

Two thirds of cases present with nephrotic syndrome

What is the diagnostic
pathology of MPGN?

Tram-track or double-contour appearance of capillary loops

What are the electron
microscopy findings in
Type I MPGN?

Subendothelial deposits

What are the electron
microscopy findings in
Type II MPGN?

Deposits in lamina densa of GBM

What is the clinical course of MPGN?	50% of patients develop chronic renal failure within 10 years.

BERGER DISEASE

What is Berger disease?	IgA nephropathy (deposition of IgA in mesangium)
What is the usual clinical picture?	Benign recurrent hematuria in kids, usually following an infection
Describe the pathogenesis of Berger disease.	Circulating IgA immune complexes in 50% of patients, leading to defective phagocytic function
What is the pathology of Berger disease?	Mesangial IgA deposition, diffuse mesangial proliferation
What is the clinical course and prognosis?	CRF in up to 50% of the patients over 20 years

HENOCH-SCHÖNLEIN PURPURA

What is Henoch-Schönlein Purpura?	A disease associated with a generalized skin rash, arthropathy, intestinal hemorrhage, hematuria, and proteinuria
What is the renal pathology of HSP?	Mild focal to diffuse mesangial proliferation; crescentic glomerular nephritis; deposition of IgA in immune complexes

URINARY TRACT OBSTRUCTION AND UROLITHIASIS

URINARY TRACT OBSTRUCTION

Name 3 clinical manifestations of urinary tract obstruction.	1. Renal colic (acute distension of ureter, usually due to stones) 2. Hydronephrosis 3. Infection
What is hydronephrosis?	Progressive dilatation of renal pelvis and calyces due to partial block of urinary outflow
Name 3 common causes of obstruction.	1. Prostatic enlargement 2. Calculi 3. Tumors

Where is the site of infection in an obstruction?	Proximal to the site of obstruction

UROLITHIASIS

What is urolithiasis?	Stones (calculi) in the urinary tract
Which sex is more often affected?	Males
Name 4 types of stones.	1. Calcium (oxalate and phosphate) 2. Ammonium magnesium phosphate (struvite) 3. Uric acid 4. Cystine
What is the most common type of stone?	Calcium oxalate (80%–85%), then calcium phosphate
Are calcium stones radiopaque?	Yes
Name 3 causes of hypercalciuria?	1. Increased absorption of Ca^{++} from GI tract 2. Increased renal excretion of calcium 3. Hypercalcemia
What are the causes of hypercalcemia?	These can be listed with the mnemonic C.H.I.M.P.A.N.Z.E.E.S. Calcium ↑: **H**yperparathyroidism, **H**yperthyroidism **I**mmobility/**I**atrogenic (thiazides) **M**alignancy/**M**ets/**M**ilk alkali syndrome **P**aget disease (bone) **A**ddison disease/**A**cromegaly **N**eoplasm (colon, lung, breast, prostate, multiple myeloma) **Z**ollinger-Ellison syndrome **E**xcessive vitamin D **E**xcessive vitamin A **S**arcoid
Are struvite stones radiopaque?	No, they are radiolucent.
What pH of urine facilitates struvite stones?	Alkaline urine caused by ammonia-producing organisms (urease positive)

Name 2 organisms that produce urease.	1. Proteus 2. Staphylococcus
What type of stones cause staghorn calculi?	Struvite (make casts of renal pelvis and calyces)
Name a common cause of uric acid stones.	Hyperuricemia secondary to gout or increased cellular turnover with malignancy (especially leukemias and myeloproliferative syndromes)
What is a major cause of cystine stones?	Impaired tubular reabsorption of cystine (cystinuria)

INFECTIONS OF THE URINARY TRACT AND KIDNEY

What are the typical offending organisms?	Colon flora, usually *E. coli*
Name 3 other infecting agents.	Proteus, pseudomonas, and staphylococcus
Name 2 methods of entry into the urinary system.	1. Hematogenous 2. External entry through urethra (vesicoureteral reflux, ascending infection)
Clinical manifestations of UTI?	Urinary frequency, dysuria, pyuria, hematuria, and bacteriuria
Name 5 predisposing factors for UTIs.	1. Obstruction of flow (prostatism, tumors) 2. Catheter insertion 3. Gynecologic abnormalities 4. Recent surgery 5. Diabetes mellitus

ACUTE PYELONEPHRITIS

List 3 significant findings.	1. Fever 2. Flank tenderness (CVA) 3. White cell casts in urine (pathognomonic)
Describe the macroscopic pathology of acute pyelonephritis.	Kidney may be enlarged; small yellowish microabscesses with hyperemic borders scattered over renal surface, granularity; and hyperemia of pelvic mucosa

What is the common microscopic pathology?

Diffuse suppurative necrosis or abscess formation within the renal parenchyma, tubular destruction; sometimes, renal papillary necrosis in apical portion of pyramids is seen, but usually in association with diabetes, sickle cell, or analgesic abuse.

CHRONIC PYELONEPHRITIS

What are the 2 forms of chronic pyelonephritis?

1. Obstructive: occurs in patients with obstruction secondary to prostatic enlargement or renal calculi.
2. Nonobstructive: probably results from derangement of vesicoureteral sphincter, causing reflux of urine and passage of bacteria from bladder to ureters.

Describe 3 diagnostic findings.

1. Coarse, asymmetric corticomedullary scarring
2. Deformity of renal pelvis and calyces
3. Tubular atrophy

Can the infectious agent in chronic pyelonephritis usually be identified?

No

What is the best diagnostic tool for chronic pyelonephritis?

Pyelograms show asymmetrically contracted kidney with deformity of caliceal system.

What is the macroscopic pathology?

Contracted kidney with irregular granular surface, atrophic parenchyma replaced by fat

Describe the microscopic pathology of chronic pyelonephritis.

Chronic inflammation of kidney and renal pelvis with papillary atrophy and fibrosis of caliceal fornices
dilated tubules, atrophy of epithelial lining, pink material in lumen giving thyroid-like appearance
marked thickening of vessel walls

What is thyroidization?

Atrophic tubules filled with eosinophilic proteinaceous casts causing an appearance similar to thyroid follicles

TUBULAR DISORDERS

What is the most common cause of acute renal failure (ARF)?	Acute tubular necrosis (ATN)
When does ATN most often lead to death?	During the initial oliguric phase
With appropriate therapy, how long does it take to recover renal function?	10–21 days
What is the most common cause of ATN?	Ischemia (toxins are second most common cause)
Name 4 causes of renal ischemia.	1. Hypotension 2. Shock due to Gram-negative sepsis 3. Trauma 4. Hemorrhage
Name several toxins that cause ATN.	Aminoglycosides, cyclosporine, mercury, lead, gold, arsenic, ethylene glycol, pesticides, carbon tetrachloride, and methyl alcohol
What are the clinical signs of ATN?	Within 24 hours of exposure to causative agent, oliguria and proteinuria develop, BUN and Cr are increased, urine serum glucose is decreased, and loss of electrolytes occurs.
What is the macroscopic appearance of the kidneys in ATN?	Enlarged, pale, swollen kidneys
Describe the microscopic appearance of the kidneys in toxic ATN.	Proximal convoluted tubules are affected. Acidophilic inclusions in tubular cells are necrotic and desquamated. Lipid deposition within cells or ballooning of cytoplasm is seen. Basement membrane is intact, distal tubules are spared.
What is the microscopic pathology in ischemic ATN?	Both distal tubules and loops of Henle are affected with necrosis of tubular cells and rupture of basement membrane.
What is the prognosis in ATN?	It depends on the etiologic agent, but most cases are reversible with complete recovery.

What is the cause of ATN associated with crush injuries?

Myoglobinuria

FANCONI SYNDROME

What is it?

Hereditary or acquired generalized dysfunction of the proximal tubules

Which substances show impaired reabsorption in Fanconi syndrome?

Glucose, amino acids, phosphate, and bicarbonate

Describe 3 clinical features.

1. Skeletal disturbances (osteomalacia, osteoporosis)
2. Acidosis
3. Dehydration

What is the pathology in Fanconi syndrome?

Flattened tubular cells, abnormal neckpiece in proximal convoluted tubule

What are the urine and serum findings?

Glycosuria, hyperphosphaturia and hypophosphatemia, aminoaciduria, and systemic acidosis

HARTNUP DISEASE

What is it?

Genetic disorder of impaired tubular reabsorption of tryptophan

What is the clinical manifestation?

Pellagra

VACUOLAR NEPHROSIS

What is it?

Presence of large vacuoles in the cytoplasm filling entire tubular cells

What is the etiology?

Hypokalemia (most common), other electrolyte imbalances, or administration of hypertonic solutions (mannitol)

The clinical signs of vascular nephrosis are most similar to what disease process?

ATN

What portions of the kidney ultrastructure can be affected?

Proximal convoluted tubule, loop of Henle, and collecting tubules

What is the prognosis of vascular nephrosis?	Recovery once osmotic disturbance is corrected.

INTERSTITIAL DISORDERS

ACUTE INTERSTITIAL NEPHRITIS

What are the 3 most common drugs that cause acute interstitial nephritis (AIN)?	1. Penicillins 2. NSAIDS 3. Diuretics
What is the probable cause of AIN?	Immune etiology
Will it resolve if the drug is stopped?	Yes
What occurs if the drug is not stopped?	Progressive renal insufficiency
Describe the pathology of AIN.	Acute interstitial inflammation
What is the characteristic finding in the urine in AIN?	Eosinophils (Hansel stain)

RENAL PAPILLARY NECROSIS (NECROTIZING PAPILLITIS)

What is it?	Ischemic necrosis of the tips of the renal papillae
Name 3 common causes of renal papillary necrosis.	1. Vascular disease related to diabetes mellitus 2. Chronic analgesic nephritis 3. Acute pyelonephritis
With what drugs is it associated?	Phenacetin, aspirin, and analgesics
What is the pathology of chronic analgesic nephritis?	Chronic inflammatory change, atrophy and loss of tubules, and interstitial fibrosis

DIFFUSE CORTICAL NECROSIS

What is it?	Acute generalized ischemic infarction of cortices of both kidneys. The medulla is spared.

With what 3 types of problems is diffuse critical necrosis commonly associated?	1. Septic shock 2. Obstetric catastrophes (abruptio placentae, eclampsia) 3. Other causes of vascular collapse

RENAL FAILURE

What differentiation must be made first?	Is it acute or chronic? (can have acute renal failure in the presence of chronic)
Describe the absolute lab findings in renal failure.	Azotemia (increased BUN and Cr)
What is uremia?	A biochemical and clinical syndrome characteristic of symptomatic renal disease

List the clinical characteristics of uremia associated with the following etiologies.

Decreased erythropoietin secretion	Anemia
Overproduction of renin	Hypertension
Inability to synthesize Vitamin D_3	Hypocalcemia
Accumulation of sulfates, phosphates, and organic acids	Acidosis
Elevation of BUN/Cr	Azotemia
Concentrating and diluting dysfunction	Abnormal control of fluid volume

PRERENAL AZOTEMIA

What is the etiology?	Decreased renal blood flow
What are predisposing conditions for prerenal azotemia?	Decreased cardiac output, Gram-negative sepsis, hemorrhage, and massive burns leading to hypovolemia
What occurs in the tubules?	Increased reabsorption of sodium and water

Describe the urine findings in prerenal azotemia.

Oliguria, concentrated urine, and decreased urinary sodium excretion

What is the BUN:Cr ratio?

Greater than 20:1 (increased reabsorption of urea with decreased GFR)

POSTRENAL AZOTEMIA

What are the causes?

Obstruction of urinary flow from stones, prostate enlargement, or bladder cancer

RENAL VASCULAR DISEASE

Name 3 types of renal vascular disease.

Aneurysm, vasculitis, and hypertension

What is renovascular hypertension?

Hypertension secondary to renal artery stenosis and its hemodynamic effects

What percentage of hypertensive cases can be attributed to renovascular hypertension?

2%–5%

Describe 2 types of renovascular narrowing.

1. Atherosclerotic narrowing of renal artery (more common in older adults)
2. Fibromuscular dysplasia of the renal artery (most common in younger women)

Define benign nephrosclerosis.

Deposition of amorphous hyaline material within the arteriolar wall, disrupting and replacing the elastic membrane and causing narrowing of the lumen. Atrophy and scarring of tubules and glomerulus results.

What is the prognosis of benign nephrosclerosis?

It may lead to renal insufficiency and cardiovascular complications.

What is malignant hypertension?

Acute and severe hypertension with an accelerated progression to serious end-organ effects; may be life-threatening

What term is used to describe renal effects of malignant hypertension?

Malignant nephrosclerosis

Describe the pathology of malignant nephrosclerosis.

1. Necrotizing arteriolitis occurs where the arteriolar medium becomes necrotic and is replaced by fibrin.
2. Hyperplastic arteriosclerosis occurs, involving the reduction of vessel diameter by intimal hyperplasia.
3. The vessel may be completely obliterated, leading to thrombosis and infarction of the parenchyma supplied by that blood vessel.

What is the prognosis of malignant nephrosclerosis?

Progression leads to renal insufficiency and death.

BENIGN TUMORS OF THE KIDNEY

Name 3 types of benign kidney tumors.

Adenoma, angiomyolipoma, and mesoblastic nephroma (benign nephroblastoma)

Which of these is a precursor lesion to renal carcinoma?

Adenoma. 10% are of adenomas considered small renal cell carcinomas of low malignant potential.

From what structures are adenomas derived?

Renal tubules

ANGIOLIPOMAS

What are the components of an angiolipoma?

Fat, blood vessels, and smooth muscle tissue

What is the pathologic appearance?

Yellow-to-gray color (depending on fat content). The cortex and medulla are equally involved.

At what age does angiolipomas usually present?

At 30–50 years of age

In which sex do angiolipomas have higher frequency?

Women are diagnosed twice as often as men.

What are the common symptoms?

Flank pain, hematuria, and hypertension

What is the treatment?

Complete resection of lesion (even if total nephrectomy required)

What syndrome is commonly associated?	Tuberous sclerosis syndrome

MESOBLASTIC NEPHROMA

What is it?	A congenital hamartoma, usually unilateral
Mesoblastic nephroma is often confused with what childhood tumor?	Wilms tumor
When is it usually diagnosed?	At < 6 months of age
Describe the pathology of a mesoblastic nephroma.	Firm, whitish surface resembling smooth muscle. The tumor lacks clear encapsulation. Interlacing bundles of mature connective tissue entrap glomeruli.
What is the treatment?	Complete resection with adequate margins

MALIGNANT TUMORS OF THE KIDNEY

What is the most common renal malignancy?	Renal cell carcinoma (hypernephroma)

RENAL CELL CARCINOMA

In what population is renal cell carcinoma most commonly found?	Men of 50–70 years of age (men:women = 2:1)
Is there a higher incidence in smokers?	Yes
What chromosome is involved in renal cell carcinoma?	Chromosome 3 (partial deletion of the short arm is frequently found)
What are the characteristic histologic cells?	Polygonal clear cells
Describe the clinical manifestations of renal cell carcinoma.	Hematuria, palpable mass, flank pain, fever, and secondary polycythemia with erythrocytosis (5%)

What is the most frequent presentation?	Hematuria
Are malignant cells detectable in the urine of a patient with renal cell carcinoma?	Rarely
In what microstructures does renal cell carcinoma develop?	Proximal or distal renal tubules
In what macroscopic portion of the kidney does renal cell carcinoma develop?	The upper pole
What is the macroscopic pathology?	The tumor protrudes from the cortex as an irregular mass with a yellow-orange appearance. Hemorrhage and necrosis are often seen.
What is the microscopic pathology of renal cell carcinoma?	Clear cells with distinct cytoplasmic membranes, abundant cytoplasm, and eccentric nuclei
What is the method of spread?	Hematogenous dissemination by invading renal veins or vena cava
Name the common metastatic sites of renal cell carcinoma.	Lungs, brain, bones, liver, adrenal glands, lymph nodes, and contralateral kidney
What is the prognosis for renal cell carcinoma?	Poor: 20% 10-year survival rate. Often it has already metastasized at the time of diagnosis.
What is the treatment?	Surgical resection with removal of adjacent lymph nodes. Radiation and chemotherapy have not been very successful.

WILMS TUMOR

What is the most common renal malignancy in children?	Wilms tumor (nephroblastoma)

What is the peak incidence?	2–4 years of age
What is the most common presentation of Wilms tumor?	Palpable flank mass causing abdominal distension (90%)
Other findings?	Hypertension, nausea, vomiting, hematuria, and leg edema
Describe the macroscopic pathology of Wilms tumor.	Large, well-delineated and well-encapsulated tumor. Grayish-white to tan in color with areas of hemorrhage and occasional cystic changes. Sharp junction between tumor and kidney.
What is the histology?	Varied—immature stroma, primitive tubules and glomeruli, and mesenchymal elements are present
What are common sites of metastatic spread of Wilms tumor?	Renal hilar and paraaortic lymph nodes, lungs, liver adrenal gland, diaphragm, retroperitoneum, and bones
What is the prognosis?	If < 2 years of age, the 5-year survival rate is good. Good prognosis with marked tubular and glomerular differentiation. Poor prognosis associated with capsular permeation, venous extension, distant metastases, nuclear pleomorphism, and abnormal mitotic features.
What is the treatment for Wilms tumor?	Surgical resection and systemic chemotherapy, supplemented by radiation to the affected area
Wilms tumor is associated with deletions of short arm of what chromosome?	Chromosome 11
What is WAGR complex?	**W**ilms tumor, **A**niridia, **G**enitourinary malformations, and mental-motor **R**etardation

CARCINOMA OF THE URINARY TRACT

Name 4 congenital anomalies of the urinary tract.	1. Bladder diverticula 2. Persistent urachus 3. Exstrophy of the bladder 4. Double ureters

What are bladder diverticula?

Pouchlike eversions of the bladder wall. They may be congenital due to failure of development of normal musculature, or acquired due to obstruction in the urethra or bladder neck.

In what sex are diverticula most commonly found?

Men

What is a persistent urachus?

A patent connection between the apex of the bladder and the umbilicus

What is exstrophy of the bladder?

Absence of the anterior musculature of the bladder

With what other developmental defects is exstrophy associated?

Anterior abdominal wall defects

TRANSITIONAL CELL CARCINOMA

What is the most common tumor of the urinary collecting system?

Transitional cell carcinoma (occurs in renal calyces, pelvic, ureter, or bladder)

What is the most common location?

Region of the trigone in the bladder

What is the most common presentation?

Painless hematuria

What is the usual method of spread of transitional cell carcinoma?

Local extension to surrounding tissues

What toxic exposures are associated with transitional cell carcinoma?

β-naphthylamine (aniline dyes), phenacetin, cigarettes, and cyclophosphamide

How is prognosis determined?

Tumors are assigned a histologic grade. Higher grade = worse prognosis.
Grade I. Rare pleomorphism and mitoses, no necrosis
Grade II. More crowding of cells, enlargement and hyperchromatism of nuclei
Grade III. Sessile, cauliflower-like appearance with necrosis and ulceration; abundant atypia and mitoses

| What is the treatment of transitional cell carcinoma? | Resection of the lesion (local or total cystectomy), followed by radiation |

SQUAMOUS CELL CARCINOMA

How common is squamous cell carcinoma (SCC) of the urinary tract?	Rare—5% of all bladder tumors
What are the causes?	Chronic inflammatory processes such as chronic bacterial infection, schistosomiasis, and renal calculi
What is the prognosis of SCC of the urinary tract?	Poor.

POWER REVIEW

Name 3 possible renal causes of a large flank mass.	1. Wilms tumor (kids) 2. Renal cell carcinoma 3. Adult PKD
Proteus infection is most likely to lead to what type of stone formation?	Struvite stones
Most common cause of nephrotic syndrome in young adults?	Membranous glomerulonephritis
What is the immunofluorescence pattern of membranous glomerular nephritis?	Granular
Glomerular crescents are the hallmark of what disease?	Rapidly progressive glomerulonephritis
In what disease would this IF pattern be seen?	Goodpasture syndrome (linear IF against anti-GBM antibodies)
Intracranial bleeding is associated with what kidney disease?	Polycystic kidney disease (associated with berry aneurysms)
What is the characteristic triad of renal cell carcinoma?	Hematuria, pain, and a flank mass

What is the most common cause of nephrotic syndrome in children?	Minimal change disease (lipoid nephrosis or nil disease)
List 2 clinical manifestations of Goodpasture syndrome.	Glomerulonephritis and pneumonitis with hemoptysis
Immune complex diseases exhibit what type of immunofluorescence pattern?	Granular IF (granular deposits of IgG or C3)
Urinalysis findings for acute glomerular nephritis?	Hematuria, RBC casts, and mild proteinuria ($<$ 2 g/day)
High urinary sodium in an oliguric patient indicates what condition?	Acute tubular necrosis
What is the most common ectopic site for the kidney?	Pelvis
What is Potter syndrome?	Bilateral (complete) renal agenesis
Name the 3 most common renal cystic diseases.	1. Adult polycystic kidney disease 2. Autosomal recessive polycystic kidney disease 3. Medullary cystic disease
List 3 causes of thickened glomerular capillary loops.	1. Deposition of immune complexes 2. Increase in GBM material (diabetes) 3. Infiltrate of abnormal material (amyloid)
Name 3 techniques used to evaluate biopsy tissue.	1. Light microscopy 2. Immunofluorescence 3. Electron microscopy
What are the diabetic effects on the kidney?	Diabetic glomerulosclerosis, arteriosclerosis, and increased susceptibility to pyelonephritis and papillary necrosis
What is Alport syndrome?	Hereditary nephritis associated with deafness
What are the clinical characteristics associated with Henoch-Schönlein purpura?	Generalized skin rash, arthropathy, intestinal hemorrhage, hematuria, and proteinuria

How does urinary obstruction present?	1. Renal colic (acute distension of ureter, usually due to stones) 2. Hydronephrosis 3. Infection
Name the 3 most common causes of urinary obstruction.	Prostatic enlargement, calculi, and tumors
Name 4 infecting agents of the urinary tract.	1. *E. coli* 2. Proteus 3. Pseudomonas 4. Staphylococcus
What is the most common cause of acute renal failure (ARF)?	Acute tubular necrosis
Name 4 causes of renal ischemia.	1. Hypotension 2. Shock due to Gram-negative sepsis 3. Trauma 4. Hemorrhage
What are the 3 most common classes of drugs that cause acute interstitial nephritis (AIN)?	1. Penicillins 2. NSAIDs 3. Diuretics
Name 4 types of renal stones.	1. Calcium (oxalate and phosphate) 2. Ammonium magnesium phosphate (struvite) 3. Uric acid 4. Cystine
Which is a precursor lesion to renal carcinoma?	Adenoma
What is the most common renal malignancy?	Renal cell carcinoma (hypernephroma)
What is the most common renal malignancy in kids?	Wilms tumor (nephroblastoma)
What is the most common tumor of the urinary collecting system?	Transitional cell carcinoma

24

Gastrointestinal Tract

MOUTH AND JAW

What causes fever blisters (cold sores)?

Herpes simplex virus type 1 (HSV-1)

When do fever blisters recur?

With febrile illness (hence the name) and with sunlight exposure, after trauma, and during menstruation

What organism causes thrush?

Candida albicans

Name 3 kinds of patients who develop thrush.

1. Children
2. Diabetic individuals
3. Immunocompromised individuals

Name 3 risk factors for oral cancer.

1. Smoking
2. Chewing tobacco
3. Alcohol consumption

What is the most common cell type of oral cancer?

Squamous cell carcinoma

Is the tongue usually involved in squamous cell carcinoma?

Yes (> 50% of cases)

What disease is often associated with acute parotitis (inflammation of the parotid gland)?

Mumps

What are the 3 characteristics of Sjögren syndrome?

1. Keratoconjunctivitis sicca (dry eyes)
2. Xerostomia (dry mouth)
3. Connective tissue disease [often rheumatoid arthritis (RA)]

What causes Sjögren syndrome?	Probably immune dysfunction
With what serious disease is Sjögren syndrome associated?	Malignant lymphoma

ESOPHAGUS

TRACHEOESOPHAGEAL FISTULAS

What is a tracheoesophageal fistula (TE)?	A congenital fistula joining the trachea and the esophagus
How does a TE fistula manifest?	With choking, regurgitation, coughing, and excessive salivation when attempting to eat. Patients may present in respiratory distress.
What is the most common type of TE malformation?	A blind upper esophagus and a fistula between the trachea and the lower esophagus (90% of patients)
What prenatal maternal condition is often associated with TE fistulas?	Maternal polyhydramnios (increased amniotic fluid) [85% of cases]
What is the treatment for a TE fistula?	Surgical correction

DIVERTICULA

Name the 2 types of esophageal diverticula.	1. True (or traction) diverticula, which consist of mucosal, muscular, and serosal layers 2. False (or pulsion) diverticula, which result from herniation of mucosa through defects in the muscular layer
Which of the 2 types of esophageal diverticula is more common?	False (pulsion) diverticula
Where do esophageal diverticula commonly occur?	Behind the cricoid cartilage in the area of the upper esophageal sphincter (Zenker diverticulum)
Zenker diverticulum is associated with what disease?	Squamous cell carcinoma of the esophagus

How might a hiatal hernia be described morphologically?	An upward sliding of the stomach through the esophageal hiatus
Describe the 2 types of hiatal hernias.	1. Sliding type: the gastroesophageal junction and a bell-shaped portion of the stomach lie above the diaphragm. The sliding type represents approximately 90% of hiatal hernias and is present in 10% of the general population and 50% of those individuals with gastroesophageal reflux disease. 2. Rolling type: a part of the gastric fundus "rolls" along the distal esophagus and through the diaphragm but the junction remains at its normal location. This type represents only about 10% of hiatal hernias.

ACHALASIA

What is achalasia?	A disorder in which the lower esophageal sphincter (LES): (1) does not completely relax, leading to increased basal tone (2) lacks propulsive peristaltic ability, resulting in a functional obstruction and leading to progressive dilation of the esophagus.
How does achalasia manifest?	Dysphagia
The pathogenesis of aphasia involves loss of what type of cells?	Myenteric ganglion cells, which are usually absent or markedly decreased in the dilated portion of the esophagus

ESOPHAGEAL VARICES

What are esophageal varices?	Dilation of the submucosal esophageal veins
What causes esophageal varices?	Portal hypertension
What major risk is associated with esophageal varices?	Bleeding

ESOPHAGEAL LACERATIONS AND RUPTURE

What is Mallory-Weiss syndrome?

Partial-thickness lacerations of the distal esophagus

What causes Mallory-Weiss syndrome?

Increased intra-abdominal pressure and failure of the LES to relax, which is usually due to retching

What individuals are predisposed to Mallory-Weiss syndrome?

Alcoholics

What is Boerhaave syndrome?

Complete rupture of the esophagus

What is a major complication of Boerhaave syndrome?

Mediastinitis

Overall, what is the most common cause of esophageal rupture?

Iatrogenic event (instrumentation)

GASTROESOPHAGEAL REFLUX DISEASE

What is the chief presenting feature of gastroesophageal reflux disease?

Heartburn

Name 6 possible causes of gastroesophageal reflux disease.

1. Hiatal hernia
2. Incompetent LES
3. Pregnancy
4. Scleroderma
5. Diabetes mellitus
6. Alcohol abuse

Name 4 complications of gastroesophageal reflux disease.

1. Esophagitis
2. Stricture
3. Ulceration
4. Barrett esophagus

NEOPLASMS OF THE ESOPHAGUS

What is Barrett esophagus?

Metaplasia of esophageal squamous epithelium to columnar cells

Why is Barrett esophagus a serious condition?

Some individuals with Barrett esophagus (3%–10%) either present with esophageal adenocarcinoma or develop this condition.

What is the most common benign neoplasm of the esophagus?

Leiomyoma

What are 4 presenting symptoms of esophageal carcinoma?

1. Anorexia
2. Dysphagia
3. Weight loss
4. Pain

What is the most common cell type in esophageal carcinoma?

Squamous cell carcinoma (70%–80%). Adenocarcinoma, which is associated with Barrett esophagus, is much less common (20%–30%).

Is esophageal squamous cell carcinoma more common in men or women?

Men, by a 4:1 ratio

What are the 2 major risk factors associated with esophageal carcinoma?

Smoking and alcohol abuse

What is the overall 5-year survival rate for esophageal carcinoma?

10%

What is the most important prognostic indicator in esophageal carcinoma?

Depth of tumor invasion. If the carcinoma is confined to the submucosa and has not spread to the lymph nodes, survival may approach 90%.

STRICTURES, RINGS, AND WEBS

What are 3 causes of esophageal strictures?

1. Reflux esophagitis (most common cause)
2. Ingestion of corrosive agents
3. Idiopathic conditions

What is Plummer-Vinson syndrome?

Upper esophageal rings and webs in association with iron deficiency anemia, atrophic glossitis, and dysphagia

Which individuals are most affected by Plummer-Vinson syndrome?

Middle-aged women. The condition rarely occurs in other individuals.

Where are Schatzki rings located?	At or close to the gastroesophageal junction
In what ways do Schatzki rings differ from Plummer-Vinson syndrome?	They show no association with female predominance or iron deficiency anemia.

INFECTIONS OF THE ESOPHAGUS

What 4 conditions may result in *Candida* esophagitis?	1. Antibiotic or immunosuppressive therapy 2. Diabetes mellitus 3. Malignancy 4. Human immunodeficiency virus (HIV) infection
What are the presenting features of *Candida* esophagitis?	Painful, white mucosal patches and difficulty swallowing
What causes herpes esophagitis?	HSV-1
Which individuals tend to develop herpes esophagitis?	Usually those who are immunosuppressed
What are the presenting features of herpes esophagitis?	Pain and difficulty swallowing without visible plaques

STOMACH

HISTOLOGY

Where are chief cells and parietal cells located?	In the body of the stomach
What substance do the chief cells produce?	Pepsinogen
What 2 important chemicals do parietal cells produce?	1. Hydrochloric acid 2. Intrinsic factor
Where is gastrin secreted?	In the antrum of the stomach (distal third), where it is made by G cells

PYLORIC STENOSIS

What is pyloric stenosis?	A narrowing of the pyloris (outflow tract) of the stomach, which is caused by hypertrophy of the circular muscular layer of the pylorus
How often does pyloric stenosis occur?	In about 1/200 live births (0.5%)
What individuals develop pyloric stenosis?	Boys. Pyloric stenosis, which often affects first-born males with a family history of the condition, is 3 times more common in boys than in girls.
What is the classic presentation of pyloric stenosis?	A male infant with projectile vomiting during the first 6 weeks of life

GASTRITIS

What features characterize acute gastritis (also known as erosive gastritis)?	Inflammation of the stomach lining with edema, erythema, erosions, ulcers, leukocyte infiltration, and occasionally hemorrhage and necrosis
Name 3 causes of acute gastritis.	1. Nonsteroidal anti-inflammatory drugs (NSAIDs) 2. Cigarette smoking 3. Alcohol
What are the 2 types of chronic gastritis?	Type A and type B
Distinguish types A and B on the basis of site of occurrence.	Type A involves the body of the stomach and characteristically spares the antrum, whereas type B begins in the antrum and spreads to the body of the stomach.
What causes type A gastritis?	Autoimmune changes involving circulating antibodies to intrinsic factor and parietal cells
Type A gastritis is associated with what 3 diseases?	1. Hashimoto thyroiditis 2. Addison disease 3. Pernicious anemia (due to loss of intrinsic factor)
What causes type B chronic gastritis?	*Helicobacter pylori* infection

ULCERS

What is a Curling ulcer?

An acute gastric ulcer caused by the severe physiologic stress of extensive burns (thick Curling iron burn)

What is a Cushing ulcer?

An acute gastric ulcer resulting from the severe physiologic stress of central nervous system (CNS) trauma

What causes the 2 types of stress ulcers—Curling ulcer and Cushing ulcer?

Hypoxia of the stomach mucosa

How does peptic ulcer disease (PUD) differ from acute gastritis?

PUD implies a more chronic course than the ulcers associated with acute gastritis.

Is PUD more common in men or women?

Men. Although any individual can develop PUD, the disease classically presents in middle-aged men.

Where do PUDs most commonly occur?

The vast majority of PUDs (98%) occur in the stomach or the proximal duodenum, but they can develop anywhere in the gastrointestinal (GI) tract. Duodenal ulcers are slightly more common than gastric ulcers. The most common site of occurrence of gastric ulcers is the lesser curvature of the antrum.

Are gastric ulcers caused by increased secretion of gastric acid?

No. Although acid and pepsin must be present for ulcers to form, levels are typically low in individuals with gastric PUD. However, typically high amounts are found in those with duodenal ulcers.

What is involved in the pathogenesis of gastric ulcers?

The picture is unclear. Many factors appear to lower gastric mucosal resistance and predispose to ulcers (NSAIDs, *Helicobacter pylori,* bile, alcohol, cigarettes).

What blood group puts individuals at increased risk for duodenal ulcers?

Blood group O

Describe how gastric ulcers appear macroscopically.

As punched-out holes 2–4 cm in diameter that penetrate into the muscularis propria, with clean, smooth bases

Describe how gastric ulcers appear microscopically.

Active lesions have 4 layers: surface fibrin, an inflammatory layer characterized by neutrophilic infiltration, a zone of granulation tissue, and a fibrous scar with blood vessels.

What are the 3 dangers associated with untreated ulcers?

1. **H**emorrhage—most common (25%–33% of cases)
2. **O**bstruction—may result from scarring
3. **P**erforation—may result in peritonitis or erosion of adjacent structures (e.g., pancreas)

"HOP"

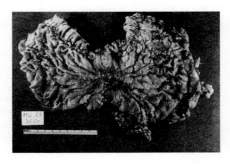

What is the treatment for PUD?

1. Medical: drugs to decrease gastric acidity as well as antibiotics and bismuth to eradicate *Helicobacter pylori*
2. Surgical: vagotomy to decrease gastric acid secretion or remove the ulcerative area

NEOPLASMS OF THE STOMACH

Benign tumors

What are the most common benign gastric epithelial tumors?

Hyperplastic polyps (80%–90% of cases)

Describe how hyperplastic ulcers appear macroscopically.

As single or multiple ulcers < 1 cm in diameter

Describe how hyperplastic ulcers appear microscopically.

As a proliferation of elongated and dilated glands lined with mucus-type cells

What accounts for almost all benign gastric epithelial tumors that are *not* hyperplastic ulcers?

Adenomas

Describe how adenomas appear macroscopically.

Usually as solitary, sessile structures that are > 2 cm in diameter. However, they may be smaller and/or pedunculated.

Describe how adenomas appear microscopically.

As villous, tubular, or tubulovillous proliferations of dysplastic epithelial cells

Malignant tumors

What individuals develop stomach cancer?

Any person may acquire the disease, but typical patients are men > 50 years of age. Incidence is high in Japan, Finland, and Iceland. Stomach cancer is more common in people with blood group A.

Do dietary factors lead to an increased incidence of stomach cancer?

Yes. High amounts of nitrosamines (used as preservatives in smoked fish, meat, and pickled vegetables) are associated with increased risk. Excessive salt intake and reduced amounts of fruits and vegetables are also risk factors.

Infection with what organism is associated with an increased risk of stomach cancer?

Helicobacter pylori

In addition to *Helicobacter pylori* infection, what are 2 predisposing factors for stomach cancer?

1. Achlorhydria
2. Chronic atrophic gastritis with or without pernicious anemia

What is the most common malignancy of the stomach?

Adenocarcinoma (> 95% of cases)

Where in the stomach is adenocarcinoma most common?

Antrum or prepyloric area (usually not the fundus)

What are the symptoms of adenocarcinoma of the stomach?

None may be present. However, if symptoms do occur, they are usually similar to those of PUD (e.g., pain, anorexia, melena, anemia, weight loss).

How is adenocarcinoma of the stomach diagnosed?

By taking a biopsy of all ulcers observed endoscopically

Name the 3 morphologic variants of adenocarcinoma of the stomach.

1. Polypoid (fungating)
2. Ulcerated
3. Infiltrating (diffuse)

What is linitis plastica?

A variant of stomach cancer in which there is no luminal mass but almost the entire gastric wall is thickened with tumor. (Linitis plastica = leather bottle.)

What is a Virchow node?

A supraclavicular node that may be involved in metastatic stomach cancer

What is a Krukenberg tumor?

Bilateral involvement of the ovaries that may occur in metastatic stomach cancer

Name 3 malignant tumors that can be found in the stomach.

1. Lymphoma
2. Leiomyosarcoma
3. Carcinoid

How is mucosa-associated lymphoid tumor (MALT) related to gastric lymphomas?

Most primary gastric lymphomas are a type of MALToma.

MISCELLANEOUS

What is Ménétrier disease?

Extreme enlargement of the rugae of the stomach, which is often associated with a protein-losing enteropathy

Describe the appearance of the stomach in patients with Zollinger-Ellison syndrome.

Hyperplasia of the parietal and chief cells due to the increased secretion of gastrin from a gastrinoma

What is a bezoar?

A concentration of accumulated swallowed material in the stomach, which is usually composed of vegetable matter or hair

SMALL INTESTINE

DIVERTICULA

What is the most common congenital anomaly of the small intestine?

Meckel diverticulum, which affects 2% of the general population

What is the embryologic origin of Meckel diverticulum?

It is a remnant of the vitelline (omphalomesenteric) duct.

Is Meckel diverticulum a true diverticulum?

Yes, because it contains all layers of the bowel wall

What causes ulceration and bleeding in Meckel diverticulum?

Acid-secreting gastric mucosa, which are present in 50% of cases

Where is Meckel diverticulum located?

In the ileum, within 2 feet of the ileocecal valve

How long is Meckel diverticulum?

Usually about 2 inches

ISCHEMIC BOWEL DISEASE

What pathologic changes are involved in ischemic bowel disease?

Infarction, necrosis, and hemorrhage of the small bowel due to ischemia

What parts of the bowel are most often affected in ischemic bowel disease?

Splenic flexure and the rectosigmoid junction

What causes ischemic bowel disease?

Cardiac failure, usually an atherosclerotic occlusion of at least 2 major mesenteric vessels

Name 3 other causes of ischemic bowel disease besides cardiac failure.

1. Shock
2. Embolism
3. Atherosclerosis

CROHN DISEASE

What is Crohn disease?

A chronic inflammatory disease that may involve any part of the GI tract but most commonly affects the ileocecum, small intestine, or colon

What individuals develop Crohn disease?

Primarily persons in the second or third decade of life. The condition is also more common in people of Jewish descent.

What proportion of individuals with Crohn disease eventually develop cancer of the small intestine or colon?

Crohn disease leads to cancer of the small intestine or colon in 3% of affected persons.

What are 5 clinical manifestations of Crohn disease?

1. Abdominal pain
2. Diarrhea
3. Fever
4. Intestinal obstruction
5. Malabsorption

Is the inflammation in Crohn disease limited to the mucosa and submucosa?

No. Crohn disease is transmural, unlike ulcerative colitis.

Are granulomas present in Crohn disease?

Yes (40% of cases), unlike in ulcerative colitis

What are "skip" lesions?

Characteristic segments of affected bowel separated by areas of normal intestine. They occur in Crohn disease but not in ulcerative colitis.

What is characteristic in a gross specimen of small intestine affected by Crohn disease?

A cobblestone appearance, caused by elevation of the mucosa because of submucosal edema

Is the rectum involved in Crohn disease?

Infrequently, unlike in most all (98%) of cases of ulcerative colitis

Is the anus involved in Crohn disease?

Often. Rarely is it affected in ulcerative colitis.

OBSTRUCTION

What are the 2 most common causes of small bowel obstruction?

1. Adhesions from previous surgery
2. Hernias

What is intussusception?

A telescoping of bowel, usually in the terminal ileum

What causes intussusception?

In children, it is usually a result of enlarged Peyer patches during a viral infection, which act as a leading point. In adults, an intraluminal tumor is usually the cause.

What is volvulus?	Twisting of bowel around its mesenteric base
What is meconium ileus?	Failure of infants to pass their first stool
With what disease is meconium ileus associated?	Cystic fibrosis
What is gallstone ileus?	A condition, usually found in elderly women, in which gallstones erode through the gallbladder wall into the small intestine and cause an impaction in the terminal ileum and obstruction
What do intussusception, volvulus, meconium ileus, and gallstone ileus have in common?	They are all causes of bowel obstruction.

NEOPLASMS OF THE SMALL INTESTINE

What percentage of GI tumors occur in the small bowel?	About 5%
What percentage of GI tumors in the small bowel are malignant?	About 50%
What is the most common benign tumor of the small intestine?	Adenoma
Where do adenomas most commonly occur?	Near the ampulla of Vater
What are the 3 most common malignant tumors of the small bowel?	1. Adenocarcinoma 2. Lymphoma 3. Carcinoid
What is another name for carcinoid tumors?	APUDomas (amine precursor uptake and decarboxylase)
From what cells are carcinoid tumors derived?	Gut neuroendocrine cells
Where are carcinoid tumors most often found?	Appendix Small bowel (usually ileum)

Rectosigmoid region
Remainder of the colon

What are 4 characteristics of carcinoid syndrome?

1. Flushing
2. Diarrhea
3. Bronchospasm
4. Pulmonic valvular lesions

What causes carcinoid syndrome?

Production by the tumor of vasoactive amines such as serotonin, bradykinin, and histamine

What is the most common extranodal site of lymphoma?

GI tract (usually stomach or small bowel)

Are lymphomas of the GI tract usually low-grade or high-grade?

High-grade—large cell, immunoblastic, Burkitt, or lymphoblastic types

MALABSORPTION SYNDROMES

What is involved in the development of a malabsorption syndrome?

Impairment of the transport of food and nutrients from the lumen of the intestine to the portal and lymphatic circulations

What results from a malabsorption syndrome?

Abnormal fecal excretion of protein, carbohydrates, or fat

What are the 3 aspects of a malabsorption syndrome?

1. Decreased absorptive capacity
2. Maldigestion
3. Transport abnormalities

What causes celiac disease (nontropical sprue)?

Gluten sensitivity

How is the diagnosis of celiac disease made?

Small intestinal biopsy, which shows blunting of the villi

What is the treatment for celiac disease?

A gluten-free diet

What is tropical sprue?

A malabsorptive disease that is probably of infectious origin. Histologic findings are similar to those in nontropical sprue, but villous atrophy is less uniform.

What is Whipple disease?

A multisystem disease that may affect any

	organ but characteristically presents with malabsorption.
What causes Whipple disease?	A bacterial infection, probably with the bacillus *Tropheryma whippelii*. The patient's macrophages may have a lysosomal defect that prevents killing of the ingested bacteria.
What structures does light microscopy of an intestinal biopsy of a patient with Whipple disease reveal?	Foamy histiocytes that are periodic acid–Schiff–positive
What structures does electron microscopy of an intestinal biopsy of a patient with Whipple disease characteristically reveal?	Bacteria-like inclusions
What is a disaccharidase deficiency?	A condition in which a disaccharide cannot be digested due to the lack of one or more enzymes
What is the most common disaccharidase deficiency?	Lactase deficiency
Where are the disaccharidases normally located?	At the mucosal brush border
What histologic findings are characteristic in disaccharidase deficiency?	Biopsies are histologically unremarkable.

LARGE INTESTINE

HIRSCHPRUNG DISEASE

What is Hirschprung disease?	A dilation of the colon due to a congenital failure of development of the ganglion cells of the myenteric and submucosal plexuses
Where does the dilation occur in Hirschprung disease?	Proximal to the aganglionic segment

What is the treatment for the functional colonic obstruction that results from Hirschprung disease?	Surgical resection of the aganglionic segment of bowel
With what other congenital anomaly is Hirschprung disease associated?	Trisomy 21 or Down syndrome

NECROTIZING ENTEROCOLITIS

Why is necrotizing enterocolitis well known?	It is the most common GI tract emergency in neonates.
What group of children develops necrotizing enterocolitis?	Infants of low birth weight who are born prematurely
What characteristics of the bowel in necrotizing enterocolitis are evident on gross appearance?	Hemorrhage, necrosis, mucosal edema, and neutrophilic infiltration

DIVERTICULA

What are diverticula?	Pockets of mucosa and submucosa that have herniated through the muscular layer of bowel
Do colonic diverticula represent true diverticula?	No. Colonic diverticula are herniations of mucosa.
Where do diverticula usually occur?	Sigmoid colon (> 90% of the time). Herniations occur between mesenteric and antimesenteric taeniae, because penetration of the blood vessels in this region causes weak spots.
Who develops diverticular disease?	Mostly older people (> 50 years of age) who live in Western countries
What is diverticulosis?	The presence of multiple diverticula but no inflammation
What is diverticulitis?	Acute inflammation of diverticula

VASCULAR ANOMALIES OF THE LARGE INTESTINE

What is angiodysplasia?　　An arteriovenous malformation, which involves areas of vascular dilation in the colon

Where are lesions in angio-dysplasia most commonly found?　　Cecum and ascending colon (> 80% of the time)

Why is angiodysplasia so important?　　These arteriovenous malformations are one of the main causes of GI bleeding in patients > 60 years of age.

In what venous plexus do hemorrhoids occur?　　Anorectal submucosal plexus

Are hemorrhoids common?　　Yes. They occur in 50% of individuals > 50 years of age.

COLITIS

Ulcerative colitis

What is ulcerative colitis?　　An inflammatory disorder of the colon of unknown etiology

What are 3 pathologic find-ings characteristic of ulcerative colitis?
1. Inflammation and ulceration of the mucosa
2. Crypt abscesses
3. Pseudopolyps (remnants of previous ulceration)

What clinical complaints are characteristic of ulcer-ative colitis?　　Bleeding and diarrhea

Name 3 complications of ulcerative colitis.
1. Toxic megacolon
2. Perforation of the colon
3. Carcinoma of the colon

Name 4 extraintestinal manifestations of ulcerative colitis.
1. Arthritis
2. Iritis
3. Sclerosing cholangitis
4. Erythema nodosum and pyoderma gangrenosum (skin disorders)

Pseudomembranous colitis

What is pseudomembranous colitis?

Inflammation of the colon with grayish, superficial mucosal exudates consisting of necrotic, adherent mucosal debris and neutrophils. The lesions resemble mushroom-shaped jellyfish.

What is the most common cause of pseudomembranous colitis?

Overgrowth of *Clostridium difficile*, which usually occurs in patients who have been taking antibiotics

What classic antibiotic is associated with pseudomembranous colitis?

Clindamycin. However, other antibiotics can cause the disease.

What antibiotics are used to treat pseudomembranous colitis?

Metronidazole or vancomycin

NEOPLASMS OF THE LARGE INTESTINE

Polyps

What is a "polyp"?

Any circumscribed protuberance into the bowel lumen or an elevation of the intestinal surface

What is the difference between a sessile polyp and a pedunculated polyp?

Pedunculated polyps have a narrow stem, while sessile polyps have a broad attachment

What are the 3 types of nonmalignant polyps?

1. Hyperplastic
2. Inflammatory
3. Hamartomatous

Are hyperplastic polyps worrisome?

They should not be, because they pose no risk. However, they are often mistaken for adenomatous polyps.

Are hyperplastic polyps common?

Yes (30%–60% of all colorectal polyps). They are present in 75% of individuals > 40 years of age, where they are usually incidental findings.

Describe how hyperplastic polyps appear macroscopically.

Usually as pink or gray, teardrop-shaped, sessile structures

Describe how hyperplastic polyps appear microscopically.

As elongated crypts with an epithelial lining

What are inflammatory polyps?

Polyps consisting of lymphoid hyperplasia, remnants of mucosa, and granulation tissue

What individuals develop inflammatory polyps?

Persons with chronic inflammatory bowel disease

What is Peutz-Jeghers syndrome?

An autosomal dominant disorder characterized by multiple hamartomatous polyps in the GI tract, as well as mucocutaneous melanin pigmentation

Describe how Peutz-Jeghers polyps appear macroscopically.

As pedunculated or sessile, firm, and lobulated polyps

Describe how Peutz-Jeghers polyps appear microscopically.

As an increased number of relatively normal crypts separated by muscularis mucosa

Are the polyps in Peutz-Jeghers syndrome associated with an increased risk of GI carcinomas?

Yes; 10%–20% of patients develop GI carcinoma before 40 years of age.

Peutz-Jeghers syndrome puts individuals at increased risk for what other forms of cancer?

Stomach, ovarian, cervical, and breast carcinoma

Hamartomatous polyps may be of what other kind?

Juvenile (retention) polyps, which may occur singly or multiply or as a polyposis syndrome

Why are juvenile polyps known as retention polyps?

Microscopically, retention polyps appear as cystically dilated mucin-containing glands in which the mucin is "retained."

How is juvenile polyposis inherited?

As an autosomal dominant trait. (The condition may also occur spontaneously.)

Are patients with juvenile polyposis at increased risk for colon cancer?

Yes. Between 15% and 20% of affected individuals develop colon cancer at a mean age of 34 years.

Are adenomatous polyps benign?

No. They are true neoplasms.

Are adenomatous polyps common?

Yes. They account for 40%–70% of all colorectal polyps. Adenomatous polyps are present in 65% of individuals > 65 years old and in about 15% of the adult population.

What presenting features are associated with adenomatous polyps?

The lesions are usually asymptomatic but may cause bleeding (e.g., melena or hematochezia).

Describe the cytologic features of adenomatous polyps.

"Picket-fence" arrangement of cells with elongated hyperchromatic nuclei, which may show prominent nucleoli; an increased nuclear-to-cytoplasmic ratio; and nuclear stratification. About 5% of these polyps harbor adenocarcinoma that invades through the muscularis mucosae.

Name the 3 histologic types of adenomatous polyps.

1. Tubular
2. Villous
3. Tubulovillous

Which is the most common type of adenomatous polyp?

Tubular (about 75% of all polyps)

Describe how tubular polyps appear macroscopically.

As small, smooth, round, < 1 cm in diameter, and pedunculated

Describe how tubular polyps appear microscopically.

As a proliferation of tubules, with < 20% of the lesion having a villous architecture

What is the second most common histologic type of adenomatous polyps?

Tubulovillous (about 15% of polyps)

Describe how tubulovillous polyps appear microscopically.

With villous architecture (20%–50% of polyps)

Which of the 3 types of adenomatous polyps has the greatest malignant potential?

Villous adenomas, which become malignant in < 30% of cases

Describe how villous adenomas appear macroscopically.

Larger than tubular adenomas in size, they are shaggy and cauliflower-like appearance and usually sessile.

Describe how villous adenomas appear microscopically.

Most polyps have > 50% villous architecture.

Colorectal cancer

What is the most common colorectal malignancy?

Adenocarcinoma, which constitutes 95% of all primary colorectal malignancies

The peak incidence of adenocarcinoma occurs at what age?

In the seventh decade. Only 20% of cases occur before 50 years of age.

Which condition is more common—rectal cancer or colon cancer?

Rectal cancer is more common in men, and colon cancer is more common in women.

Name 5 factors that predispose individuals to colorectal cancer?

1. Inherited multiple polyposis syndrome
2. Adenomatous polyps
3. Ulcerative colitis
4. Family history
5. High-fat, low-fiber diet

Why is diet important in the etiology of colorectal cancer?

It is believed that high-fat diets may increase the anaerobic gut flora, leading to higher concentrations of secondary bile acids, which may be carcinogens. Decreased amounts of fiber causes increased gut transit time, thus adding to the time that potential carcinogens are in contact with epithelium.

Where are colorectal cancers usually located?

About 70% occur in the sigmoid, rectum, or rectosigmoid region, and the remainder are distributed throughout the colon.

What is the incidence of synchronous lesions (presence of another distinct carcinoma in the GI tract at the same time)?

About 2%

What is the incidence of metachronous lesions (another distinct cancer occurring at a different time)?

About 5%

What are the presenting features of rectosigmoid lesions?

Obstruction or overt rectal bleeding

Describe rectosigmoid lesions in terms of their gross appearance.

Ulcerated, annular plaques (usually). Sometimes the characteristic "napkin-ring" lesions cause obstruction.

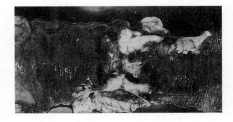

Describe the presenting features of right-sided lesions in colorectal cancer.

Occult GI blood loss, anemia, or iron deficiency

Describe how right-sided lesions appear macroscopically.

Usually as fungating, polypoid masses

What are the 2 chief determinants of prognosis in colorectal cancer?

1. Depth of mural invasion
2. Status of pericolorectal nodes

Characterize the Dukes stages of colorectal cancer.

Stage A—limited to mucosa
Stage B1—limited to muscularis propria; − nodes
Stage B2—beyond muscularis propria; − nodes
Stage C1—limited to muscularis propria; + nodes
Stage C2—beyond muscularis propria; + nodes
Stage D—distant metastases
Note: The number describes depth, and the letter indicates nodal status.

What is the approximate 5-year survival rate for each of the following stages of colorectal cancer?

Stage A	100%
Stage B1	85%
Stage B2	75%
Stage C1	65%
Stage C2	45%
Stage D	5%

How is colorectal cancer treated?

Primarily by surgical resection. Adjunctive radiation and chemotherapy are used in rectal cancer, and patients with stage C colon cancer are given 5-fluorouracil and levamisole.

What is familial adenomatous polyposis?

An autosomal dominant condition characterized by more than 100 to 1000 adenomas throughout the colon

What percentage of patients with familial adenomatous polyposis will develop cancer?

100% (if untreated)

What is the treatment for familial adenomatous polyposis?

Prophylactic resection of the colon

What is Gardner syndrome?

An autosomal dominant condition in which patients have numerous adenomatous polyps, osteomas, and soft tissue tumors

What is Turcot syndrome?

Adenomatous polyps and tumors of the CNS

DISEASES OF THE VERMIFORM APPENDIX

What individuals develop appendicitis?

Young adults most commonly, but the condition can occur in anyone who has an appendix. The lifetime risk is 7%.

What causes appendicitis?

Obstruction of the appendix (two-thirds of cases due to fecaliths), leading to ischemia and bacterial infection

What are the presenting features of appendicitis?

The disease is extremely variable. It is usually marked by periumbilical or right lower quadrant pain, fever, anorexia, nausea and vomiting, and leukocytosis.

Describe the histologic appearance associated with appendicitis.

Acute inflammatory infiltrate extending from the mucosa through the wall of the appendix, with possible mural necrosis, perforation, and abscess formation

What is the most common tumor of the appendix?

Carcinoid

POWER REVIEW

What is the most common cause of esophageal stricture?

Prolonged gastric acid reflux

What often causes projectile, nonbilious vomiting in infants?

Congenital pyloric stenosis

What is a Cushing ulcer?

A stress ulcer associated with a CNS injury

What is a Curling ulcer?

A stress ulcer associated with severe burns

An ulcer on the greater curvature of the stomach is suspicious for what disease?

Gastric cancer

What must be performed on any gastric ulcer visible with an endoscope?

Biopsy

With what disease are nitrosamines associated?

Stomach carcinoma

What is the most common primary site in the GI tract for lymphoma?

Stomach

Which of the following is associated with the following conditions—Crohn disease or ulcerative colitis?

Increased risk of colorectal cancer	Ulcerative colitis
Transmural involvement	Crohn disease
Cobblestone appearance	Crohn disease
Rectal involvement	Ulcerative colitis
"Skip" lesions	Crohn disease
Crypt abscesses	Ulcerative colitis
Granulomas	Crohn disease
What is the "rule of 2s" in Meckel diverticulum?	Present in 2% of population About 2 inches long Within 2 feet of the ileocecal valve 1/2 contain heterotopic gastric or pancreatic tissue or both.
What is the most common small bowel malignancy?	Adenocarcinoma
What is the most common APUDoma?	Carcinoid tumor
What features are characteristic of the carcinoid syndrome?	**B**ronchospasm **F**lushing **D**iarrhea **R**ight-sided heart lesions "B FDR"
What causes carcinoid syndrome?	Vasoactive peptides such as serotonin released from APUDomas
In Hirschsprung disease, where does the dilation occur?	In the colon proximal to the aganglionic segment
In celiac disease, what does a biopsy of the bowel show?	Villous atrophy

Where in the colon are diverticula usually found?

In the sigmoid colon

What is the difference between diverticulosis and diverticulitis?

Diverticulosis is the presence of diverticula.
Diverticulitis is the presence of inflamed diverticula.

What causes pseudomembranous colitis?

Usually *Clostridium difficile* infection following broad-spectrum antibiotic therapy

Are hyperplastic colon polyps premalignant?

No

Are most adenomatous polyps of tubulovillous histology?

No; 75% are tubular.

What adenomatous polyps are most likely to become malignant?

Villous polyps; about 30%–40% of these lesions become malignant.

For what tumor is the appendix famous?

Carcinoid tumors

25

Liver, Biliary Tract, and Exocrine Pancreas

LIVER

NORMAL STRUCTURE AND FUNCTION

What are the functions of the liver?

Synthesis of serum proteins (except immunoglobulins), intermediary metabolism storage, catabolism, detoxification, and excretion

What is unique about the blood supply of the liver?

This organ has a dual blood supply—from the portal vein and the hepatic artery.

Which vessel supplies most of the blood to the liver?

The portal vein (60%–70%)

What constitutes a portal triad?

1. Portal vein
2. Hepatic artery
3. Bile duct

CONGENITAL ANOMALIES OF THE LIVER

What are the 2 types of congenital hepatic cysts?

1. Communicating
2. Noncommunicating

What is another name for communicating cysts?

Caroli disease

Caroli disease is character-ized by dilation of what structures?

Intrahepatic bile ducts, due to obstruction and weak duct walls

With what conditions do patients with Caroli disease present?

Recurrent episodes of cholangitis and occasionally bacteremia in the first few decades of life

Describe how the cysts in Caroli disease appear macroscopically.

The cysts are 1–4 cm in diameter and are often separated by normal segments of duct.

What cancer may complicate Caroli disease?

Cholangiocarcinoma, in about 10% of patients

How do noncommunicating cysts differ from those of Caroli disease?

Noncommunicating cysts do not communicate with the biliary tree

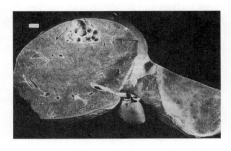

With what conditions do patients with noncommunicating cysts present?

These cysts are often incidental findings; patients may complain of abdominal pain.

ACUTE HEPATITIS

Name 6 general causes of acute hepatic dysfunction.

1. Viruses
2. Chemicals
3. Alcohol consumption
4. Ischemia
5. Congestion
6. Extrahepatic biliary obstruction

With what conditions do patients with acute hepatitis present?

Nausea, vomiting, fever, anorexia, abdominal pain, jaundice, and dark urine

What are typical laboratory findings in acute hepatitis?

Elevated transaminase levels, often increased bilirubin, and/or a slight elevation of alkaline phosphatase

Which transaminase is more elevated in viral hepatitis?

Alanine aminotransferase (ALT)

Which transaminase is higher in alcoholic hepatitis?	Aspartate aminotransferase (AST)
What is fulminant hepatic failure?	Hepatic failure with encephalopathy, a rare but often fatal complication of acute hepatitis
What is hepatorenal syndrome?	Unexplained renal failure associated with liver disease
Can kidneys in hepatorenal syndrome be used as transplants?	Yes. Nothing is wrong with the kidneys in this disorder, which is likely caused in part by ↓ renal blood flow and ↓ glomerular filtration rate (GFR).

Viral hepatitis

What is the most common cause of posttransfusion hepatitis?	Hepatitis C virus (HCV)
What is the most common cause of traveler's hepatitis?	Hepatitis A virus (HAV)
What is the most common viral cause of fulminant hepatitis?	Hepatitis B virus (HBV)
What is the only DNA-containing hepatitis virus?	HBV
How is HAV transmitted?	By the fecal–oral route
How is HBV transmitted?	By parenteral, sexual, or perinatal routes. Body fluid transmission plays a role.
How is HCV transmitted?	By the parenteral route or perhaps the sexual route. Body fluid transmission plays a role.
Which 2 hepatitis viruses are associated with an increased risk of hepatocellular carcinoma?	HBV and HCV
Which hepatitis virus is associated with the greatest risk of progression to chronic hepatitis?	HCV (50%–70%)

What is unique about hepatitis D virus (HDV)?

HDV is a "delta agent" that cannot cause infection by itself but must be associated with HBV. HDV makes HBV infection worse.

Describe the gross appearance of the liver in the setting of acute viral hepatitis.

The liver is swollen and red with a bulging capsule, or it may be green or yellow due to cholestasis. Necrotic foci may be present.

What are the 2 basic histologic features of viral hepatitis?

1. Ballooning degeneration due to hepatocyte swelling
2. Acidophilic degeneration

What is spotty (focal) necrosis?

Necrosis of individual hepatocytes. This is the most common lesion of acute viral hepatitis.

What is confluent necrosis?

Necrosis of adjacent groups of hepatocytes

What is lobular disarray?

A disordered appearance of the lobule due to necrosis, regeneration, and inflammation

Chemical hepatitis

What is predictable hepatotoxicity?

Hepatotoxicity resulting from an agent that is intrinsically hepatotoxic and injurious to most people

What are the 2 groups of agents that cause predictable hepatotoxicity?

1. Direct hepatotoxins
2. Indirect hepatotoxins

What is the difference between direct and indirect hepatotoxins?

Direct hepatotoxins cause damage by direct, nonselective physiochemical effects that destroy the structure of cells.
Indirect hepatotoxins cause harm by interfering with a specific metabolic pathway or structural process.

Name 2 common indirect hepatotoxins.

1. Alcohol
2. Acetaminophen

How is chemical hepatitis treated?

By removal of the offending agent

Table 25–1.
Drug or Toxin-Induced Hepatotoxicity: Types of Hepatic Injury and Selected Causative Agents

Primary Type of Injury	*Example*
Hepatocellular	
Acute hepatitis	Isoniazid, ketoconazole
Focal, spotty	Zone 1: inorganic phosphorus
Zonal°	Zone 3: acetaminophen, carbon tetrachloride, halothane
Chronic hepatitis or cirrhosis	Isoniazid, methyldopa, methotrexate
Steatosis	
Macrovesicular	Ethanol, methotrexate
Microvesicular	Tetracycline, valproate
Steatohepatitis	Ethanol, amiodarone
Cholestasis	Erythromycin, OCS, androgens
Neoplasm	
Hepatocellular adenoma	OCS
Hepatocellular carcinoma	Thorium dioxide (Thorotrast)
Intrahepatic bile ducts	
Chronic cholestasis	Chlorpromazine, amitryptiline
Cholangiocarcinoma	Thorium dioxide (Thorotrast)
Vascular	
Sinusoidal dilatation	OCS, cytotoxic drugs
Veno-occusive disease	Pyrrolizidine alkaloids, cytotoxic drugs
Hepatic or portal vein thrombosis	OCS
Peliosis hepatis	Androgens, estrogens, azathioprine
Angiosarcoma	Thorium dioxide (Thorotrast), polyvinyl chloride, arsenic androgens
Granulomas	Allopurinol, phenytoin, quinidine

OCS = oral contraceptive steroids.
°The same agents that cause zonal acute hepatitis may also cause massive hepatic necrosis.

CHRONIC HEPATITIS

What is the definition of chronic hepatitis?	Hepatic necroinflammation that lasts for at least 6 months
What are the 3 major forms of chronic hepatitis?	1. (Chronic) persistent 2. (Chronic) active 3. (Chronic) autoimmune (lupoid)
What characterizes chronic persistent hepatitis?	Inflammatory infiltrate limited to the portal tract, with an intact limiting plate.

Inflammation, fibrosis, and necrosis are minimal.

What characterizes chronic active hepatitis?

Portal and periportal inflammation and piecemeal necrosis. Cirrhosis is common.

What pathologic processes are involved in piecemeal necrosis?

Degeneration and necrosis of hepatocytes at the limiting plate

Is chronic autoimmune hepatitis more frequent in women or men?

Women

What causes chronic immune hepatitis?

Its etiology is unknown.

What type of white blood cells (WBCs) usually predominate in the infiltrate of autoimmune hepatitis?

Plasma cells

OTHER INFECTIONS OF THE LIVER

What is the most common cause of pyogenic hepatic abscesses?

Biliary obstruction and subsequent ascending cholangitis

What is the most common causative organism in pyogenic hepatic abscesses?

Escherichia coli. However, half of all cases are polybacterial.

Do patients with pyogenic hepatic abscesses have jaundice?

No. Jaundice affects only about one-third of patients.

What conditions are associated with pyogenic hepatic abscesses?

Fever, right upper quadrant pain, malaise, anorexia, night sweats, and rigors

Where in the liver are pyogenic abscesses most common?

Right lobe

What is the treatment for pyogenic hepatic abscesses?

In otherwise healthy individuals, antibiotics alone may suffice. If not, drainage, either open or percutaneous, may be necessary.

What is the most frequent extraintestinal complication of amebiasis?

Amebic hepatic abscess

How are amebic hepatic abscesses diagnosed?

Serologic tests (> 90% sensitive)

If one amebic abscess is present, are there usually more?

Sometimes; multiple abscesses occur in 50% of cases.

What cells are present in pyogenic hepatic abscesses in great numbers but are rare in amebic hepatic abscesses?

Neutrophils

What is the treatment for amebic hepatic abscesses?

Metronidazole

What is the most common cause of hepatic cysts worldwide?

Echinococcosis

What causes echinococcosis?

Cestodes (tapeworms) of the genus *Echinococcus*

What animal is the definitive host of *Echinococcus*?

Dogs. Humans become infected by swallowing eggs in the stool of infected dogs.

How do the worms reach the liver?

Oncospheres (larvae) invade the intestinal mucosa and reach the liver through the portal venous system.

With what conditions do patients with echinococcosis present?

Abdominal pain (usually), as well as occasional generalized allergic reaction and shock

What type of leukocytosis may be seen in echinococcosis?

Peripheral eosinophilia (25% of cases)

ALCOHOLIC LIVER DISEASE

What is the most common form of liver disease in the United States?

Alcoholic liver disease, which affects over 10 million Americans

What types of liver disease may result from chronic alcohol consumption?

Steatosis (fatty liver), alcoholic hepatitis, cirrhosis

How much alcohol does it take to cause liver disease?

Usually about 80 g/day (i.e., 8 beers, 1 L of wine, or 1/2 pint of whiskey) for several years, although the amount varies

What kind of hepatotoxin is alcohol?

Indirect

What are the clinical signs of steatosis?

Usually only hepatomegaly; sometimes abdominal discomfort

What are the clinical signs of alcoholic hepatitis?

Nausea, vomiting, jaundice, hepatomegaly, a high AST-to-ALT ratio, and possible hepatic encephalopathy

Describe the appearance of the liver in steatosis.

Yellow-tan, massively enlarged, and fatty, with granulomas

Describe the appearance of the liver in alcoholic hepatitis.

Ballooning (hydropic) degeneration with scattered acidophilic bodies

What are Mallory bodies (Mallory hyalin)?

Clumps, strands, or rings of eosinophilic hyalin in the cytoplasm of hepatocytes. These structures are found in 50%–75% of individuals with alcoholic hepatitis.

How can affected individuals become free of steatosis?

Stop drinking alcohol. This resolves the condition.

What is the overall mortality rate from alcoholic hepatitis?

15%–30%

What percentage of patients with alcoholic hepatitis who continue to drink will progress to cirrhosis within 2 years?

About 33%

What percentage of patients with alcoholic hepatitis who do *not* continue to drink will eventually progress to cirrhosis?

About 20%

CIRRHOSIS

Name the 3 pathologic characteristics of cirrhosis.

1. Disorganization of hepatic architecture
2. Scarring
3. Nodule formation

How is cirrhosis classified?

Usually morphologically, on the basis of nodule size

Name the 3 types of cirrhosis.

1. Micronodular
2. Macronodular
3. Mixed macromicronodular

What is the most common cause of micronodular cirrhosis?

Alcohol consumption

Name 4 other causes of micronodular cirrhosis.

1. Hemochromatosis
2. Biliary disease
3. Hypervitaminosis A
4. Venous outflow obstruction

How small do the nodules have to be to be called micronodular?

< 3 mm

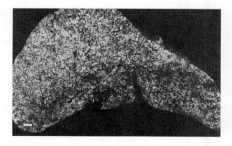

What separates the nodules in micronodular cirrhosis?

Thin, fibrous bands without portal tracts or central veins

What is the most common cause of macronodular cirrhosis?

Viral hepatitis

Name 2 other causes of macronodular cirrhosis.

1. Autoimmune hepatitis
2. Alcohol, especially after the patient has stopped drinking

Name 5 clinical signs of cirrhosis.

1. Ascites
2. Muscle wasting
3. Jaundice
4. Testicular atrophy
5. Esophageal varices

What are some other major clinical features of cirrhosis?

Hypoalbuminemia, clotting abnormalities, impaired drug detoxification, portal hypertension, and increased risk of hepatocellular carcinoma

What kind of cirrhosis is often associated with hypogonadism and gynecomastia?

Micronodular cirrhosis associated with alcohol consumption

What is genetic hemochromatosis?

A familial defect in iron absorption by the intestinal mucosa leading to markedly increased serum iron values

How is hemochromatosis related to the liver?

10%–20% of patients eventually develop hepatocellular carcinoma.

What is the pattern of inheritance of hemochromatosis?

Autosomal recessive. However, progression to symptomatic disease occurs in only about 20% of homozygotes.

Where is the iron deposited in hemochromatosis?

In many organs, most notably the heart, pancreas, and salivary glands

How is hemochromatosis treated?

With phlebotomy

Characterize Wilson disease.

An autosomal recessive disorder characterized by decreased serum ceruloplasmin and abnormal accumulation of copper in cells

The cells of which organs are most affected in Wilson disease?

Parenchymal cells of the liver and kidney, brain, and cornea

What are the characteristic markings on the cornea in Wilson disease called?

Kayser-Fleischer rings

How is Wilson disease treated?

With D-penicillamine, which chelates copper and promotes excretion of copper in the urine

Name 3 inborn errors of metabolism that may cause cirrhosis.	1. α_1-Antitrypsin deficiency 2. Glycogen storage disease 3. Galactose-1-phosphate uridyl transferase deficiency

VASCULAR DISORDERS OF THE LIVER

Define portal hypertension.	Elevation of portal vein pressure of more than 5–10 mm Hg
What results from portal hypertension?	Development of venous collaterals with varices in the veins of the esophagus, the hemorrhoidal plexus, and other sites
What is the most important complication of portal hypertension?	Bleeding from esophageal varices
What is the mortality rate for patients with bleeding esophageal varices?	50%
Name 2 other complications of portal hypertension.	1. Ascites 2. Congestive splenomegaly
On what basis are the various types of portal hypertension classified?	By where the obstruction occurs
What causes prehepatic portal hypertension?	Portal and splenic vein obstruction, which is usually due to thrombosis
Name 2 causes of intrahepatic portal hypertension.	1. Cirrhosis 2. Metastatic tumor
What causes posthepatic portal hypertension?	Congestion in the distal hepatic venous circulation due to congestive heart failure, constrictive pericarditis, tricuspid insufficiency, or Budd-Chiari syndrome
Briefly define ascites.	Abnormal accumulation of peritoneal fluid
What dangerous condition is associated with ascites?	Spontaneous bacterial peritonitis
What organism usually causes spontaneous bacterial peritonitis?	*Escherichia coli*

What are the signs of hepatic encephalopathy?	In this central nervous system (CNS) disorder resulting from portosystemic shunts, patients have alterations of consciousness, neuromuscular abnormalities, impaired intellectual functioning, and slowed brain waves.
What is asterixis?	A flapping tremor associated with hepatic encephalopathy
What is Budd-Chiari syndrome?	Thrombosis of the hepatic vein
With what conditions do patients with Budd-Chiari syndrome present?	Abdominal pain, enlarged painful liver, ascites, jaundice, and liver failure
What are the risk factors for Budd-Chiari syndrome?	Myeloproliferative disorders, hypercoagulable states, renal cancer, adrenal cancer, hepatocellular cancer, oral contraceptive use, and pregnancy
What characterizes a "nutmeg" liver?	Alternating pale portal areas and red congested centrilobular areas, which are due to a long history of right-sided heart failure
Describe how the liver in Budd-Chiari syndrome appears microscopically.	With dilation and congestion of centrilobular sinuses and efferent veins
Why is infarction of the liver rare?	The organ has a dual blood supply (hepatic and mesenteric).

REYE SYNDROME

What is another name for Reye syndrome?	Fatty liver with encephalopathy
Who develops Reye syndrome?	Children, most commonly 4–12 years of age
What causes Reye syndrome?	The syndrome typically follows a viral infection, and aspirin is implicated in > 90% of cases.
Is Reye syndrome common?	Not anymore, because children with fevers are not given aspirin

How is Reye syndrome manifested?	By encephalopathy and nonicteric hepatic dysfunction
Why is Reye syndrome called a biphasic illness?	Children have a prodromal febrile illness and then appear to recover. About 1 week later they experience an abrupt onset of vomiting and may rapidly progress to seizures, coma, and death.
What laboratory abnormalities are associated with Reye syndrome?	Serum transaminase elevation (up to > 3 times normal), serum ammonia elevation, and hypoprothrombinemia
Describe how the liver in Reye syndrome appears macroscopically.	As a yellow or white organ due to a high triglyceride content
Describe how the liver in Reye syndrome appears microscopically.	With microvesicular steatosis without necrosis or inflammation

HYPERBILIRUBINEMIA AND CHOLESTASIS

What is the definition of hyperbilirubinemia?	Serum bilirubin > 1.2 mg/dl
What is an obvious clinical sign of high bilirubin?	Jaundice
At what level of bilirubin is jaundice first noticeable?	2.0–2.5 mg/dl
What are the 2 kinds of hyperbilirubinemia?	1. Conjugated 2. Unconjugated
What are the 2 most common general causes of conjugated hyperbilirubinemia?	1. Intrinsic liver disease 2. Extrahepatic biliary obstruction
What is Dubin-Johnson syndrome?	Jaundice and conjugated hyperbilirubinemia due to a defect in hepatocytic excretion of conjugated bilirubin. (Think **D**ubin = **D**eparture defect.)
What are the typical clinical features of Dubin-Johnson syndrome?	The condition is usually asymptomatic.

Name 2 disorders of bilirubin conjugation.

1. Crigler-Najjar syndrome
2. Gilbert syndrome

What enzyme is missing in Crigler-Najjar syndrome?

Uridine diphosphate (UDP)–glucuronosyltransferase

What is the difference between type I and type II Crigler-Najjar syndrome?

Type I (complete absence of the enzyme)—more severe type; incompatible with life
Type II (partial deficiency of the enzyme)—usually causes asymptomatic jaundice

What enzyme is missing in Gilbert syndrome?

UDP-glucuronosyltransferase. (Gilbert syndrome closely resembles type II Crigler-Najjar syndrome.)

What are the typical clinical findings in Gilbert syndrome?

The disorder is often asymptomatic, but jaundice is common.

Which of the 2 inherited disorders, Gilbert syndrome or Crigler-Najjar syndrome, is more common?

Gilbert syndrome, which affects 3%–7% of the population. Crigler-Najjar syndrome is rare.

What are 2 other general causes of unconjugated hyperbilirubinemia?

1. Reduced hepatic uptake (from drugs such as rifampin)
2. Increased red blood cell (RBC) destruction

Which of the 2 types of hyperbilirubinemia is associated with cholestasis?

Conjugated hyperbilirubinemia

Describe the pathophysiology of cholestasis?

Decreased bile flow through the canaliculi with decreased hepatocytic secretion of bilirubin, bile acids, and water

With what conditions do patients with cholestasis present?

Jaundice, pruritus, increased conjugated bilirubin, and increased alkaline phosphatase values

What color is the liver in cholestasis?

Dark green or black

Microscopically, what causes this discoloration?

Bile pigments in hepatocytes and bile canaliculi

What is cholangitis?

Bile duct obstruction and ascending biliary tract infection with the presence of neutrophils

What techniques are used to determine the location of the obstruction?

CT or endoscopic retrograde cholangiopancreatography (ERCP)

NEOPLASMS OF THE LIVER

Benign tumors

What is the most common benign tumor of the liver?

Hemangioma, which is found in about 1% of routine autopsies

Describe the size and gross appearance of hemangiomas.

Soft, red lesions that are 2–4 cm in diameter

Who develops hepatocellular adenoma?

Women who take birth control pills (about 90% of cases)

With what condition do patients with hepatocellular adenomas present?

Abdominal pain

What serious complication is associated with hepatocellular adenoma?

Rupture and severe intraperitoneal hemorrhage

How does hepatocellular adenoma appear microscopically?

As sheet-like cords of normal-appearing hepatocytes without bile ducts or portal tracts

Who develops focal nodular hyperplasia?

Women, typically between the ages of 30 and 50. Only about 10% of cases occur in men.

With what conditions do patients with focal nodular hyperplasia present?

Findings are incidental in 50%–80% of cases, but an abdominal mass is the most common presenting sign.

Is focal nodular hyperplasia caused by oral contraceptives?

These agents probably play a role but are not the single cause of the condition.

Describe how focal nodular hyperplasia appears macroscopically.

Usually as a solitary, subcapsular, tan nodular mass, with a diameter generally < 5 cm. Fibrous septa divide the lesion into nodules.

Describe how focal nodular hyperplasia appears microscopically.

As normal hepatocytes separated by septa that contain bile ductules and inflammatory cells

Malignant tumors

What is the most common malignancy in the liver?

Metastatic cancer, which accounts for about 98% of hepatic malignancies

What are the 4 most common primary sites of liver metastases?

1. Lung
2. Breast
3. Colon
4. Pancreas

What is the most common primary malignancy of the liver?

Hepatocellular carcinoma (hepatoma), which accounts for 80%–90% of primary malignant tumors of the liver in adults

Who is affected by hepatocellular carcinoma more often, men or women?

Men

What risk factors are associated with hepatomas?

Anything that causes chronic liver injury (usually cirrhosis, especially if associated with HBV infection)

What percentage of hepatomas occur in individuals with otherwise normal (uninjured) livers?

About 10%

What serum marker is commonly elevated in hepatomas?

Alpha-fetoprotein (AFP) [about 80% of patients]

Describe how a hepatoma appears macroscopically.

As a soft, multinodular growth or single large mass, which is gray or green (bile-stained). The tumor(s) often invade portal veins and may extend into inferior vena cava via hepatic veins.

Describe how a hepatoma appears microscopically.

As bile-producing cells that grow in a trabecular pattern

How do hepatomas metastasize?

Usually by a hematogenous route

What is the second most common primary malignancy of the liver?

Cholangiocarcinoma (bile duct carcinoma)

Is cholangiocarcinoma associated with HBV infection and cirrhosis?	Minimally. Fewer than 10% of patients have cirrhosis, and there is no association with HBV.
What causes cholangio-carcinoma?	90% of cases—idiopathic etiology 10% of cases—association with chronic ulcerative colitis (usually with primary sclerosing cholangitis), congenital hepatic fibrosis, hemochromatosis, or thorium oxide (Thorotrast) administration
When cholangiocarcinoma occurs in the Far East, with what condition is it associated?	*Clonorchis sinensis* (liver fluke) infestation
From what cells does cholangiocarcinoma originate?	Intrahepatic epithelial cells
How does a cholangio-carcinoma appear micro-scopically?	Over 95% of tumors are adenocarci-nomas, which cannot be histologically distinguished from metastatic adeno-carcinoma

BILIARY TREE

NONMALIGNANT DISEASES OF THE GALLBLADDER

What is another name for cholelithiasis?	Gallstones
What individuals are affected by gallstones?	20 million Americans (20% of all women)
Name the "4 Fs" that describe the typical indivi-dual with an increased risk for gallstones?	Fat, Female, Fertile, and Forty
What percentage of gall-stones are radiopaque?	15%
What makes up the majority of radiopaque gallstones?	Pigment stones made of insoluble calcium salts (calcium bilirubinate) and cholesterol

With what type of anemia are these gallstones associated?

Hemolytic anemia

What type of gallstones are most common?

Cholesterol gallstones

Why do cholesterol gallstones form?

The liver does not provide enough bile salts and lecithin to keep the cholesterol soluble.

Name the 2 types of cholesterol gallstones.

1. Pure cholesterol stones (> 90% cholesterol)
2. Mixed cholesterol stones (60%–90% cholesterol)

Which of the 2 types of cholesterol gallstones is more common?

Mixed, which account for about 75% of all gallstones

What are the clinical manifestations associated with cholesterol gallstones?

They are often asymptomatic. Fatty food intolerance is common.

What are 5 possible complications of cholelithiasis?

1. Obstructive jaundice
2. Biliary colic
3. Ascending cholangitis
4. Acute pancreatitis
5. Acute or chronic cholecystitis

What is acute cholecystitis?

Acute inflammation of the gallbladder

With what conditions do patients with acute cholecystitis present?

Fever, nausea, vomiting, and right upper quadrant pain

What is the most common cause of acute cholecystitis?

Over 90% of cases are due to impaction of a gallstone in the gallbladder neck or the cystic duct.

Describe the pathophysiology involved in acute cholecystitis.

After impaction, the obstruction causes an increase in intraluminal pressure with subsequent vascular compromise, necrosis, and often bacterial invasion.

What are the other causes of the remaining fraction of cases of acute cholecystitis besides gallstone impaction?

Diabetes, shock, sepsis, burns, trauma, and arteritis

What is Murphy sign?

Involuntary arrest of inspiration with deep palpation of the right upper quadrant, which is often present with cholecystitis

Describe the gallbladder in cholecystitis in terms of its gross appearance.

The organ is enlarged and discolored, and a surface exudate is often present.

What is the most serious complication of acute cholecystitis?

Perforation, which occurs in about 10% of cases

Is perforation more common in calculous or acalculous cholecystitis?

Acalculous cholecystitis

What is chronic cholecystitis?

A thickening of the gallbladder wall due to extensive fibrosis

Is chronic cholecystitis associated with gallstones?

Yes; it almost never occurs in the absence of gallstones.

What is a strawberry gallbladder?

Diffuse cholesterolosis characterized by yellow cholesterol-containing flecks in the mucosa

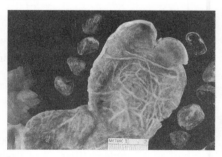

TUMORS OF THE GALLBLADDER

Are tumors of the gallbladder common?

No; they account for only about 2%–3% of all gastrointestinal (GI) malignancies.

What is the most common tumor of the gallbladder?

Adenocarcinoma

Is carcinoma of the gallbladder caused by gallstones?

This is unknown, but a relationship probably exists. Gallstones are found in about 75% of all cases of cancer of the gallbladder. However, < 1% of patients with gallstones develop cancer.

Describe how the gall-bladder tumor appears macroscopically.

As a bulky or papillary mass, which may cause diffuse wall thickening that resembles the fibrosis associated with chronic cholecystitis

Describe how the gall-bladder tumor appears microscopically.

Usually as adenocarcinoma with signs of chronic cholecystitis

DISORDERS INVOLVING THE EXTRAHEPATIC BILE DUCTS

What is a cholodochal cyst?

A congenital dilation of the biliary tract

Describe the histology of the wall of a cholodochal cyst.

Fibrous tissue containing a chronic inflammatory infiltrate

Do patients with cholo-dochal cysts have an increased risk for any particular disease?

Biliary tract carcinoma, which occurs in about 5% of cases

What is choledocholithiasis?

Gallstones in the common bile duct

With what conditions do patients with choledocholi-thiasis present?

Fever, jaundice, and pain

Which of these symptoms is the most common?

Pain occurs in 90% of patients, jaundice in 50%, and fever in 33%.

What is the most common benign tumor of the bile duct?

Adenoma

What is the most common malignant tumor of the bile duct?

Adenocarcinoma

Is carcinoma of the bile duct more or less common than carcinoma of the gallbladder?

Less common

What is the name of the tumor that arises near the confluence of the right and left hepatic ducts?	Klatskin tumor
Name 2 risk factors associated with a Klatskin tumor.	1. Ulcerative colitis 2. Primary sclerosing cholangitis
What symptoms are typical of a Klatskin tumor?	Jaundice, weight loss, and pain
How does a Klatskin tumor tend to metastasize?	Direct extension into surrounding soft tissue and invasion of local lymph nodes and the liver
What is Courvoisier law?	A palpably enlarged gallbladder is likely due to a tumor that obstructs the common bile duct rather than a gallstone. With obstruction caused by a gallstone, too much fibrosis and scarring usually prevent enlargement.

BILIARY CIRRHOSIS

What features distinguish primary biliary cirrhosis (PBC)?	A disease of middle-aged women characterized by obstructive jaundice, hypercholesterolemia, and itching
What etiologic mechanism is involved in PBC?	PBC is probably an autoimmune disease, which is associated with antimitochondrial antibodies.
What clinical features are associated with PBC?	Pruritus, jaundice, xanthoma formation, pigmentation changes, and steatorrhea
What laboratory findings are used to diagnose PBC?	1. Increased serum alkaline phosphatase 2. Increased cholesterol and triglycerides 3. Increased IgM 4. Elevated antimitochondrial antibodies
With what diseases is PBC associated?	Scleroderma, CREST syndrome, and sicca syndrome
What are the components of the CREST syndrome?	**C**alcinosis, **R**aynaud phenomenon, **E**sophageal dysfunction, **S**yndactyly, and **T**elangiectasia
What are the characteristics of the sicca syndrome?	Dry eyes and dry mouth

What is the pathophysiology of secondary biliary cirrhosis?	Extrahepatic biliary obstruction with subsequent increased pressure in the bile ducts, causing ductal and periductal inflammation

INFANTILE CHOLESTASIS AND HEPATITIS

What type of hyperbilirubinemia is present in infantile cholestasis?	Conjugated hyperbilirubinemia
What does α_1-antitrypsin do?	This protease inhibitor inhibits trypsin and elastase.
What happens to children born with an α_1-antitrypsin deficiency?	They usually develop hepatitis within 1 or 2 weeks of birth. This condition usually resolves by about 6 months of age but may later progress to cirrhosis.
What occurs in the livers of children with α_1-antitrypsin deficiency?	Proliferation of bile ductules simulates extrahepatic obstruction. With time, changes characteristic of chronic active hepatitis and cirrhosis occur.
What is the treatment for α_1-antitrypsin deficiency?	Liver transplantation for cirrhosis. (Currently, research regarding gene replacement therapy is ongoing.)
What are the 2 types of intrahepatic biliary atresia?	1. Syndromic form (Alagille syndrome) 2. Nonsyndromic form
Describe how the liver of an infant with intrahepatic biliary atresia appears macroscopically.	A near absence of interlobular bile ducts and a decreased number of portal tracts
What is the course and prognosis of intrahepatic biliary atresia?	Usually patients survive to adulthood. Pruritus is the major problem and is treated symptomatically. Fibrosis and cirrhosis are rare, and liver transplantation should be considered if they occur.

EXOCRINE PANCREAS

NORMAL STRUCTURE AND FUNCTION

What percentage of the pancreas is devoted to exocrine function?	80%

What are the 2 major pancreatic ducts called?	1. Duct of Wirsung—main duct 2. Duct of Santorini—accessory duct
What does the exocrine pancreas secrete?	2–3 L of fluid rich in amylase, lipase, and proteases daily
What is an annular pancreas?	A congenital anomaly in which a ring of pancreatic tissue at the head of the pancreas encircles the descending portion of the duodenum and causes stenosis

PANCREATITIS

What are the 2 most common causes of acute pancreatitis?	1. Alcohol consumption 2. Gallstones
Name 8 causes of acute pancreatitis aside from alcohol consumption and gallstones.	1. Trauma 2. Viral infection (mumps) 3. Pancreatic carcinoma 4. Hypertriglyceridemia 5. Drug toxicity 6. Vasculitis 7. Hyperparathyroidism 8. Scorpion bite
How do patients with acute pancreatitis present?	Nausea; vomiting; fever; and severe abdominal pain, often radiating to the back
How are Ranson criteria used?	These criteria, which are two sets of signs associated with acute pancreatitis, are used as prognostic indicators. Patients are assessed both at admission and during the first 48 hours of hospitalization.
What are Ranson criteria?	At admission: **G**lucose > 200 mg/dl, **A**ge > 55 years, **L**DH (lactate dehydrogenase) > 350 units/L, **A**ST > 250 units/L, **W**BC > 16,000/μl (remember GA LAW) During first 48 hours: **C**alcium < 8 mg/dl, **H**ematocrit decrease of 10% or more, **P**o$_2$ < 60 mm Hg, **B**UN increase of 5 or more, **B**ase deficit > 4 mEq/L, **S**equestration of > 6 L of fluid (remember C + HOBBS)

How are the Ranson criteria used as indicators of prognosis?

Presence of 1 or 2 criteria: mortality rate almost zero
Presence of 3 or 4 criteria: mortality rate about 15%
Presence of 5 or 6 criteria: mortality rate nearly 50%
Presence of at least 7 criteria: mortality rate almost 100%

Describe how the inflamed pancreas appears macroscopically.

As an edematous gland with areas of hemorrhage, necrosis, and chalky fat necrosis

Describe how the inflamed pancreas appears microscopically.

With cloudy-appearing cells that have a neutrophilic infiltrate, often with basophilic calcium salts and foamy macrophages

What are the 5 possible complications of acute pancreatitis?

1. Hemorrhage
2. Necrosis
3. Abscess formation
4. Diabetes
5. Pseudocyst formation

Why is a pseudocyst not a true cyst?

This fluid-filled "cyst" is not lined with epithelium.

What is the most common cause of chronic pancreatitis?

Alcohol consumption

Briefly describe what happens to the pancreas in chronic pancreatitis.

Chronic irritation leads to fibrosis and calcification.

NEOPLASMS OF THE PANCREAS

What is the most common malignancy of the pancreas?

Adenocarcinoma

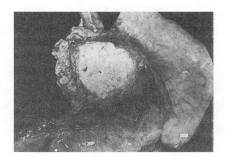

Where in the pancreas does adenocarcinoma most often occur?

Head (about 70%)
Body (10%–15%)
Tail (5%–10%)

Is adenocarcinoma a common pancreatic tumor?

It is the 4th leading cause of cancer death in men and the 5th in women, with the occurrence of about 25,000 new cases annually in the United States.

In which groups of people is pancreatic cancer more common?

Individuals who smoke cigarettes and those who drink alcohol

How do patients with pancreatic cancer present?

Usually the tumor is well advanced by the time patients complain of abdominal pain radiating to the back, weight loss, anorexia, and obstructive jaundice due to common bile duct compression.

What does Trousseau sign represent?

Migratory thrombophlebitis. It is occasionally associated with pancreatic cancer.

POWER REVIEW

What is the difference between communicating and noncommunicating hepatic cysts?

By definition, communicating cysts communicate with the biliary tree, whereas noncommunicating cysts do not.

At what serum level of bilirubin is jaundice first noticeable?

2–2.5 mg/dl

Is conjugated or unconjugated hyperbilirubinemia associated with cholestasis?

Conjugated hyperbilirubinemia

What inborn error of metabolism is associated with conjugated hyperbilirubinemia?

Dubin-Johnson syndrome

What is cholangitis?

Ascending biliary tract infection marked by neutrophil infiltration into the large bile ducts

Which is more elevated in viral hepatitis, AST or ALT?

ALT

Which is more elevated in alcoholic hepatitis, AST or ALT?	AST
What is wrong with the kidneys in hepatorenal syndrome?	Nothing; they will function if transplanted.
What is the most common cause of traveler's hepatitis?	HAV
What is the most common cause of posttransfusion hepatitis?	HCV
What is the meaning of the term "lobular disarray"?	The disordered appearance of the liver in hepatitis after necrosis, regeneration, and inflammation of the lobules have taken place
What should you recommend to clear up the steatosis of alcoholic hepatitis?	Stop drinking alcohol
What causes nutmeg liver?	Chronic passive congestion (often from heart failure)
What conditions are characteristic of Reye syndrome?	Acute encephalopathy and nonicteric hepatic dysfunction
What is the classic triad of Reye syndrome?	Elevated transaminase, elevated plasma ammonia, and hypoprothrombinemia
What disease is associated with pruritus and elevated serum antimitochondrial antibody titers?	PBC
What is the treatment for genetic hemochromatosis?	Phlebotomy
What is the most common cause of micronodular cirrhosis?	Alcohol consumption
What is the most common cause of macronodular cirrhosis?	Viral hepatitis

What condition causes asterixis?	Hepatic encephalopathy
What is the most common pathogen in spontaneous bacterial peritonitis?	*Escherichia coli*
What is the most common pathogen in a pyogenic hepatic abscess?	*Escherichia coli*
What is the major difference between pyogenic liver abscesses and amebic liver abscesses with regard to infiltrate?	Neutrophils, which are present in the infiltrate of pyogenic abscesses but not in that of amebic abscesses
What is a Kayser-Fleischer ring?	A ring of copper-containing pigment at the periphery of the cornea in patients with Wilson disease
What is Budd-Chiari syndrome?	Thrombotic occlusion of the hepatic vein that may lead to liver failure
What individuals develop hepatocellular adenomas?	Women who take oral contraceptive pills (at least 90% of cases)
What benign liver tumor is characterized by a lesion divided by fibrous septa?	Focal nodular hyperplasia
What accounts for the majority of liver malignancies?	Metastatic tumors
What is a common complication of cirrhosis associated with HBV infection?	Hepatocellular carcinoma
What microscopic finding in liver tumors is diagnostic of hepatocellular carcinoma?	Bile canaliculi
What hepatic malignancy is not associated with HBV infection?	Cholangiocarcinoma
What percentage of gallstones are radiopaque?	About 15%

Name the "4 Fs" of gallstones.	Fat, Fertile, Female, and Forty
What type of stone is the most common?	A mixed cholesterol stone
What is the most common cause of acute cholecystitis?	Stones in the gallbladder neck or cystic duct
Are gallstones associated with carcinoma of the gallbladder?	Yes; they are present in about 75% of gallbladders with carcinoma.
What is choledocholithiasis?	Gallstones in the common bile duct
What are the 2 most common causes of acute pancreatitis?	1. Alcohol consumption 2. Gallstones
Why is a pseudocyst not a true cyst?	It has no epithelial lining.
Where in the pancreas is cancer most commonly found?	The head of the gland

26

Endocrine System

Name the 3 sites where endocrine regulation occurs.

1. Hypothalamus
2. Pituitary gland
3. Target organs

How is the endocrine system regulated?

By positive and negative feedback systems

What happens if these feedback systems malfunction?

Endocrinopathies from overproduction or undersecretion of various hormones

HYPOTHALAMUS

What are the 2 roles of the hypothalamus?

1. Center for regulation of the endocrine and nervous systems
2. Secretion of releasing or inhibiting factors that invoke specific hormonal responses

Describe the effect of each of the following hormones of the hypothalamus on the pituitary gland.

    Thyrotropin-releasing hormone

Stimulates release of thyrotropin

    Corticotropin-releasing hormone

Stimulates release of adrenocorticotropin

    Prolactin-inhibiting factor

Inhibits the release of prolactin

Name 4 conditions that produce lesions in the hypothalamus.

1. Hamartomas
2. Neoplasms
3. Trauma
4. Inflammation (e.g., sarcoidosis)

PITUITARY GLAND

What are the 2 parts of the pituitary gland?

1. Adenohypophysis (anterior pituitary)
2. Neurohypophysis (posterior pituitary)

ANTERIOR PITUITARY AND RELATED DISORDERS

Name the 5 types of cells of the anterior pituitary.	1. Somatotrophs 2. Corticotrophs 3. Gonadotropins 4. Lactotropes 5. Nonsecretory cells
What substances do somatotrophs secrete?	Growth hormones (somatomedins)
Corticotrophs secrete pro-opiomelanocortin (POMC), which splits into what 2 products?	1. Adrenocorticotropic hormone (ACTH) 2. Beta-lipotropin
Beta-lipotropin splits into what 3 products?	1. Endorphins 2. Enkephalins 3. Beta-melanocyte–stimulating hormone
What 2 hormones do gonadotropins secrete?	1. Follicle-stimulating hormone (FSH) 2. Luteinizing hormone (LH)
What substance do lactotropes secrete?	Prolactin

Give the staining pattern for each of the following cells.

Somatotrophs	Acidophilic with hematoxylin and eosin
Corticotrophs	Basophilic
Gonadotrophs	Basophilic to chromophobic
Lactotropes	Acidophilic to chromophilic
Nonsecretory cells	As chromophobes (mostly)

Hyperfunction of the anterior pituitary

Name the 3 kinds of anterior pituitary hyperfunctioning.	1. Prolactinoma with hyperprolactinemia 2. Somatotropic adenoma with hypersecretion of growth hormone (GH) 3. Corticotropic adenoma and hypersecretion of ACTH

What is the most common pituitary tumor?

Prolactinoma with hyperprolactinemia

What are the presenting features of prolactinomas?

Amenorrhea and galactorrhea

Name 3 causes of prolactinomas.

1. Hypothalamic lesions
2. Medications that interfere with dopamine (prolactin inhibitory factor) secretion
3. Estrogen therapy

What is the second most common type of pituitary tumor?

Somatotropic adenoma with hypersecretion of GH

How does this somatotropic adenoma present clinically?

It depends on the developmental age of the individual. If skeletal epiphyseal plates are open, gigantism results. If epiphyseal plates are closed, acromegaly results.

Describe physical features associated with acromegaly.

Coarsening of the facies, thickening of lips, and enlargement and swelling of hands and feet

What metabolic disorder is associated with acromegaly?

Diabetes mellitus, because hypersecretion of GH affects glucose tolerance

What condition is seen with hypercortisolism?

Cushing disease or Cushing syndrome

What is the difference between Cushing disease and Cushing syndrome?

Cushing disease classically refers to hypercortisolism due to a corticotropic adenoma, most often a basophilic adenoma.
Cushing syndrome refers to hypercortisolism regardless of cause (i.e., ectopic ACTH production by a tumor).

Hypofunction of the anterior pituitary

What type of anterior pituitary hypofunction occurs most commonly?

Generalized panhypopituitarism

What may cause panhypopituitarism?

Any condition that destroys the pituitary gland. Possibilities include the following:

Tumor of pituitary
Tumor of neighboring structure
Metastasis, infarction, or irradiation
Granulomatous disease (sarcoidosis)
Empty sella syndrome

How does infarction of the pituitary occur?

As a result of shock and hemorrhage in childbirth. The hypopituitarism is called postpartum pituitary necrosis.

What is another name for this hypopituitarism?

Sheehan syndrome

What is the empty sella syndrome?

Absence or destruction of the pituitary

What is the etiology of empty sella syndrome?

Unknown

How is empty sella syndrome diagnosed?

By radiologic examination

What results in an isolated deficiency of GH in children?

Pituitary dwarfism from growth retardation

What results in an isolated deficiency of GH in adults?

Increased insulin sensitivity with hypoglycemia, decreased muscle strength, and anemia

Tell what condition(s) occur as a result of isolated deficiency of gonadotropin in the following individuals:

    Preadolescent children

Retarded sexual maturation

    Men

Loss of libido, impotence, and loss of muscular mass, and decreased facial hair

    Women

Amenorrhea and vaginal atrophy

What condition results in isolated deficiency of thyroid-stimulating hormone (TSH)?

Secondary hypothyroidism

What condition results in isolated deficiency of ACTH?	Secondary adrenal failure

POSTERIOR PITUITARY AND RELATED DISORDERS

What is the function of the posterior pituitary?	To store and release 2 hypothalamic hormones: oxytocin and vasopressin (also called antidiuretic hormone, ADH)
What is the function of oxytocin?	To stimulate uterine contractions and initiate lactation
What is the function of vasopressin?	To regulate the maintenance of serum osmolality by promoting water retention through action on the renal collecting duct

Hyperfunction of the posterior pituitary

What disorder involves ADH?	Syndrome of inappropriate ADH (SIADH) secretion
What are the clinical features of SIADH?	Retention of water with consequent dilutional hyponatremia and inability to dilute the urine
How does SIADH occur?	Most commonly by ectopic production of ADH by nonendocrine tumors
What tumor commonly produces this SIADH?	Small-cell carcinoma of the lung
What else can cause SIADH besides small-cell carcinoma?	Intracranial trauma; infection; and certain antineoplastic drugs (e.g., cyclophosphamide, vincristine)

Hypofunction of the posterior pituitary

What metabolic disorder results from a deficiency of vasopressin secretion?	Diabetes insipidus
What are the clinical features of diabetes insipidus?	Excretion of large volumes of dilute urine (polyuria) with dehydration and insatiable thirst
What conditions cause diabetes insipidus?	Local tumors, radiation, cranial vascular lesions, trauma, or surgery lead to com-

pression or destruction of the posterior pituitary.

PITUITARY TUMORS

What is the most common anterior pituitary tumor?	Adenoma
What is a rare tumor of the anterior pituitary?	Carcinoma
What are the effects of anterior pituitary tumors?	Functional tumors: Possible hyper-secretion of a particular hormone Nonfunctional tumors: Possible mass effects such as vision loss or palsies as a result of cranial nerve damage
Can a tumor secrete more than 1 hormone?	Yes
Describe the histology of most pituitary tumors.	The tumors are usually composed of groups or nests of uniform, cytologically bland cells encompassed by a delicate vascular network.
What is a craniopharyngioma?	A benign childhood tumor derived from the Rathke pouch (not a true pituitary tumor)
Describe the histologic appearance of a craniopharyngioma.	The nests of squamous cells in a loose stroma closely resemble the appearance of embryonic tooth bud enamel organs. They are often cystic.
How is a craniopharyngioma detected?	Radiographically, because of calcification

THYROID GLAND

How much does the normal thyroid weigh?	20–30 g
What is the clinical presentation of thyroid disease?	A palpable mass or pain in the thyroid gland, or occurrence of symptoms referable to abnormal thyroid hormone levels
What is the most common thyroid anomaly?	Thyroglossal duct cyst

What is a thyroglossal duct cyst?	A remnant of the thyroglossal duct

GOITER

What is goiter?	A nonspecific term for thyroid enlargement, which may occur in euthyroid, hypothyroid, or hyperthyroid states. It is not used for inflammatory or neoplastic conditions.
Name 7 causes of thyroid enlargement.	1. Inborn errors of thyroid hormone biosynthesis 2. Nutritional iodine deficiency 3. Goitrogenic substances 4. Nontoxic nodular goiter 5. Diffuse toxic goiter (Graves disease) 6. Thyroiditis 7. Neoplasms
What is the most common cause of goiter worldwide?	Iodine deficiency
How large can the thyroid become in goiter?	> 500 g
Describe the gross characteristics of goiter.	Marked enlargement in a diffuse or nodular pattern
Describe the histologic characteristics of goiter.	Variable, from large, distended masses of colloid lined with flattened cells to smaller follicles with cuboidal or columnar cells
Name the 4 different categories of goiter.	1. Nontoxic goiter 2. Toxic goiter 3. Endemic thyroid 4. Nodular goiter
What is the difference between nontoxic and toxic goiter?	Nontoxic goiter: goiter without hormone dysfunction Toxic goiter: goiter associated with hyperthyroidism
Why does the thyroid gland enlarge in nontoxic goiter?	As the result of repeated or continual hyperplasia in response to a deficiency in thyroid hormone

What substance is deficient in the diet where goiter is endemic?	Iodine
Define nodular goiter.	A goiter in which hemorrhage within the large thyroid follicles and a secondary fibrous reaction has occurred.
What is the difference between a "hot" and a "cold" thyroid nodule?	Hot nodule: functional status, which is signified by increased uptake of radioactive intravenous ^{131}I Cold: nonfunctional status, which is signified by decreased uptake of radioactive intravenous ^{131}I

HYPERTHYROIDISM

What are the clinical signs of hyperthyroidism?	1. Nervousness, restlessness, and fine tremor 2. Palpitations and tachycardia 3. Fatigue and muscle weakness 4. Diarrhea and weight loss, with an intact appetite 5. Heat intolerance 6. Menstrual abnormalities (amenorrhea or oligomenorrhea)
What condition is most commonly associated with hyperthyroidism?	Diffuse toxic goiter (Graves disease)
What are 7 causes of hyperthyroidism other than Graves disease?	1. Functioning thyroid adenoma or carcinomas 2. Pituitary tumors that secrete thyrotropin 3. Choriocarcinomas that secrete thyrotropin-like substances 4. Exogenous administration of thyroid hormone 5. Plummer syndrome 6. Pituitary hyperfunction 7. Struma ovarii
What is the pathogenesis of hyperthyroidism?	Circulating antibodies stimulate TSH receptors on follicular cells of the thyroid and cause deregulated production of thyroid hormones.

What is the etiology of hyperthyroidism?

It is unknown but presumed to be immunologic.

In which group of individuals is hyperthyroidism most common?

Young females

The incidence of hyperthyroidism is increased in what individuals?

HLA-DR3–positive and HLA-B8–positive individuals

What are the most common symptoms of hyperthyroidism?

1. Nervousness and sweating
2. Tachycardia
3. Weight loss
4. Exophthalmos (sometimes)

How does the thyroid appear microscopically in hyperthyroidism?

Diffuse severe hyperplasia of the follicular epithelium is apparent, with small follicles that contain little colloid. Follicular cells are tall and columnar with enlarged nuclei. The stroma shows marked vascularity, and lymphocytic infiltrates are common.

HYPOTHYROIDISM

What 4 laboratory abnormalities are characteristic of hypothyroidism?

1. Decreased serum triiodothyronine (T_3) and thyroxine (T_4)
2. Increased serum TSH
3. Increased serum cholesterol
4. Decreased T_3 resin uptake

Hypothyroidism is manifested in adults by what condition?

Myxedema

Hypothyroidism is manifested in children by what condition?

Cretinism

What are 4 causes of myxedema?

1. Previous therapy for hyperthyroidism, including surgery, irradiation, or drugs
2. Hashimoto thyroiditis
3. Iodine deficiency
4. Primary idiopathic myxedema

Which of these 4 causes is most common in the United States?

Previous therapy for hyperthyroidism

What are the clinical characteristics of myxedema?

1. Lethargy
2. Cold intolerance
3. Constipation
4. Modest weight gain
5. Dry skin
6. Sparse coarse hair with thinning of lateral third of eyebrows
7. Menorrhagia
8. Lowered pitch of voice
9. Bloated appearance with edema of the subcutaneous tissue
10. Increase in the relaxation phase of deep tendon reflexes

Is hypothyroidism more common in women or men?

Women

What are 5 causes of cretinism?

1. Iodine deficiency
2. Deficiency of enzymes necessary for synthesis of thyroid hormones
3. Maldevelopment of the thyroid gland
4. Failure of the fetal thyroid to descend from its origin at the base of the tongue
5. Transplacental transfer of antithyroid antibodies from a mother with autoimmune disease

What are the characteristics of cretinism?

1. Severe mental retardation
2. Impaired physical growth with retarded bone development and dwarfism
3. Large tongue
4. Protuberant abdomen

THYROIDITIS

What are the 4 types of thyroiditis?

1. Acute suppurative thyroiditis
2. Subacute (granulomatous) thyroiditis
3. Chronic thyroiditis (Hashimoto thyroiditis)
4. Riedel struma (Riedel disease)

What causes acute suppurative thyroiditis?

Bacterial infection of the thyroid gland

What individuals are most commonly affected by acute suppurative thyroiditis?

Young children or debilitated adults

Is acute suppurative thyroiditis a common disorder?

No

What is subacute thyroiditis (de Quervain or granulomatous thyroiditis)?

A self-limited disorder characterized by painful swelling of the thyroid and transient hypothyroidism. Recovery occurs in 1–3 months.

Subacute thyroiditis constitutes what percentage of all thyroid disease?

About 2%

How does subacute thyroiditis present?

With sudden neck pain that radiates to the jaw or ear. Fever and malaise may also be present.

What is characteristic of subacute thyroiditis on gross examination?

A slightly enlarged thyroid, with involved areas that are firm and poorly defined, resembling carcinoma

What are the histologic characteristics of subacute thyroiditis?

Early stages: degeneration of follicular epithelium → colloid leakage (initial hyperthyroidism) → inflammatory response → granulomatous tissue → gland destruction → hypothyroidism
Late stages: regeneration of follicles, usually from the edges of the most affected areas

How does chronic thyroiditis (Hashimoto thyroiditis) present?

Patients are in a euthyroid or hypothyroid state.

Describe the gross pathology of the thyroid gland in chronic thyroiditis.

The thyroid gland is firm and moderately enlarged (size: 2–4× normal), with accentuated lobulation and bulging of individual lobules. At the end stage of Hashimoto thyroiditis, the gland can appear small and fibrotic.

Describe the microscopic appearance of the thyroid gland in chronic thyroiditis.

The follicles are small and atrophic, with sparse or absent colloid. Infiltration by lymphocytes and plasma cells with formation of germinal centers occurs. Fibrosis is present in varying degrees.

What causes chronic thyroiditis?

The etiology is unknown.

What is Riedel disease?

A connective tissue proliferation that involves the thyroid gland

Riedel disease is associated with what pathologic changes?

Fibrosing processes in the retroperitoneum, the orbit, and the mediastinum, which all suggest a systemic collagenosis

What clinical condition is a concern in Riedel disease?

Growth of the thyroid gland such that it compresses surrounding structures and obstructs the airway

Describe the appearance of the thyroid gland in Riedel disease on gross examination.

The gland is woody or iron-hard. Tissue planes are obliterated, and abnormal tissue is adherent to surrounding structures.

Describe the appearance of the thyroid gland in Riedel disease on microscopic examination.

Fibrous tissue replaces thyroid tissue. Vasculitis may be present.

MALIGNANT TUMORS OF THE THYROID GLAND

What are the 4 types of thyroid carcinomas, with the percent of cases of malignant thyroid cancer each represents?

1. Papillary carcinoma (60%)
2. Follicular carcinoma (20%)
3. Medullary carcinoma (10%)
4. Undifferentiated or anaplastic carcinoma (10%)

How does papillary adenocarcinoma of the thyroid present?

As a painless, anterior neck mass

Individuals of what age(s) are most commonly affected by this papillary adenocarcinoma?

The cancer has a bimodal distribution; patients in the first peak are under 40, and those in the second peak are in their 50s or 60s.

What are the histologic features of papillary adenocarcinoma of the thyroid?

Papillary projections into gland-like spaces
Tumor cells with characteristic "ground glass nuclei"
Psammoma bodies (in 40% of papillary carcinomas), which are laminated calcific spherules

What is the prognosis for patients with papillary adenocarcinoma?

The carcinoma exhibits extremely slow growth, and the 10-year survival rate is about 95%.

How does follicular adeno-carcinoma of the thyroid present?

As a nodule. Invasion of blood vessels is common and causes metastases to the brain, lung, and bones.

What is the prognosis for patients with follicular adenocarcinoma?

If invasion is limited to the capsule, the prognosis is good, with a 5-year survival rate of 85%. The outlook is dependent on the extent of invasion.

How does medullary carcinoma of the thyroid present?

With high serum calcitonin, because C cells retain their ability to make calcitonin

Individuals of what age are affected by medullary carcinoma of the thyroid?

Usually > 40 years

From where does medullary carcinoma arise?

In the upper lateral two-thirds of the thyroid, where parafollicular (C) cells are in high concentration

With what condition is this medullary carcinoma associated?

Multiple endocrine neoplasia (MEN) types 2A and 2B

Describe the appearance of medullary carcinoma of the thyroid on gross examination.

A hard, grayish-white to yellowish-tan, usually well-demarcated mass

Describe the appearance of medullary carcinoma on microscopic examination.

Tumor cells clustered in solid or irregular groups and separated by a hyaline, amyloid-containing stroma

What is the prognosis for patients with medullary carcinoma of the thyroid?

The overall 5-year survival rate is 50%. The cancer can metastasize both by lymphatics and blood vessels.

Individuals of what age are affected by anaplastic carcinoma of the thyroid?

> 60 years (almost exclusively)

What other thyroid condition may lead to this anaplastic carcinoma?

Goiter; > 50% of affected patients have a long history of goiter

How does anaplastic carcinoma of the thyroid appear clinically?

As a rapidly growing mass that may compress the trachea and compromise the airway

How does this anaplastic carcinoma appear on gross examination?	As invasion into adjacent areas of thyroid gland and neck
How does this anaplastic carcinoma appear on microscopic examination?	As large tumor cells and pleomorphism
What is the prognosis for patients with anaplastic carcinoma of the thyroid?	The outlook is poor; the tumor is nearly always fatal in 1 to 2 years.

PARATHYROID GLANDS

Describe the parathyroid glands.	4 small glands located at the inferior and superior poles of the thyroid gland that have a total weight of 120–150 mg
Are the parathyroid glands always attached to the thyroid?	About 5% of people have parathyroid tissue at ectopic sites.
From where do the superior parathyroid glands arise?	The fourth branchial arch
From where do the inferior parathyroid glands arise?	The third branchial arch
What happens to the parathyroid glands with increasing age?	The cellularity of gland decreases, and the ratio of cells to fat becomes 1:1.
What is the function of parathyroid hormone (PTH)?	Maintenance of calcium homeostasis in conjunction with vitamin D, calcitonin, and the kidney
To what does PTH respond?	Plasma concentration of ionized calcium

HYPERTHYROIDISM

What is involved in primary hyperparathyroidism?	Increased secretion of PTH by parathyroid gland(s). The hallmark of the condition is hypercalcemia.
What are the symptoms of hypercalcemia?	None if the condition is mild. As calcium levels increase, patients develop gastrointestinal (GI) complaints, as well as musculoskeletal, cardiovascular, neuro-

psychiatric, and urinary symptoms.
Hypercalcemia can be lethal.

What are the clinical features of primary hyperparathyroidism?

1. Osteitis fibrosa cystica: cystic changes in bone due to osteoclastic resorption
2. Metastatic calcification in various tissues, especially the kidneys (nephrocalcinosis)
3. Renal calculi
4. Peptic duodenal ulcer

What pathologic features are associated with primary hyperparathyroidism?

Solitary parathyroid adenomas (60%–80% of patients)
Primary hyperplasia (enlargement of all 4 parathyroid glands) [10%–25% of patients]

What laboratory findings are associated with primary hyperparathyroidism?

1. Hypercalcemia and hypercalciuria
2. Decreased serum phosphorus, decreased tubular reabsorption of phosphorus, and increased serum alkaline phosphatase
3. Increased serum PTH

What is secondary hyperparathyroidism?

An increase in serum PTH due to renal failure and constant calcium wasting

What pathology is characteristic of secondary hyperparathyroidism?

Diffuse chief cell or clear-cell hyperplasia

What are the clinical features of secondary hyperparathyroidism?

Symptoms of underlying disease (usually), with possible development of soft tissue calcification and osteosclerosis

How is tertiary hyperparathyroidism related to the primary and secondary forms of the thyroid disease?

Secondary hyperparathyroidism causes persistently elevated PTH due to refractory hyperplasia (serum calcium is corrected but fails to regulate PTH secretion). Tertiary disease can be viewed as a combination of primary and secondary hyperparathyroidism.

HYPOPARATHYROIDISM

Name 4 causes of hypoparathyroidism.

1. Iatrogenic disease resulting from thyroid surgery
2. Radioiodine therapy

3. Radical neck dissection
4. Congenital thymic hypoplasia
   (DiGeorge syndrome)

What are the clinical mani-festations of hypopara-thyroidism?

1. Hypocalcemia, causing increased neuromuscular excitability and tetany
2. Hyperphosphatemia

PARATHYROID TUMORS

What is the most common parathyroid neoplasm?

Parathyroid adenoma

Are malignant parathyroid tumors common?

No; they account for 1%–3% of all cases of hyperparathyroidism

What is the presenting feature of malignant para-thyroid tumors?

Severe hypercalcemia

ENDOCRINE PANCREAS

What cells in the pancreas have endocrine function?

Islets of Langerhans

Describe the islets of Langerhans in terms of appearance and location.

Appearance: rounded cellular masses that contain several types of endocrine cells
Location: scattered throughout the pancreas but most numerous in its distal part or tail

Name the cells that make up the islets of Langerhans and name the substance produced by each cell type.

1. Beta cells: insulin
2. Alpha cells: glucagon
3. Other cells: somatostatin, vasoactive intestinal polypeptide (VIP), and other hormones

What are the disorders of the endocrine pancreas?

Insulin-dependent diabetes mellitus (IDDM, juvenile-onset, or type I diabetes)
Non–insulin-dependent diabetes mellitus (NIDDM, adult-onset, or type II diabetes)

Which type of diabetes is more common?

Non–insulin-dependent diabetes

INSULIN-DEPENDENT DIABETES MELLITUS

What causes insulin-dependent diabetes mellitus?	Failure of insulin synthesis by beta cells of the islets of Langerhans
At what age does insulin-dependent diabetes mellitus occur?	Early in life, usually before 30 years of age
What are the presenting features of insulin-dependent diabetes mellitus?	Polyuria, polydipsia, and weight loss despite increased appetite
Individuals with what characteristics are more likely to lead insulin-dependent diabetes mellitus?	1. Positive family history 2. HLA-DR3–positive and HLA-DR4–positive status 3. Specific point mutation at HLA-DQ gene
What metabolic condition results from sustained levels carbohydrate intolerance with hyperglycemia?	Ketoacidosis
Why does ketoacidosis occur?	Increased catabolism of fat with production of ketone bodies
What substances make up ketone bodies?	Beta-hydroxybutyric acid and acetoacetic acid

NON–INSULIN-DEPENDENT DIABETES MELLITUS

What is non–insulin-dependent diabetes mellitus?	Increased insulin resistance, most often associated with mild to moderate obesity
What findings are characteristic of non–insulin-dependent diabetes mellitus?	1. Normal or increased plasma insulin concentration 2. Mild carbohydrate intolerance that does not usually require insulin for control
Can ketoacidosis develop in non–insulin-dependent diabetes mellitus?	Yes, but it is uncommon and usually precipitated by unusual stress such as infection or surgery.
What are the complications of diabetes mellitus?	Kidney: glomerular sclerosis leading to end-stage renal disease

Eyes: diabetic retinopathy (retinal
exudates, edema, hemorrhages, and
microaneurysms of small vessels),
which can lead to blindness; cataract
formation

Cardiovascular: increased atherosclerosis
in blood vessels, including the
coronary, cerebral, mesenteric, renal,
and femoral arteries; increased risk of
myocardial infarction (MI); peripheral
vascular insufficiency; capillary
basement membrane thickening

Nervous system: peripheral and
autonomic neuropathies

Skin: xanthomas, increased skin infections
(e.g., furuncles, abscesses); increased
fungal infection

ENDOCRINE PANCREATIC TUMORS

**What are the 5 types of
islet cell tumors?**

1. Insulinoma (beta cell tumor)
2. Gastrinoma
3. Glucagonoma (alpha cell tumor)
4. VIPoma
5. Nonfunctioning islet cell tumor

**What is the most common
type of islet cell tumor?**

Insulinoma

What is an insulinoma?

A benign (90% of cases) or malignant
(10% of cases) islet cell tumor characterized by markedly increased secretion of
insulin

**What clinical characteristics
are associated with insuli-
nomas?**

The Whipple triad:
1. Episodic hypoglycemia
2. Central nervous system (CNS) dysfunction related to hypoglycemia
3. Dramatic reversal of CNS symptoms
by administration of glucose

**How can endogenous
insulin production and
exogenous insulin produc-
tion be distinguished?**

By calculating the level of C-peptide. C-
peptide is a fragment of the proinsulin
molecule cleaved in commercial
preparations.

Define a gastrinoma.

Often a malignant tumor (60%–70% of
cases), a gastrinoma secretes gastrin,

leading to stimulation and hyperplasia of the gastric parietal cells. It can be found in extrapancreatic sites.

With what condition is a gastrinoma associated?

Zollinger-Ellison syndrome

What are the characteristic features of Zollinger-Ellison syndrome?

1. Marked gastric hypersecretion of hydrochloric acid
2. Recurrent peptic ulcer disease (PUD)
3. Hypergastrinemia

What is a glucagonoma?

A tumor of alpha cell origin that produces glucagon

How does glucagon affect glucose levels?

It increases them.

What are the presenting features of glucagonoma?

1. Diabetes
2. Necrotizing skin lesions
3. Stomatitis
4. Anemia

What is a VIPoma?

A VIP-producing islet cell tumor that causes watery diarrhea, hypokalemia, achlorhydria, or the WDHA syndrome

What is another name for WDHA syndrome?

Verner-Morrison syndrome or pancreatic cholera

Are VIPomas serious?

Yes; 80% are classified as malignant and can be fatal.

What are nonfunctioning islet cell carcinomas?

Tumors that produce no hormone but can be malignant and stimulate adeno-carcinoma

Name the presenting features of nonfunctioning islet cell carcinomas.

1. Obstructive jaundice
2. Hepatic metastasis
3. Large mass in abdomen

ADRENAL GLANDS

ANATOMY AND HISTOLOGY

What are the 2 distinct parts of the adrenal glands?

1. Adrenal cortex
2. Adrenal medulla

Describe the anatomy and function of the adrenal cortex.

It is composed of 3 zones, which all produce steroid hormones:
1. Zona glomerulosa (outermost part): produces mineralocorticoids (e.g., aldosterone)
2. Zona fasciculata (middle part): produces glucocorticoids (e.g., cortisol)
3. Zona reticularis (innermost part): produces androgens and progestins

What is the functional cell of the adrenal medulla and what does it produce?

The chromaffin cell, which produces catecholamines (e.g., epinephrine)

Name the 4 general categories of adrenal cortex—related disorders.

1. Hypercortisolism
2. Hyperaldosteronism
3. Adrenogenital syndromes
4. Adrenocortical insufficiency

HYPERCORTISOLISM

What syndrome results from prolonged exposure to an excess of glucocorticoids?

Cushing syndrome

How is Cushing syndrome classified in terms of etiology?

ACTH-dependent causes
Non–ACTH-dependent causes

Describe the ACTH-dependent causes of Cushing syndrome.

1. Iatrogenic: excessive doses of ACTH or a synthetic analog
2. Pituitary: hypersecretion of ACTH causing bilateral adrenocortical hyperplasia (Cushing disease)
3. Ectopic ACTH syndrome: secretion of ACTH by a malignant or benign tumor of nonendocrine origin

Describe the non–ACTH-dependent causes of Cushing syndrome.

1. Iatrogenic: administration of excessive doses of corticosteroids
2. Adrenal: Adenoma or carcinoma of the adrenal cortex

What are the clinical features of hypercortisolism?

Truncal obesity with "buffalo hump," rounded facies, abdominal striae, and thinning of skin
Mild hypertension

Increased susceptibility to infection
Osteoporosis
Mild glucose intolerance and mild
electrolyte changes (hypokalemia)

In Cushing disease, what pattern of fluctuation do plasma cortisol levels normally exhibit?

Diurnal variation (high in the morning, low in the evening)

What group of people are more commonly affected by adrenal adenomas?

Women (80% of cases)

What is the most common cause of Cushing syndrome in children?

Adrenal carcinoma

How are malignant adrenal neoplasms diagnosed?

By demonstration of distant metastases—the only criterion—because of the frequent absence of the usual morphologic criteria (mitotic activity and vascular or capsular invasion)

What happens to the contralateral adrenal gland in the presence of a functioning adenoma or carcinoma?

It becomes grossly and functionally atrophic.

What nonendocrine tumor accounts for the majority of cases of ectopic ACTH syndrome?

Small-cell (oat-cell) carcinoma of the lung

What are the presenting features of ectopic ACTH syndrome?

Usually electrolyte disturbances, because the typical Cushing syndrome features have not yet had time to develop

Table 26–1.
Incidence of Adrenal Lesions in Cushing Syndrome

Adrenal Lesion	Incidence (%)	
	Adults	Children
Hyperplasia	81	35
Adenoma	9	14
Carcinoma	10	51

HYPERALDOSTERONISM

Define Conn syndrome.

Primary hyperaldosteronism due to a lesion of the adrenal gland that produces excess aldosterone

What is the most common cause of Conn syndrome?

A benign aldosterone-producing adrenocortical adenoma

What other conditions besides adrenal adenomas can cause Conn syndrome?

Hyperplasia of zone glomerulosa
Adrenocortical carcinomas (rarely)

What are the clinical features of Conn syndrome?

1. $\uparrow$ Na^+ and $\downarrow$ K^+
2. Increased total plasma volume
3. Increased renal artery pressure
4. Inhibition of renin secretion

Define secondary hyperaldosteronism.

Hyperaldosteronism due to extra-adrenal causes related to hypersecretion of renin

What conditions cause hypersecretion of renin?

Renal hypertension
Edematous states (e.g., cirrhosis, nephrotic syndrome, or cardiac failure)

ADRENOGENITAL SYNDROMES

Describe adrenogenital syndromes.

Disorders resulting from congenital adrenal hyperplasia due to an inborn enzyme defect that inhibits cortisol synthesis

What biochemical sequence of events occurs in congenital adrenal hyperplasia?

Inhibition of cortisol synthesis $\rightarrow$ feedback overproduction of ACTH $\rightarrow$ adrenal hyperplasia and overproduction of adrenal hormones (not affected by enzyme deficiency)

Name the 2 most common enzyme deficiencies and the syndromes they cause.

1. 21-Hydroxylase deficiency: salt-losing syndrome
2. 11-Hydroxylase deficiency: Eberlein-Bongiovanni syndrome

Do adrenogenital syndromes occur in adults?

Yes; adrenal virilism can occur in adults with adrenal hyperplasia, adrenal carcinoma, and adrenal adenomas.

ADRENOCORTICAL INSUFFICIENCY

What condition occurs as a result of destruction of the adrenal cortex?	Primary adrenal insufficiency
What is another name for primary adrenal insufficiency?	Addison disease
What causes primary adrenal insufficiency?	Most often, idiopathic adrenal atrophy (probably autoimmune)
Describe the course of acute primary adrenal insufficiency.	Rapidly progressive adrenal crisis that presents as shock
Individuals with what condition often develop acute primary adrenal insufficiency?	Septicemia
What bacteria has a propensity to cause adrenal crisis?	Meningococcal species
What is the clinical syndrome of acute primary adrenal insufficiency called?	Waterhouse-Friderichsen syndrome
With what condition is Waterhouse-Friderichsen syndrome associated?	Disseminated intravascular coagulation
What are the clinical features of chronic adrenal insufficiency?	Increased skin pigmentation Malaise and weight loss Decreased serum sodium, chloride, glucose, and bicarbonate; increased serum potassium Hypotension Loss of body hair Menstrual irregularities
In Addison disease, what anatomic and pathologic changes occur in the adrenal cortex?	Adrenal cortex loses its normal 3-layered architecture, and adrenocortical cells become islets surrounded by fibrous tissue.

What disease was once a major contributor to primary adrenal insufficiency?	Tuberculosis (TB). Tuberculous granulomas caused over 50% of adrenal failures before effective treatment.

ADRENAL MEDULLA

Pheochromocytomas

What are pheochromocytomas?	An uncommon chromaffin cell tumor
Where do pheochromocytomas occur?	Medulla (90% of tumors) Extra-adrenal (in other neural crest–derived tissue) [10% of tumors]
Are pheochromocytomas benign or malignant?	Mostly benign (90%)
What are the clinical features of pheochromocytomas?	Initial excess catecholamine–caused symptoms: Paroxysmal or sustained hypertension, angina, cardiac arrhythmias, headache, and carbohydrate intolerance Late-stage features: cerebrovascular accident, congestive heart failure with pulmonary edema, and ventricular fibrillation
What laboratory findings are associated with pheochromocytomas?	Elevated urinary vanillylmandelic acid and norepinephrine levels
Describe pheochromocytomas in terms of their gross appearance.	Circumscribed gray to brown tumors 1–4 cm in size
Describe pheochromocytomas in terms of their microscopic appearance.	Nests and cords of large cells with voluminous cytoplasm. Nuclear atypia and multiple nuclei can be seen.
With what 2 disorders are pheochromocytomas sometimes associated?	1. MEN type 2A or 2B 2. Neurofibromatosis or von Hippel-Lindau disease
What are the organs of Zuckerkandl?	Embryonic chromaffin cells around the abdominal aorta that normally atrophy during childhood

What is the relationship between pheochromocytomas and the organs of Zuckerkandl?	These chromaffin cells are a major site of extra-adrenal pheochromocytomas.

Neuroblastomas

What are neuroblastomas?	Highly malignant catecholamine-producing solid tumors
How common are neuroblastomas?	Neuroblastomas occur most often in early childhood. Neonatal malignancies (15%–50% of cases) Childhood malignancies (7%–14% of cases)
Are neuroblastomas more common in boys or girls?	Boys
What are frequent sites of neuroblastomas other than the adrenal medulla?	Cervical, thoracic, and abdominal sympathetic ganglia
How are neuroblastomas diagnosed?	By finding abnormal quantities of catecholamines in the urine (89% of patients)
Describe the appearance of neuroblastomas on gross examination.	Nodular with a grayish surface and usually within a pseudocapsule, with areas of necrosis, hemorrhage, and calcification
Describe the appearance of neuroblastomas on microscopic examination.	Highly cellular, with cells arranged in broad sheets that can form rosette patterns. A large number of mitotic figures are often found.
What finding is pathognomonic for neuroblastomas?	Presence of rosettes plus neurofibril formation on microscopic examination
What is the prognosis for patients with neuroblastomas?	5-year survival rates vary from 30% for wide metastatic disease to 85% for localized disease. The younger the age, the better the prognosis.

MULTIPLE ENDOCRINE NEOPLASIA (MEN) SYNDROMES

What are MEN syndromes?	Autosomal dominant syndromes characterized by neoplasia (benign or

malignant), hyperplasia of one or more endocrine glands, or both

What is another name for MEN type 1?

Wermer syndrome

What features are characteristic of MEN type 1?

1. Parathyroid hyperplasia
2. Pancreatic islet cell tumor
3. Pituitary tumor
Remember PPP (3 Ps—parathyroid, pancreas, and pituitary), and think "P" for primary, as in the first kind of MEN (type 1).

How can MEN type 1 present?

With its pancreatic component: Zollinger-Ellison syndrome, hyperinsulinism, or pancreatic cholera

What is another name for MEN type 2?

Sipple syndrome (MEN type 2A)

Describe the characteristic features of Sipple syndrome.

Medullary carcinoma of the thyroid
Pheochromocytoma
Hyperparathyroidism due to hyperplasia or tumor
"MPH"

Describe the characteristic features of MEN type 3 (type 2B).

1. Pheochromocytoma
2. Medullary thyroid carcinoma
3. Multiple mucocutaneous neuromas
4. Marfanoid body habitus
"P MMM"
Note: Hyperparathyroidism is not evident.

POWER REVIEW

How is the endocrine system regulated?

Positive and negative feedback systems

What are the 2 roles of the hypothalamus?

1. Center for regulation of the endocrine and nervous systems
2. Secretion of releasing or inhibiting factors that invoke specific hormonal responses

Name the 5 types of cells of the anterior pituitary.

1. Somatotrophs
2. Corticotrophs

3. Gonadotropins
4. Lactotropes
5. Nonsecretory cells

What is the most common pituitary tumor?

Prolactinoma

Acromegaly occurs as a result of what process?

Hypersecretion of GH

What is Sheehan syndrome?

Infarction of the pituitary during the shock and hemorrhage of childbirth

What results in isolated deficiency of ACTH?

Secondary adrenal failure

What 2 hormones does the posterior pituitary store and release?

1. Oxytocin
2. Vasopressin (also called ADH)

What are the clinical features of SIADH?

Retention of water with consequent dilutional hyponatremia and inability to dilute the urine

What tumor commonly produces SIADH?

Small-cell carcinoma of the lung

What does a deficiency of vasopressin secretion cause?

Diabetes insipidus

What is the most common anterior pituitary tumor?

Adenoma

What is a craniopharyngioma?

A benign childhood tumor derived from the Rathke pouch

What is the most common thyroid anomaly?

Thyroglossal duct cyst

What is the most common cause of goiter in the world?

Iodine deficiency

What is the difference between nontoxic and toxic goiter?

Nontoxic goiter: without hormone dysfunction
Toxic goiter: associated with hyperthyroidism

What is the causal mechanism in Graves disease?

Circulating antibodies stimulate TSH receptors on follicular cells of the thyroid, causing deregulated production of thyroid hormones.

What laboratory abnormalities are associated with hypothyroidism?

1. Decreased serum T_3 and T_4
2. Increased serum TSH
3. Increased serum cholesterol
4. Decreased T_3 resin uptake

What are the characteristics of cretinism?

1. Severe mental retardation
2. Impaired physical growth with retarded bone development and dwarfism
3. Large tongue
4. Protuberant abdomen

What characterizes subacute thyroiditis (de Quervain or granulomatous thyroiditis)?

A self-limited disorder characterized by painful swelling of the thyroid, transient hypothyroid, and recovery in 1–3 months

What is the most common malignant tumor of the thyroid gland?

Papillary carcinoma

From where do the inferior parathyroid glands arise?

The third branchial arch

What is the function of PTH?

Maintenance of calcium homeostasis, in conjunction with vitamin D, calcitonin, and the kidney

What metabolic disorder is the hallmark of primary hyperparathyroidism?

Hypercalcemia

Name 4 causes of hypoparathyroidism.

1. Iatrogenic from thyroid surgery
2. Radioiodine therapy
3. Radical neck dissection
4. Congenital thymic hypoplasia (DiGeorge syndrome)

What is the most common parathyroid neoplasm?

Parathyroid adenoma

What cells in the pancreas have endocrine function?

Islets of Langerhans

What causes IDDM?

Failure of insulin synthesis by the beta cells of the islets of Langerhans

What happens with sustained levels of carbohydrate intolerance with hyperglycemia?

Ketoacidosis

Describe the kidney complications of diabetes.

Glomerular sclerosis leading to end-stage renal disease

What islet cell tumor occurs most commonly?

Insulinoma

What is the Whipple triad seen in insulinoma?

1. Episodic hypoglycemia
2. CNS dysfunction related to hypoglycemia
3. Dramatic reversal of CNS symptoms by administration of glucose

From where does the adrenal medulla originate?

Neural crest cells

What are the clinical features of hypercortisolism?

Truncal obesity with "buffalo hump," rounded facies, abdominal striae, and thinning of skin
Mild hypertension
Increased susceptibility to infection
Osteoporosis
Mild glucose intolerance and mild electrolyte changes (hypokalemia)

What nonendocrine tumor accounts for the majority of cases of ectopic ACTH syndrome?

Small-cell (oat-cell) carcinoma of the lung

What name is given to primary hyperaldosteronism due to a lesion of the adrenal gland that produces excess aldosterone?

Conn syndrome

What condition results from destruction of the adrenal cortex?

Primary adrenal insufficiency (Addison disease)

What bacteria has a propensity to cause adrenal crisis?

Meningococcal species

What is another name for meningococcal adrenal crisis?

Waterhouse-Friderichsen syndrome

What are the laboratory findings in pheochromocytoma?

Elevated urinary vanillylmandelic acid and norepinephrine levels

Describe the features of MEN type 2A.

1. Hyperparathyroidism due to hyperplasia or tumor
2. Pheochromocytoma
3. Medullary carcinoma of the thyroid

27

The Musculoskeletal System

BONES

ANATOMY

Name the 3 main functions of bone.
1. Mechanical stability
2. Mineral storage
3. Hematopoiesis

Macroscopically, name 2 types of bone.
Cortical bone and cancellous bone

Which type of bone is more dense and compact?
Cortical bone

What covers the cortex?
Periosteum

What is the main purpose of cortical bone?
It provides mechanical stability.

Where is cancellous bone found?
At the ends of long bones, in the medullary canal

Name the transverse cartilage plate present in a growing child.
Epiphysial plate (also known as physis or growth plate)

Name the 3 anatomic structures defined in relation to the physis.
Epiphysis, metaphysis, and diaphysis

How do long bones develop?
By endochondral ossification

How do flat bones develop?
By intramembranous ossification

Describe the main difference between endochondral and intramembranous ossification.
Intramembranous ossification lacks a cartilaginous phase.

What are the 4 types of bone cells?	1. Osteoprogenitor cell 2. Osteoblast 3. Osteocyte 4. Osteoclast
Describe the role of the osteoprogenitor cell.	The osteoprogenitor cell gives rise to an osteoblast.
What cells make bone tissue?	Osteoblasts
What is an osteocyte?	Osteoblasts that are embedded in bone matrix and isolated in lacunae
What cells resorb bone tissue?	Osteoclasts
How do osteoclasts resorb bone?	By the action of lysosomes and hydrolytic enzymes
What 3 hormones are integral to bone growth and development?	Parathyroid hormone (PTH), calcitonin, and vitamin D

CONGENITAL BONE DISEASES

Osteogenesis imperfecta

What is osteogenesis imperfecta?	A group of heritable diseases characterized by abnormal type I collagen
How many types of osteogenesis imperfecta are there?	4 (types I to IV)
What is the usual clinical presentation of osteogenesis imperfecta?	Multiple fractures, often with minimal trauma
Besides bone, what else is affected in osteogenesis imperfecta?	Teeth, skin, and eyes
What are the characteristic eye findings in osteogenesis imperfecta?	Blue sclerae

What are the radiographic findings in osteogenesis imperfecta?	Thin and osteopenic bones, often with many foci of fracture callus

Osteopetrosis

What is osteopetrosis?	An inherited disorder characterized by abnormally dense bone
What causes osteopetrosis?	Failure of osteoclastic cells by an unknown mechanism
What are 2 other names for osteopetrosis?	Marble bone disease; Albers-Schönberg disease
Why the name "marble bone" disease?	Bones look short and block-like, and are radiodense, like marble.
What is the common clinical presentation of osteopetrosis?	Multiple fractures
Why are multiple fractures common in osteopetrosis?	Although bone is hyperdense, it is intrinsically disorganized. Consequently, it is weaker.
What are 2 common conditions associated with osteopetrosis?	1. Anemia due to decreased marrow space 2. Blindness, deafness, and other cranial nerve involvement due to narrowing of neural foramina
What are the 2 variants of osteopetrosis?	Autosomal recessive; autosomal dominant
Which is more severe?	The autosomal recessive variant is fatal in infancy.

METABOLIC BONE DISORDERS

Osteoporosis

What is osteoporosis?	A decrease in bone mass
What causes osteoporosis?	Impaired synthesis or increased resorption of bone matrix
Name 5 states with which osteoporosis is associated.	1. Postmenopause 2. Physical inactivity

3. Hypercorticism
4. Hyperthyroidism
5. Calcium deficiency

Describe the pathophysiology associated with osteoporosis of the elderly.

A continuous loss of bone occurs at the trabecular and cortical layers due to increased resorption.

What commonly prescribed drug induces osteopenia?

Steroids

What commonly results from osteopenia?

Fractures

What are the calcium and phosphorus levels in the blood in patients with osteoporosis?

Normal

What is seen radiographically in patients with osteoporosis?

Diffuse radiolucency of bone

What is the treatment for osteoporosis?

No cure. Calcium supplements, exercise, and estrogen therapy (in some patients) help reduce the risk, however.

BONE ABNORMALITIES WITH HORMONAL DISORDERS

Hyperparathyroidism

What is the effect of PTH on bone?

It stimulates the active phase of bone remodeling.

What are the 2 main causes of hyperparathyroidism?

Parathyroid hyperplasia and parathyroid adenoma

What are the 2 clinical features of hyperparathyroidism?

Bone pain and hypercalcemia

What are the significant laboratory values in hyperparathyroidism?

Calcium > 11.5 mg/dL; phosphorus < 2.0 mg/dL

What is seen on bone histologic examination in hyperparathyroidism?

An increased number of osteoclasts

After bone is resorbed, what replaces it?	Fibrous tissue
What abnormality is often seen in the fibrous tissue?	Hemosiderin pigment
What are the fibrous tissue lesions called?	Brown tumors
How is hyperparathyroidism treated?	By removal of the parathyroid lesion

Hypoparathyroidism

How does hypoparathyroidism affect bone?	It decreases the turnover rate.
What is the most common reason for hypoparathyroidism?	Surgical removal of parathyroid glands
What are the clinical signs of hypoparathyroidism?	Signs of hypocalcemia, including soft tissue ossification and calcification, abnormal dentition, and otosclerosis
What is seen on bone histologic examination in hypoparathyroidism?	Active osteoblasts and lack of osteoclasts
What is the treatment for hypoparathyroidism?	Administration of PTH or vitamin D

BONE ABNORMALITIES WITH NUTRITIONAL DISORDERS

Osteomalacia

What is osteomalacia?	A bone abnormality caused by defective calcification of osteoid matrix
What causes osteomalacia?	Vitamin D deficiency
In what age group does osteomalacia typically occur?	Adults
What can osteomalacia mimic radiographically?	Osteoporosis
How is osteomalacia diagnosed?	By bone biopsy

What is the treatment for osteomalacia?

Correct vitamin D deficiency

What is osteomalacia called when secondary to renal disease?

Renal osteodystrophy

Rickets

Define rickets.

Bone abnormality caused by defective calcification of osteoid matrix and increased thickness of epiphysial growth plates

What causes rickets?

Vitamin D deficiency

Describe the difference between rickets and osteomalacia.

Osteomalacia occurs in adults, rickets in children. Because bone growth is not complete in patients with rickets, skeletal deformities are common.

What are 6 clinical manifestations of rickets?

1. Craniotabes: thickening and softening of occipital and parietal bones
2. Late closing of fontanelles
3. Rachitic rosary: costochondral swelling
4. Harrison groove: depression of insertion site of diaphragm into rib cage
5. Pigeon breast: protrusion of sternum
6. Short stature caused by spinal deformity

What is the treatment for rickets?

Correction of vitamin D deficiency

Scurvy

Define scurvy.

Bone abnormality characterized by impaired osteoid matrix formation

What causes scurvy?

Vitamin C (ascorbic acid) deficiency

How does vitamin C deficiency lead to impaired bone formation?

Failure of proline and lysine hydroxylation required for collagen synthesis

Name 3 clinical characteristics of scurvy.

1. Subperiosteal hemorrhage
2. Osteoporosis
3. Epiphysial cartilage not replaced by osteoid

Why does subperiosteal hemorrhage occur?	Because of increased capillary fragility
What is seen on bone histologic examination in scurvy?	Decreased trabecular bone mass and abnormal osteoblasts
What is the treatment for scurvy?	Correction of vitamin C deficiency

INFECTIONS OF BONES

Pyogenic osteomyelitis

What is pyogenic osteomyelitis?	Infection of the medullary and cortical portions of the bone, including the periosteum
What bones are commonly affected:	
In children?	Long bones
In adults?	Vertebrae
What is the usual causative organism of pyogenic osteomyelitis:	
In children?	*Staphylococcus aureus*
In newborns (2 organisms)?	Group B β-hemolytic streptococci; *Escherichia coli*
In sickle cell anemia patients?	*Salmonella* organisms
In intravenous (IV) drug users?	*Pseudomonas* organisms
How do the causative bacteria spread in the body?	Hematogenously
In adults, what is the usual cause of pyogenic osteomyelitis?	Complications from surgery and compound fractures
What portion of the bone is most commonly involved initially?	Metaphysis

Name 3 reasons for persistent pyogenic osteomyelitis.

1. Necrotic bone acting as a locus (sequestrum) for persistent infection
2. Pyogenic exudate compressing vascular supply of bone
3. Inflammation in relatively avascular areas of bone

Name 2 clinical symptoms of pyogenic osteomyelitis.

Fever, local bone pain

What are significant laboratory test values in pyogenic osteomyelitis?

Marked leukocytosis, fever, and increased sedimentation rate

What is a localized infection surrounded by granulation tissue called?

Brodie abscess

How is a Brodie abscess treated?

Drain or debride the abscess; administer antibiotics.

How frequently do flare-ups occur with chronic osteomyelitis?

It varies, with intervals of months to years.

Tuberculous osteomyelitis

What is tuberculous osteomyelitis?

Bone infection due to spread of tuberculous organisms

How are the tuberculous organisms spread?

Hematogenously

What is tuberculous osteomyelitis with spinal involvement called?

Pott disease

What other bones does tuberculous osteomyelitis affect?

Hip, long bones, and bones of the hands and feet

What happens to affected bone?

Progressive destruction, with little ossification

HISTIOCYTOSIS X

What is histiocytosis X?

A group of disorders affecting other organ systems in addition to bone. It is

characterized by proliferation of
histiocytic cells.

**Histiocytic cells are similar
to what epidermal cells?**

Langerhans cells

**What are characteristic
markers of histiocytic cells?**

Birbeck granules

**What do Birbeck granules
look like?**

Tennis rackets

**Name 3 variants of histio-
cytosis X.**

1. Eosinophilic granuloma
2. Hand-Schüller-Christian disease
3. Letterer-Siwe disease

Eosinophilic granuloma

**What is characteristic of
eosinophilic granuloma?**

Histiocytic proliferation with inflammatory cells, including many eosinophils

**What is the clinical presen-
tation of eosinophilic
granuloma?**

Solitary bone lesion

**Does extraskeletal involve-
ment occur?**

Yes, commonly in the lung

What is the prognosis?

Best of all variants of histiocytosis X.
Lesions sometimes heal without
treatment.

Hand-Schüller-Christian disease

**What is characteristic of
Hand-Schüller-Christian
disease?**

Histiocytic proliferation with inflammatory cells

What is affected?

Bone, liver, spleen, and other tissues

**What population is
affected?**

Children < 5 years

**List the classic triad of
Hand-Schüller-Christian
disease.**

1. Skull lesions
2. Diabetes insipidus
3. Exophthalmos

What is the prognosis?

Better than Letterer-Siwe, worse than
eosinophilic granuloma

Letterer-Siwe disease

What is characteristic of Letterer-Siwe disease?

Widespread histiocytic proliferation

What population is affected?

Infants

What are 5 clinical findings in Letterer-Siwe disease?

1. Hepatosplenomegaly
2. Lymphadenopathy
3. Pancytopenia
4. Pulmonary involvement
5. Recurrent infections

What is the course of Letterer-Siwe disease?

Aggressive and fatal

CYSTIC BONE LESIONS

Unicameral bone cysts

What is another name for unicameral bone cysts?

Solitary bone cysts

What is the cause?

Unknown

What population is affected?

Young males

What portion of bone is usually affected?

Distal ends of long bones

Name 3 clinical signs of unicameral bone cysts.

1. Pain
2. Soft tissue swelling
3. Occasional fractures

What is seen on radiography of unicameral bone cysts?

Radiolucent area with smooth, thin cortex

What is their appearance on gross pathology?

Multiloculated cavity

What is the treatment for unicameral bone cysts?

Curettage with insertion of bone chips

What is the prognosis?

Excellent, with few recurrences

Aneurysmal bone cysts

What population is affected by aneurysmal bone cysts?	Females in 2nd to 3rd decade of life
What portion of bone is usually affected?	Metaphysis of long bones; vertebrae
Name the 2 clinical signs of aneurysmal bone cysts.	Pain; soft tissue swelling
What is seen on radiography of aneurysmal bone cysts?	Circumscribed zone of rarefaction, with extension into soft tissues
What is the size range of aneurysmal bone cysts?	Up to 20 cm
What is the gross pathology of aneurysmal bone cysts?	Bone is greatly distorted with irregular outlines. It appears spongy, with cystic spaces of various sizes.
Give 2 histologic differential diagnoses.	1. Giant cell tumor of bone 2. Telangiectatic osteosarcoma
How are aneurysmal bone cysts treated?	Removal of entire lesion with insertion of bone chips
What is the prognosis?	Recurrences occur 20% to 30% of the time.

BENIGN NEOPLASMS OF BONE

Fibrous dysplasia

Fibrous dysplasia most commonly affects what bones?	Ribs, femur, tibia, maxilla
Is fibrous dysplasia monostotic or polyostotic?	80% monostotic; 20% polyostotic
Polyostotic lesions are part of what syndrome?	Albright syndrome
What bone complications occur in fibrous dysplasia?	Deformity secondary to repeated fractures

Describe the radiographic appearance.	Well-defined zones of rarefaction surrounded by narrow rims of sclerotic bone
Describe the major histologic feature of fibrous dysplasia.	Proliferation of fibroblasts, which produce a dense collagenous matrix

What is the treatment:

For monostotic lesions?	Curettage or local resection
For polyostotic lesions?	Conservative (nonsurgical), because lesions stop growing after puberty

Osteochondroma

What is another name for osteochondroma?	Exostosis
Define osteochondroma.	Bony growth covered by a cartilaginous cap
What is osteochondroma's claim to fame?	Most common benign tumor of bone
Where does the tumor originate?	In the metaphysis
What are the 2 most frequent locations?	Distal femur; proximal tibia
What population is most commonly affected?	Males < 25 years
Does it undergo transformation to a malignant tumor?	Rarely
Describe the clinical symptoms.	Pain and compression of adjacent structures
What is the prognosis?	Excellent. Resection is usually curative.

Giant cell tumor

What is giant cell tumor?	Benign tumor characterized by multinucleated giant cells and fibrous stroma

Where does the tumor originate?	Epiphysis of long bones
What are the 2 most frequent locations?	Distal femur; proximal tibia
How does giant cell tumor appear radiographically?	Soap bubble appearance
What population is most commonly affected?	Females 20 to 40 years
What is the course?	Although benign, it is locally aggressive.
What is the prognosis?	Frequently recurs after local curettage.

Enchondroma

What is enchondroma?	Benign intramedullary cartilaginous neoplasm
Where does enchondroma most frequently occur?	Hands and feet
What population is most commonly affected?	All age groups

Osteoma

What is osteoma?	Benign tumor of mature bone
What are the 2 most frequent locations?	Skull; facial bones
What population is most commonly affected?	Males of any age
Osteoma occurring as multiple lesions, with intestinal polyps and soft tissue tumors, is known by what name?	Gardner syndrome
What are the clinical features of osteoma?	It is asymptomatic, unless drainage of paranasal sinus is blocked.
What is the prognosis?	Excellent. Resection is curative.

Osteoid osteoma

What is osteoid osteoma?	Neoplastic proliferation of osteoid and fibrous tissue
What are the most frequent locations of osteoid osteoma?	Ends of diaphysis of femur or tibia
What population is most commonly affected by osteoid osteoma?	Males < 25 years
What are the clinical features of osteoid osteoma?	Increasing pain, worse at night, relieved by aspirin
How does osteoid osteoma appear radiographically?	Central radiolucent area surrounded by sclerotic bone
What is the central radiolucent area called?	Nidus
What is in the nidus, microscopically?	Osteoblasts, calcification, and multinucleate giant cells
What is the prognosis for osteoid osteoma?	Excellent. Resection of nidus and sclerotic bone is curative.

Osteoblastoma

Name the 2 most frequent locations of osteoblastoma.	Vertebrae and long bones
What population is most commonly affected?	Males < 30 years
What are the clinical features of osteoblastoma?	Usually none
Radiographically, how does osteoblastoma appear?	Well-circumscribed lesion surrounded by sclerotic bone
What treatment allows the best prognosis?	Results are excellent when the lesion is removed by curettage.

MALIGNANT NEOPLASMS OF BONE

Osteosarcoma

Give another name for osteosarcoma.	Osteogenic sarcoma

State its claim to fame.

Osteosarcoma is the most common primary malignant tumor of bone.

Define osteosarcoma.

Malignant osteoid and bone-producing neoplasm

What causes osteosarcoma?

The cause is unknown.

Name the 2 most frequent locations of osteosarcoma.

Distal femur and proximal tibia

What population is most commonly affected?

Males 10 to 20 years old

What are the clinical features?

Pain, swelling, and pathologic fractures

What are the significant laboratory values?

A 2- to 3-fold increase in alkaline phosphatase values

Radiographically, elevation of periosteum is called what?

Codman triangle

How does tumor spread?

Hematogenously

Name 4 factors predisposing to osteosarcoma.

1. Paget disease
2. Ionizing radiation
3. Bone infarcts
4. Familial retinoblastoma

How does osteosarcoma appear on gross pathology?

Large necrotic and hemorrhagic mass

What is the microscopic appearance of osteosarcoma?

Malignant stroma containing osteoid and bone

How is osteosarcoma treated?

Surgical amputation of affected limb, and adjunctive chemotherapy

What is the prognosis for osteosarcoma?

Poor; 5-year survival rate is 5% to 20%.

Chondrosarcoma

What is chondrosarcoma?

Malignant cartilaginous neoplasm

Name the 4 most frequent locations of chondrosarcoma.

Proximal femur, proximal humerus, pelvis, spine

What population is most commonly affected?	Males 30 to 60 years old
Name 3 clinical features of chondrosarcoma.	Pain, swelling, and presence of mass for several years
Radiographically, how does chondrosarcoma appear?	Cortical destruction with occasional medullary involvement
From what 2 preexisting cartilaginous tumors can chondrosarcoma arise?	1. Multiple familial osteochondromatosis 2. Multiple enchondromatosis
How does chondrosarcoma appear on gross pathology?	Lobulated white or gray mass, with mucoid material and calcification
What is chondrosarcoma's microscopic appearance?	Poorly developed cartilage cells with anaplastic cells
What is the treatment for chondrosarcoma?	Total resection, if possible
What is the prognosis for chondrosarcoma?	Chondrosarcoma is slow growing, but has a high tendency to recur; 10-year survival rate is 50% to 60%.

Ewing sarcoma

What is Ewing sarcoma?	Undifferentiated round cell malignant tumor
In what 4 areas does Ewing sarcoma occur most often?	Long bones, pelvis, scapula, ribs
What population is most commonly affected?	Males < 15 years
What are the clinical features?	Pain, swelling, and presence of mass for several years
How does Ewing sarcoma appear radiographically?	Destructive appearance
What does subperiosteal reactive new bone resemble?	Onion skin
The early phase of Ewing sarcoma mimics what other disease?	Acute osteomyelitis

What genetic defect is present in Ewing sarcoma?	11, 22 translocation
Where does Ewing sarcoma arise?	Undifferentiated mesenchymal cells of the medullary cavity
How does Ewing sarcoma appear on gross pathology?	Hemorrhagic and necrotic destruction of medullary cavity
Microscopically, what is seen with Ewing sarcoma?	Undifferentiated small round cells in sheets or cords
How is Ewing sarcoma treated?	Amputation of limb; possibly chemo-therapy
What is the prognosis?	Poor. Malignant course with early metastases; the 5-year survival rate is 0% to 12%.

MISCELLANEOUS BONE DISEASES

Osteitis deformans

Give another name for osteitis deformans.	Paget disease of the bone
Define osteitis deformans.	Bone disease characterized by abnormal bony architecture with increases in osteoblastic and osteoclastic activity, and a "high turnover rate"
Name the 5 most common locations of osteitis deformans.	Spine, pelvis, skull, femur, and tibia
What population is most commonly affected?	Elderly persons
What causes osteitis deformans?	Cause is unknown; an infectious nature is postulated.
Describe the clinical features of osteitis deformans.	Pain, fracture, and skeletal deformities; deafness when skull involved; short stature when spine involved
Is osteitis deformans monostotic or polyostotic?	Both

Microscopically, how does osteitis deformans appear?	Marked medullary fibrosis; disorganization of normal trabecular pattern
What is the treatment for osteitis deformans?	Calcitonin or one of the diphosphonates
Why these drugs?	They decrease resorption, and thus decrease the high turnover rate.

Avascular necrosis

What is avascular necrosis?	Necrosis of bone, usually the femoral head, caused by infarction
Give 3 possible causes of avascular necrosis.	1. Emboli 2. Decompression syndrome ("the bends") 3. Sickle cell anemia
Radiologically, what is seen with avascular necrosis?	Reparative foci replacing necrotic bone
With what other conditions is avascular necrosis commonly associated?	1. Alcoholism 2. Corticosteroid treatment 3. Hyperuricemia 4. Systemic lupus erythematosus (SLE) 5. Trauma
What is the treatment for avascular necrosis?	Hemiarthroplasty
When avascular necrosis occurs in the femoral head of children, what is it called?	Legg-Calvé-Perthes disease

POWER RECALL

Name the 3 main functions of bone.	1. Mechanical stability 2. Mineral storage 3. Hematopoiesis
Macroscopically, name 2 types of bone.	1. Cortical bone 2. Cancellous bone
Name the 3 anatomic structures defined in relation to the physis.	1. Epiphysis 2. Metaphysis 3. Diaphysis

What cells resorb bone tissue?

Osteoclasts

What is osteogenesis imperfecta?

A group of heritable diseases characterized by abnormal type I collagen

What causes osteopetrosis?

Failure of osteoclastic cells by an unknown mechanism

Describe the common clinical presentation of osteopetrosis.

Multiple fractures. Although bone is hyperdense, it is intrinsically disorganized, and weaker.

Define osteoporosis.

A decrease in bone mass

Name 5 states associated with osteoporosis.

1. Postmenopause
2. Physical inactivity
3. Hypercorticism
4. Hyperthyroidism
5. Calcium deficiency

What reduces the risk of osteoporosis?

Calcium supplements, exercise, and in some cases, estrogen therapy

What is the effect of PTH on bone?

It stimulates the active phase of bone remodeling.

What causes osteomalacia?

Vitamin D deficiency

What is rickets?

Bone abnormality resulting from defective calcification of osteoid matrix and increased thickness of epiphysial growth plates. It is caused by vitamin D deficiency.

State the difference between rickets and osteomalacia.

Osteomalacia occurs in adults, rickets in children.

What causes scurvy?

Vitamin C (ascorbic acid) deficiency

What is the usual causative organism of osteomyelitis:

In children?

Staphylococcus aureus

In newborns (2 organisms)?

Group B β-hemolytic streptococci; *Escherichia coli*

In sickle cell anemia patients?	*Salmonella* organisms
In IV drug users?	*Pseudomonas* organisms
What are characteristic markers of the cells in histiocytosis X?	Birbeck granules
Name 3 variants of histiocytosis X.	1. Eosinophilic granuloma 2. Hand-Schüller-Christian disease 3. Letterer-Siwe disease
Describe the gross pathology of aneurysmal bone cysts.	Bone is greatly distorted with irregular outline, and appears spongy with cystic spaces of various sizes.
What is an exostosis, and by what other name is it known?	Bony growth covered by a cartilaginous cap. Also called osteochondroma.
What is the most common benign tumor of bone?	Exostosis
What is a giant cell tumor?	Benign tumor characterized by multi-nucleated giant cells and fibrous stroma
Name the 2 most common locations of an osteoma.	Skull; facial bones
What is the central radiolucent area in an osteoid osteoma called?	Nidus
Name the most common primary malignant tumor of bone.	Osteosarcoma
What population is most commonly affected by osteosarcoma?	Males, 10 to 20 years
Radiographically, elevation of periosteum is called?	Codman triangle
Name the 4 most common locations of chondrosarcoma.	Proximal femur, proximal humerus, pelvis, spine

What is Ewing sarcoma?   Undifferentiated round cell malignant tumor

What is Paget disease?   Bone disease characterized by abnormal bony architecture with increases in osteoblastic and osteoclastic activity and a "high turnover rate"

What is avascular necrosis?   Necrosis of bone, usually the femoral head, caused by infarction

JOINTS

ANATOMY

What is a joint?   An articulation between two or more bones

Name 2 types of joints.   Synovial (diarthrodial) joint; synarthrosis

Which type of joint allows for more movement?   Synovial joint

Synovial joints

How are synovial joints classified?   By the type of movement they permit

Name 4 types of synovial joints.
1. Uniaxial joint
2. Biaxial joint
3. Polyaxial joint (ball and socket)
4. Plane joint

Give an example of a plane joint.   Patella

What lines synovial joints?   The synovium

Does the synovium line the entire joint?   No, the articular cartilage is devoid of synovium.

What are the 3 functions of the synovium?
1. Regulates transport of nutrition in and out of the joint through joint fluids
2. Secretes substances (i.e., hyaluronate, lysosomal enzymes) that maintain the joint
3. Lubricates the joint

What are the 3 major constituents of articular cartilage?	1. Water 2. Proteoglycans 3. Type II collagen

Synarthrosis

What is a synarthrosis?	A joint that permits little movement
Name 4 types of synarthroses.	1. Symphysis 2. Synchondrosis 3. Syndesmosis 4. Synostosis
Describe a symphysis.	Union of two bones joined by fibro-cartilage and ligaments
Give an example of a symphysis.	Symphysis pubis
Describe a synchondrosis.	Union of bones with articular cartilage, but lacking a joint cavity
Give an example of a synchondrosis.	Sternal manubrial joint
Describe a syndesmosis.	Union of bones by only fibrous tissue
Give an example of a syndesmosis.	Cranial sutures
Describe a synostosis.	Pathologic bony connection between two bones
Give an example of a synostosis.	Spinal ankylosis

OSTEOARTHRITIS

What is osteoarthritis?	Chronic, noninflammatory joint disease characterized by progressive degeneration of articular cartilage with new bone formation subchondrally and at the affected joint
What is another name for osteoarthritis?	Degenerative joint disease (DJD)
State its claim to fame.	It is the most common type of arthritis.

Is DJD more common in males or females?

Females

At what age does osteoarthritis typically occur?

After 50 years

Name 3 factors implicated in the pathogenesis of DJD.

1. Increased load on cartilage
2. Decreased resilience of cartilage
3. Increased stiffness of bone adjacent to cartilage

What 2 types of joints are most commonly affected by DJD?

1. Weight-bearing joints
2. Posterior interphalangeal (PIP) and distal interphalangeal (DIP) joints of the upper extremity

What is the earliest histologic change seen in DJD?

Loss of proteoglycans from surface of articular cartilage

Anatomically, what is the next stage of DJD?

Fibrillation (development of cracks) in articular cartilage

Development of cracks results in what?

Eburnation

Describe eburnation.

Thick, shiny, smooth areas of subchondral bone due to loss of overlying cartilage

What forms when the eburnated bone cracks, allowing synovial fluid to reach the subchondral bone?

Subchondral bone cysts

What happens after subchondral bone cysts form?

Osteophyte (bony spur) formation, usually at the lateral portion of the joint

What is another name for osteophytes at:

The DIP joints?

Heberden nodes

The PIP joints?

Bouchard nodes

What are 4 radiologic findings in DJD?

1. Decreased joint space
2. Increased thickness of subchondral bone
3. Subchondral bone cysts
4. Osteophytes

Name 2 types of DJD.	Primary osteoarthritis; secondary osteoarthritis

What is the cause of:

Primary osteoarthritis?	Unknown
Secondary osteoarthritis?	Occurs in joints with known damage from trauma, metabolic factors, or inflammatory disorders
Which is more common, primary or secondary?	Secondary osteoarthritis
What is the treatment for DJD?	Exercise, weight loss, and supportive measures early; total joint replacement when disabling

RHEUMATOID ARTHRITIS

What is rheumatoid arthritis?	A chronic inflammatory arthritis primarily affecting synovial joints
What is the most likely cause of rheumatoid arthritis?	Autoimmune
What population is most commonly affected by rheumatoid arthritis?	Females ages 25 to 50
What is often present in serum?	Rheumatoid factor
What is rheumatoid factor?	An immunoglobulin with anti-IgG Fc specificity
Do titers of rheumatoid factor correspond to severity of disease?	Yes. There is a direct correlation.
What are the 4 stages of rheumatoid arthritis?	1. Acute inflammatory reaction 2. Hyperplasia and hypertrophy of synovial lining cells 3. Pannus (granulation tissue) extension 4. Fibrosis, contracture, and deformity from destruction

Describe a pannus.

A vascularized mass consisting of lymphocytes and plasma cells surrounding areas of necrosis.

What 3 initial symptoms, not related to joint involvement, are often present in patients with rheumatoid arthritis?

Fatigue, fever, and malaise

What joints are most frequently involved?

PIP and metacarpophalangeal (MCP) joints of hands and feet

What is the distribution of joint involvement?

Bilateral and symmetrical

When do the joints most commonly hurt?

In the morning or after inactivity

What chronic changes of the fingers occur with rheumatoid arthritis?

Ulnar deviation

In later stages of rheumatoid arthritis, what happens to the joints?

Ankylosis

Name 4 common extra-articular manifestations of rheumatoid arthritis.

1. Pericarditis
2. Pleuritis
3. Vasculitis
4. Amyloidosis

What is the treatment for rheumatoid arthritis?

Aspirin and corticosteroids are first-line treatments.

What is the prognosis for rheumatoid arthritis?

Recurrences and exacerbations occur. The disease ultimately is debilitating.

SPONDYLOARTHROPATHIES

What is spondyloarthropathy?

A group of arthritides similar to rheumatoid arthritis, but lacking rheumatoid factor

Name 4 types of spondyloarthropathy.

1. Ankylosing spondylitis
2. Reiter syndrome
3. Psoriatic arthritis
4. Enteropathic arthritis

Genetically, what is common among individuals with spondyloarthropathy?	A high incidence of HLA-B27 (class I histocompatability antigen)

Ankylosing spondylitis

What is ankylosing spondylitis?	An inflammatory arthropathy of the vertebral column and sacroiliac joint
Is ankylosing spondylitis more common in males or females?	It is more common in males.
At what age does ankylosing spondylitis occur?	Peak incidence is 20 years of age.
What percentage of patients are HLA-B27 positive?	> 90%
Eventually, what occurs in patients with ankylosing spondylitis?	Bony fusion of the vertebral bodies

Reiter syndrome

What is Reiter syndrome?	The triad of urethritis, conjunctivitis, and arthritis
Reiter syndrome resembles what other type of arthritis?	Rheumatoid arthritis
Over 50% of patients with Reiter syndrome develop what kind of skin lesions?	Keratoderma blennorrhagicum
Where do the skin lesions appear?	On the palms, soles, and trunk
What is the course of Reiter syndrome?	In 75% to 80% of patients, disease remits within 1 year.

Psoriatic arthritis

What is psoriatic arthritis?	Inflammatory arthritis associated with psoriasis
What percentage of patients with psoriasis develop psoriatic arthritis?	7% to 10%

What is the prognosis of psoriatic arthritis?	Disease is usually mild, and slowly progressive.

Enteropathic arthritis

What is enteropathic arthritis?	Inflammatory arthritis associated with inflammatory bowel disease (IBD)
What percentage of patients with IBD get arthritis?	10% to 20%
Does bowel resection relieve enteropathic arthritis?	It does in ulcerative colitis, but not in Crohn disease.

GOUT

Define gout.	Deposition of urate crystals in joints and other tissues
What population most commonly is affected by gout?	Middle-aged men
What causes gout?	Hyperuricemia due to an error of purine metabolism
What is the inheritance pattern?	Autosomal recessive
What causes the pain of gout?	Intense inflammatory response to the urate crystals
What joint does gout most commonly affect?	Metatarsophalangeal (MTP) joint of the great toe
What is gout in the MTP joint called?	Podagra
What often precipitates an attack of gout?	A large meal or alcohol intake
When do attacks of gout usually first occur?	At night
What are serum uric acid levels in patients with gout?	> 6 mg/dL

Name the deposits of urate surrounded by fibrous connective tissue.	Tophi
Give 2 common locations for tophi.	1. Helix and antihelix of ear 2. Achilles tendon
What other organ system is often affected by deposition of crystals?	Kidneys
What characterizes urate crystals at biopsy?	They are negatively birefringent under polarized light.

What is the treatment:

To reduce swelling and pain?	Colchicine
For prophylaxis?	Probenecid and allopurinol

CHONDROCALCINOSIS (PSEUDOGOUT)

What is chondrocalcinosis?	An inflammatory reaction in cartilage
What causes chondro-calcinosis?	Calcium pyrophosphate dihydrate (CPPD) crystal deposition
What population is affected by chondrocalcinosis?	Elderly persons
What abnormality predisposes to deposition of CPPD?	High levels of inorganic pyrophosphate in joints
What does chondrocal-cinosis resemble clinically?	Gout (hence the name "pseudogout")
Are metatarsophalangeal joints affected?	Usually not
How is the diagnosis of chondrocalcinosis made?	Biopsy of synovial fluid shows leukocytes with CPPD crystals.
What is characteristic of CPPD crystals at biopsy?	They are weakly birefringent under polarized light.

INFECTIOUS ARTHRITIDES

Gonococcal arthritis

What is gonococcal arthritis?	An acute inflammatory arthritis caused by gonococci
State the claim to fame of gonococcal arthritis.	It is the most common form of bacterial arthritis.
Is gonococcal arthritis monoarticular or poly-articular?	Monoarticular
What population is pre-disposed to gonococcal arthritis?	Sexually active persons between the ages of 20 and 40
What joint does gonococcal arthritis most commonly affect?	The knee
How does the spread of gonococci occur?	Hematologically
What is the clinical presen-tation of gonococcal arthritis?	Pain, swelling, tenderness, and limitation of motion in affected joint

How does gonococcal arthritis appear on radio-graphs:

Early?	Fluid accumulation
Late?	Destruction of articular surface
What is the treatment for gonococcal arthritis?	Antibiotics

Tuberculous arthritis

What is tuberculous arthritis?	A chronic inflammatory arthritis caused by spread of tuberculosis
What population does tuberculous arthritis most commonly affect?	Children

What is the clinical presentation of tuberculous arthritis?

It is similar to gonococcal arthritis, but presents late, after joint destruction has occurred.

What is present in cultures of fluid aspirated from patients with tuberculous arthritis?

Thick, purulent material and acid-fast bacilli

What is the treatment for tuberculous arthritis?

Anti-tuberculosis drugs

Lyme disease

What is Lyme disease?

Arthritis caused by the spirochete *Borrelia burgdorferi*

How is the spirochete transmitted?

In the eastern United States, by the tick *Ixodes dammini;* in the western United States, by the tick *I. pacificus*

Is Lyme disease mono-articular or polyarticular?

Polyarticular

What joints does Lyme disease affect?

The knees and other large joints

What is the characteristic skin lesion in Lyme disease?

Erythema chronicum migrans

Describe erythema chronicum migrans.

Slowly spreading, with characteristic "bull's-eye" lesions

How is the diagnosis of Lyme disease made?

IgM serum antibodies to *B. burgdorferi*

What is the treatment for Lyme disease?

Antibiotics

POWER RECALL

Name 2 types of joints.

Synovial (diarthrodial) joint; synarthrosis

Name 4 types of synovial joints.

1. Uniaxial joint
2. Biaxial joint
3. Polyaxial joint (ball and socket)
4. Plane joint

What lines synovial joints?   Synovium

Name 4 types of synarthroses.
1. Symphysis
2. Synchondrosis
3. Syndesmosis
4. Synostosis

Define osteoarthritis (degenerative joint disease; DJD).   A chronic, noninflammatory joint disease characterized by progressive degeneration of articular cartilage with new bone formation subchondrally and at the affected joint

What population does DJD most commonly affect?   Females > 50 years

What joints does DJD most commonly affect?
1. Weight-bearing joints
2. PIP and DIP joints of the upper extremity

What are the 4 typical findings in DJD?
1. Decreased joint space
2. Increased thickness of subchondral bone
3. Subchondral bone cysts
4. Osteophytes

What is rheumatoid arthritis?   A chronic inflammatory arthritis, of probable autoimmune origin, primarily affecting synovial joints

What population does rheumatoid arthritis most commonly affect?   Females 25 to 50 years

What is often present in serum of patients with rheumatoid arthritis?   Rheumatoid factor

What is present in the joint space of rheumatoid arthritis patients?   A pannus

What joints are most commonly involved in rheumatoid arthritis?   PIP and MCP joints of hands and feet

What is spondyloarthropathy?   A group of arthritides similar to rheumatoid arthritis but lacking RF

Name 4 types of spondylo-arthropathy.	1. Ankylosing spondylitis 2. Reiter syndrome 3. Psoriatic arthritis 4. Enteropathic arthritis
Genetically, what is common among those with spondyloarthropathy?	A high incidence of HLA-B27 (class I histocompatability antigen)
Eventually, what happens in ankylosing spondylitis?	Bony fusion of the vertebral bodies
What is Reiter disease?	The triad of urethritis, conjunctivitis, and arthritis
Define gout.	Deposition of urate crystals in joints and other tissues, caused by hyperuricemia
What joint does gout most commonly affect?	Metatarsophalangeal joint of the great toe
Define pseudogout.	An inflammatory reaction in cartilage caused by calcium pyrophosphate dihydrate (CPPD) crystal deposition
What is characteristics of crystals at biopsy:	
In gout?	Negatively birefringent under polarized light
In pseudogout?	Weakly birefringent under polarized light
Name the most common form of bacterial arthritis.	Gonococcal arthritis
Describe the clinical presentation of infectious arthritides.	Pain, swelling, tenderness, and limitation of motion in affected joint
What causes Lyme disease?	*Borrelia burgdorferi*
What skin lesion is characteristic of Lyme disease?	Erythema chronicum migrans

SKELETAL MUSCLE

ANATOMY

Are skeletal muscles considered upper or lower motor neurons?	Lower
Several myofilaments constitute one what?	Myofibril
What surrounds each myofibril?	Sarcoplasmic reticulum
Name the functional unit of the myofibril.	Sarcomere
In the myofibril, what anchors the thin actin filaments?	Z-band
What is the dark band appearing where the actin filaments surround the myosin filament?	A-band
What does the M line represent?	Zone of intermolecular bridging of myosin
Describe the 2 myofiber types.	
Type I?	Dark muscle (red), slow twitch
Type II?	White muscle, fast twitch
How do type II fibers react to training?	Hypertrophy
What muscle fibers are more important for:	
Marathon runners?	Type I
Sprinters?	Type II
Are any human muscles composed exclusively of one fiber type?	No

CONGENITAL MYOPATHIES

How do newborns with congenital myopathies usually present?	Hypotonia, decreased deep tendon reflex, and decreased muscle mass
What is necessary to distinguish congenital myopathies from muscular dystrophies?	Muscle biopsy, to look for histologic change

Central core disease

What muscle fibers does central core disease affect?	Type I
What is the histologic appearance of central core disease?	Degeneration of organelles from the central portion of type I fibers
What does the central core anomaly resemble?	Target cells from denervation atrophy of muscles
What is the course of central core disease?	Typically, the patient becomes ambulatory, but never develops normal muscle strength.

Rod myopathy

What is another name for rod myopathy? Why?	Nemaline myopathy. When first described, the rod-shaped clusters looked tangled and threadlike.
What fibers does rod myopathy affect?	Type I
Where do the rod-shaped structures appear?	Sarcoplasm
What is the course of disease?	Rod myopathy varies from mild and nonprogressive to a severe, progressive form.
In severe cases of rod myopathy, what causes death?	Respiratory failure

Myotubular myopathy

What fibers does myotubular myopathy affect?	Type I

What is another name for myotubular myopathy?	Central nuclear myopathy
Describe the histologic appearance of myotubular myopathy.	Type I fibers contain a round central pale zone or a single central nucleus.
Why is it called "myo-tubular"?	The fibers look like the myotube stage in the embryonic development of normal skeletal muscle.
What is the course of disease?	Myotubular myopathy is slowly progressive.

Mitochondrial myopathy

What is the mode of transmission of mitochondrial myopathy?	Maternally transmitted mitochondrial DNA abnormalities
Describe the histologic appearance of mitochondrial myopathy.	Ragged, red muscle fibers
What problems are associated with mitochondrial myopathy?	Multiple mitochondrial enzyme or coenzyme defects

MUSCULAR DYSTROPHIES

What are muscular dystrophies?	A group of diseases characterized by progressive degeneration of skeletal muscles
How do muscular dystrophies typically present?	With weakness and muscular wasting
How are muscular dystrophies usually differentiated?	1. Age of onset 2. Muscle groups involved 3. Mode of inheritance
What is usually used as a marker for progression of disease?	Creatine phosphokinase (CPK) levels

Duchenne muscular dystrophy

State the claim to fame of Duchenne muscular dystrophy.	It is the most common of all muscular dystrophies.

What population does Duchenne muscular dystrophy affect?

It is exclusive to males.

What is the mode of inheritance of Duchenne muscular dystrophy?

X-linked

What percentage of cases result from new mutations?

33%

Genetically, what causes Duchenne muscular dystrophy?

A deletion on the short arm of the X chromosome

What does this gene code for?

Dystrophin. The deficiency of this trace protein causes the disease.

State the most popular theory about the cause of Duchenne muscular dystrophy.

Dystrophin-deficient muscles lack the normal interaction between the sarcolemma and the extracellular matrix, leading to increased osmotic fragility.

Describe the earliest pathologic changes in Duchenne muscular dystrophy.

Irregular foci of regenerating and degenerating muscle fibers

Name the 3 histologic findings in Duchenne muscular dystrophy.

1. Variation in muscle fiber size
2. Necrosis of individual muscle fibers
3. Replacement of necrotic fibers by fibrofatty tissue

Clinically, at what age does weakness usually present?

1 to 4 years

Where is the weakness first noted?

Proximal muscle groups

What happens later, usually in the calf muscles?

Compensatory hypertrophy, followed by pseudohypertrophy

At what age do patients with Duchenne muscular dystrophy usually die?

In their teens

What usually causes death in patients with Duchenne muscular dystrophy?

1. Weakness of respiratory muscles
2. Cardiac arrhythmia due to myocardial involvement

Becker muscular dystrophy

What does Becker muscular dystrophy resemble?

Duchenne muscular dystrophy

Is Becker muscular dystrophy more or less severe than Duchenne muscular dystrophy?

Less severe

What causes Becker muscular dystrophy?

Abnormality in dystrophin. It is truncated, and consequently less functional.

Myotonic dystrophy

Define myotonic dystrophy.

Weakness associated with inability to relax muscles when contracted (myotonia)

What is the mode of inheritance of myotonic dystrophy?

Autosomal dominant

Myotonic dystrophy is more common in what age group?

Adults

At a genetic level, what correlates with the severity of myotonic dystrophy?

Trinucleotide repeat segment

With what 3 other conditions is myotonic dystrophy often associated?

1. Cataracts
2. Testicular atrophy in males
3. Baldness in males

Facioscapulohumeral muscular dystrophy

What 3 muscle groups are involved in facioscapulohumeral muscular dystrophy?

1. Muscles of facial expression
2. Muscles surrounding the scapula
3. Muscles attaching to the humerus

What is the course of facioscapulohumeral muscular dystrophy?

Slow and nondisabling. Patients have a normal life expectancy.

What is the mode of inheritance of facioscapulohumeral muscular dystrophy?

Autosomal dominant

MUSCULAR ATROPHIES

Name 2 types of muscular atrophy.	Denervation atrophy; disuse atrophy

Denervation atrophy

What is denervation atrophy?	Muscle atrophy due to interruption in the nerve supply
What muscle fibers are involved in denervation atrophy?	Types I (red) and II (white)
What do fibers often look like on cross section?	Target fibers, with a central area darker than the periphery, resembling a bull's-eye
What happens after reinnervation?	Fiber type grouping, where clusters of type I are adjacent to clusters of type II
What congenital, denervating atrophy disease is autosomal recessive and often causes death in the first year of life?	Werdnig-Hoffman disease (infantile spinal muscular atrophy)

Disuse atrophy

What patients are predisposed to disuse atrophy?	Immobilized patients
What fibers does disuse atrophy usually affect?	Type II
Describe the histologic appearance of disuse atrophy.	Angular atrophy
With what 2 entities are biopsies from patients with disuse atrophy often confused?	1. Upper motor neuron disease 2. Corticosteroid toxicity

MYASTHENIA GRAVIS

What is myasthenia gravis?	Autoimmune disease characterized by muscle weakness

What do the autoantibodies attack?

Acetylcholine receptors of the neuro-muscular junction

Does myasthenia gravis affect males or females?

It affects females twice as often.

Name 3 causes of muscle weakness and easy fatigability.

1. Partially blocked acetylcholine receptor sites
2. Decreased number of acetylcholine receptors
3. Widened synapse space

Myasthenia gravis is often associated with tumors or hyperplasia of what organ?

The thymus

What is the overall mortality for myasthenia gravis?

10%

Myasthenia gravis often improves with what class of drugs?

Anticholinesterases

Name 2 other treatments for myasthenia gravis.

1. Thymectomy
2. Corticosteroids

POWER RECALL

What is a sarcomere?

The functional unit of the myofibril

Describe the 2 myofiber types.

Type I fibers are dark muscle (red), slow twitch. Type II fibers are white muscle, fast twitch.

Marathon runners have more of what muscle fiber?

Type I

How do newborns with congenital myopathies usually present?

Hypotonia, decreased deep tendon reflex, and decreased muscle mass

Name 4 congenital myopathies.

1. Central core disease
2. Rod myopathy
3. Myotubular myopathy
4. Mitochondrial myopathy

What gives central core disease its name?

Degeneration of organelles from the central portion of type I fibers.

What fibers are affected in rod myopathy?

Type I

In rod myopathy, where do the rod-shaped structures appear?

Sarcoplasm

What is the course of myotubular myopathy?

Slowly progressive

What is the mode of transmission of mitochondrial myopathy?

Maternally transmitted mitochondrial DNA abnormalities

What are muscular dystrophies?

A group of diseases characterized by progressive degeneration of skeletal muscles

What is the marker for progression of muscular dystrophy?

Creatine phosphokinase levels

Name 4 types of muscular dystrophy.

1. Duchenne muscular dystrophy
2. Becker muscular dystrophy
3. Myotonic dystrophy
4. Facioscapulohumeral muscular dystrophy

What causes Duchenne muscular dystrophy?

A deletion on the short arm of the X chromosome results in lack of dystrophin.

Name 3 histologic changes in Duchenne muscular dystrophy.

1. Variation in muscle fiber size
2. Necrosis of individual muscle fibers
3. Replacement of necrotic fibers by fibrofatty tissue

What happens in the calf muscles of patients with Duchenne muscular dystrophy?

Compensatory hypertrophy, followed by pseudohypertrophy

Describe Becker muscular dystrophy.

A mild form of Duchenne muscular dystrophy

What is myotonic dystrophy?

Weakness associated with inability to relax muscles when contracted (myotonia)

Name 2 types of muscular atrophy.

Denervation atrophy; disuse atrophy

In denervation atrophy, what do fibers often resemble on cross section?

Target fibers

What fibers are usually affected in disuse atrophy?

Type II

What is myasthenia gravis?

Autoimmune disease characterized by muscle weakness

What do autoantibodies attack in patients with myasthenia gravis?

Acetylcholine receptors of the neuro-muscular junction

28

Skin

Describe the following terms.

Macule	Flat, nonpalpable, < 1 cm in diameter
Papule	Raised, palpable, < 1 cm in diameter
Patch	Flat (like a macule), > 1 cm in diameter
Plaque	Palpable (like a papule), > 1 cm in diameter
Vesicle	Fluid-containing blister, small (< 0.5 cm)
Bulla	Fluid-containing blister, large (> 0.5 cm)
Pustule	Blister that contains pus
Crust	Dried exudate from vesicle, bulla, or pustule
Hyperkeratosis	Thickening of stratum corneum; occurs in warts
Acanthosis	Thickening of epidermis (stratum spinosum), often from chronic irritation (e.g., a callus)
Spongiosis	Epidermal intercellular edema with widening of intercellular spaces; occurs in poison ivy
Lichenification	Accentuation of skin markings; may be caused by scratching

COMMON SKIN DISEASES

CONTACT DERMATITIS

What is contact dermatitis? Irritation of the skin caused by contact with agents that act either as antigens in

487

cell-mediated hypersensitivity or as direct irritants

What kind of contact dermatitis is typical after yard work?

Poison ivy

ACNE VULGARIS

What is acne vulgaris?

An inflammatory reaction of the pilosebaceous apparatus

Describe the 2-fold theory of the pathogenesis of acne vulgaris.

1. Hyperplastic sebaceous glands accumulate debris under a keratinous plug in an outer hair follicle. This causes distention and eventual rupture into surrounding dermis, with subsequent inflammatory reaction.
2. The anaerobic bacterium *Corynebacterium acnes* makes the reaction worse, but its exact role is unknown.

Name 4 possible causes of acne vulgaris.

1. Genetic component
2. Diet
3. Stress
4. Inadequate cleansing

When are flare-ups common in women?

Prior to menstruation

What is the treatment for acne vulgaris?

Tetracycline and vitamin A derivatives

PSORIASIS

What is psoriasis?

Chronic, recurrent, inflammatory process characterized by erythematous papules and plaques, with characteristic silvery scaling and sharply demarcated lesions

What is the etiology of psoriasis?

Likely genetic. It is thought to be autosomal dominant with incomplete penetrance.

What areas of the body does psoriasis most often affect?

Scalp, sacrum, and extensor surfaces of elbows and knees

| **Name a painful association.** | Psoriatic arthritis is a severe, destructive rheumatoid-like arthritis most commonly occurring in the fingers. |

PEMPHIGUS VULGARIS

Define pemphigus vulgaris.	An acantholytic, autoimmune disorder characterized by formation of intra-epidermal bullae
What causes pemphigus vulgaris?	IgG autoantibodies directed against an epidermal intercellular cement substance
Name 2 major complications of pemphigus vulgaris.	Infection; fluid loss

BULLOUS PEMPHIGOID

| **What is bullous pemphigoid?** | An autoimmune disorder characterized by autoantibodies to epidermal basement membrane. It is similar to pemphigus vulgaris, but not as severe. |
| **Which blisters rupture more easily, those of pemphigus vulgaris or bullous pemphigoid?** | Pemphigus vulgaris blisters rupture more easily because they are more superficial. |

KERATIN PRODUCTION DISORDERS

VERRUCA VULGARIS

| **What is verruca vulgaris?** | Common warts, which are firm, well-circumscribed growths due to hyper-keratosis, acanthosis, and papillomatosis. They are most commonly found on the fingers, but can occur anywhere on skin or mucosa. |
| **What is the etiology of verruca vulgaris?** | Human papillomavirus (HPV), which is often found in nuclei of vacuolated cells with clear cytoplasm and hyperchromatic nuclei (koilocytes) |

CONDYLOMA ACUMINATUM

| **Describe condyloma acuminatum.** | Large cauliflower-like masses around genital and anal regions, formed by fusion of smaller verrucous nodules |

What causes condyloma acuminatum?	HPV
How is this lesion transmitted?	Sexually
How is condyloma acuminatum treated?	Resection
What do you see under the microscope?	Koilocytes

MOLLUSCUM CONTAGIOSUM

What virus causes the characteristic dome-shaped papules of molluscum contagiosum?	A DNA poxvirus
Who gets molluscum contagiosum, and how?	Children get it most often. It is transmitted by direct contact.

SEBORRHEIC KERATOSIS

Describe seborrheic keratosis.	A brownish, slightly raised, verrucous, well-circumscribed lesion on the trunk, face, or arm
What is another name for seborrheic keratosis, and why?	Senile keratosis, because it is common in the elderly
What is a distinguishing characteristic of seborrheic keratosis?	Its "stuck-on" appearance

NONMALIGNANT PIGMENTED LESIONS

EPHELIS

What is ephelis?	A freckle
What causes ephelis?	An increase in melanin in the basal layer of the epidermis (in the keratinocytes)

LENTIGO MALIGNA

What is lentigo maligna?	A dark, pigmented macule with whitish,

hypopigmented borders that are due to melanocyte regression

Who gets lentigo maligna, and where?

Older people get them, predominantly on the face and neck (sun-exposed areas).

Describe the histology of lentigo maligna.

Increased number of clustered melanocytes with varying degrees of atypia

To what malignant process is lentigo maligna a precursor?

Lentigo maligna melanoma

NEVI

What is a nevocytic (nevocellular) nevus?

A mole. They are hyperpigmented areas composed of melanocytes and nevus cells.

Describe the 3 histologic types of nevi.

1. Intradermal: confined to dermis; cells in clusters, often not pigmented
2. Compound: cells are in the dermis and the epidermal-dermal junction
3. Junctional: cells confined to epidermal-dermal junction

Name 2 characteristics of a blue nevus.

1. Present at birth (usually on buttocks, face, or arm)
2. Formed by foci of fibroblastic, dendritic, pigmented cells

Why are they blue?

Because they are located deep in the dermis

What is "juvenile melanoma"?

A misnomer. Refers to a Spitz nevus, which is a reddish brown nodule occurring primarily in children. It is characterized by spindle-shaped cells and may be confused with melanoma, but is not malignant.

What is a dysplastic nevus?

A disorderly proliferation of melanocytes, dermal fibrosis, and often dermal lymphocytic infiltration. It appears atypical and is irregularly pigmented.

Is a dysplastic nevus malignant?

It is nonmalignant, but may transform into malignant melanoma.

SKIN MALIGNANCIES

BASAL CELL CARCINOMA

Describe the gross appearance of basal cell carcinoma.	Pearly papule; may have raised, "rolled borders" with central ulceration or depression. Usually occurs on sun-exposed areas (e.g., head, neck, ears, nose).
Describe the microscopic appearance of basal cell carcinoma.	Clusters of cells with oval nuclei and little cytoplasm; nuclei of cells at the periphery of the tumor have a characteristic palisade arrangement (Fig. 28–1).

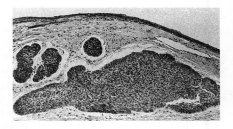

Does basal cell carcinoma metastasize?	Rarely. It is almost always cured by surgical resection, but may be locally aggressive.

SQUAMOUS CELL CARCINOMA

What is the metastasis rate of squamous cell carcinoma?	< 5%
Where does squamous cell carcinoma occur?	Sun-exposed skin; most frequently on face and back of hands, but can be anywhere on skin or mucous membranes
Which squamous cell carcinomas are more likely to metastasize?	Those arising in areas other than sun-exposed skin
From what kind of lesion does squamous cell carcinoma usually originate?	Actinic keratosis
What does the common presenting lesion look like?	A scaling, indurated, ulcerated nodule

MELANOMA

From what cells does melanoma arise?

Nevus cells or melanocytes

Name the 4 types of malignant melanoma.

1. Superficial spreading
2. Nodular
3. Lentigo maligna
4. Acral-lentiginous

Describe the 2 growth phases of malignant melanoma.

1. Radial: usually the initial phase; the lesion grows in all directions, but mostly laterally in the epidermis and the papillary zone of the dermis. These lesions do not metastasize and cure is common.
2. Vertical: growth extends into the reticular dermis or beyond. Prognosis is determined largely by depth of invasion.

Which type of malignant melanoma is the most common?

Superficial spreading

How does superficial spreading melanoma typically present?

As an enlarging pigmented nodule on the trunk and shoulders

Which type of malignant melanoma occurs on the palms, soles, and genitals of dark-skinned people?

Acral-lentiginous

Which type of malignant melanoma most often develops from an existing lesion?

Lentigo maligna melanoma. It arises from lentigo maligna.

Which type of malignant melanoma has the worst prognosis? Why?

Nodular. It usually presents in the vertical growth phase.

What are the 5 levels of malignant melanoma invasion?

1. Tumor cells are limited to the epidermis.
2. Tumor cells invade the papillary dermis.
3. Tumor cells fill the papillary dermis.

4. Tumor cells invade the reticular dermis.
5. Tumor extends through the skin into the subcutis.

What is the Breslow level?   0.76 mm of thickness. Lesions with invasion less than this have excellent cure rates.

HYPOPIGMENTATION DISORDERS

What causes albinism?   Failure of otherwise normal melanocytes to produce pigment

Name 4 problems associated with albinism.
1. Actinic keratosis
2. Malignant melanoma
3. Basal cell carcinoma
4. Squamous cell carcinoma

What is vitiligo?   An acquired loss of melanocytes in discrete areas of skin, producing white patches

MISCELLANEOUS SKIN DISORDERS

What is an inclusion cyst?   An epidermal nodule lined by stratified squamous epithelium and filled with keratin

What is an acrochordon?   A skin tag or fibroepithelial polyp; most common on the face or eyelids, trunk, neck, or axilla

What is a xanthoma?   A yellowish papule composed of focal dermal collections of lipid-laden histiocytes

With what are xanthomas associated?   Hypercholesterolemia

What is a keloid?   An abnormal proliferation of the connective tissue of scars, which results in large, raised lesions

POWER REVIEW

How does contact dermatitis occur?   Either by direct chemical injury, or an agent may act as an antigen in a type IV hypersensitivity reaction.

How is acne treated?

Tetracycline or vitamin A derivatives

What do the lesions of psoriasis look like grossly?

Erythematous papules and plaques with silvery scaling and sharply demarcated lesions

What body areas are most often involved in psoriasis?

Extensor surfaces of the elbows and knees, scalp, sacrum

Which blisters rupture more easily: those of bullous pemphigoid or pemphigus vulgaris?

Pemphigus vulgaris, because these bullae are more superficial

Which disease is worse, pemphigus vulgaris or bullous pemphigoid?

Pemphigus vulgaris

What is the characteristic microscopic appearance of cells infected with HPV?

Hyperchromatic nuclei in vacuolated cells

What are these vacuolated cells called?

Koilocytes

How is molluscum contagiosum passed from one child to another?

By direct contact

What lesion on older people has a characteristic "stuck-on" appearance?

Seborrheic keratosis

What causes freckles?

Increased melanin in the keratinocytes

What are the 3 histologic types of mole?

1. Intradermal
2. Compound
3. Junctional

What is the most common skin malignancy?

Basal cell carcinoma

What does basal cell carcinoma look like?

Rolled borders, central depression or ulceration, pearly papule

From what kind of lesion do most squamous cell malignancies arise?

Actinic keratoses

What are the 4 types of malignant melanoma?

Superficial spreading, nodular, lentigo maligna, and acral-lentiginous

Which is the most common malignant melanoma?

Superficial spreading

Which is the worst malignant melanoma to have?

Nodular. It usually presents in the vertical growth phase.

What is the Breslow level?

0.76 mm. Lesions with less than this depth of invasion have an excellent prognosis.

What usually causes a xanthoma?

High cholesterol levels

What group of people is most likely to get keloids?

African-Americans

29

Soft Tissues

Define "soft tissues."	Tissues of nonvisceral origin that lie between the skeleton and the dermis
Give 6 examples of soft tissue.	1. Fat 2. Blood vessels 3. Nerves 4. Paraganglia 5. Muscles 6. Connective tissue

PSEUDOTUMORS

What is a pseudotumor?	A mass due to a reaction to tissue injury
Is a pseudotumor a true neoplasm?	No
Name 4 materials found in pseudotumors.	1. Hemosiderin 2. Hemorrhage 3. Inflammatory cells 4. Myofibroblasts
What are the 8 types of pseudotumors?	1. Hematoma 2. Fat necrosis 3. Foreign-body granuloma 4. Xanthogranuloma 5. Myxoma 6. Pseudosarcomatous (nodular) fasciitis 7. Proliferative myositis 8. Myositis ossificans
How does a hematoma appear microscopically?	Many histiocytes, fibroblasts, endothelial cells, and white blood cells lining proliferating capillaries
What is fat necrosis?	A disruption of fat cells with subsequent release of fatty esters into surrounding tissues

What is fat necrosis usually due to?	A traumatic insult
Explain a foreign-body granuloma.	Foreign material incites a reaction of giant cells, which wall off the foreign body.
Where are xanthogranulomas most often found?	The retroperitoneum
Of what materials are xanthogranulomas composed?	Predominantly lipid, histiocytes, fibroblasts, and giant cells
What is the difference between fat necrosis and a xanthogranuloma?	A xanthogranuloma contains "foam cells," but fat necrosis does not.
What is a "foam cell"?	A lipid-filled histiocyte
What is a myxoma?	A benign, whitish tumor composed of proteoglycans and spindle cells
What are the 3 most common sites for myxoma?	1. Jaw 2. Thighs 3. Shoulder

SOFT TISSUE NEOPLASMS

BENIGN NEOPLASMS

What is the most common soft tissue tumor?	Lipoma
What is a lipoma?	An encapsulated mass of adipose tissue that lacks the lobulations of normal fat
What is a hemangioma?	Clusters of small or large blood channels lined by normal-appearing endothelial cells
What are the 2 types of hemangioma?	Capillary (small); cavernous (large)
What is a keloid?	A hypertrophic, post-traumatic scar in the dermis
In what group of people are keloids most common?	African-Americans

What are 2 types of nerve sheath tumors?	Neurofibroma; neurilemmoma (schwannoma)
What is von Recklinghausen disease?	A disorder in which multiple neurofibromas occur in association with café au lait spots on the skin
How is von Recklinghausen disease inherited?	Autosomal dominant
What is a leiomyoma?	A benign neoplasm of the smooth muscle
What is another name for a uterine leiomyoma?	Uterine fibroid
What is a rhabdomyoma?	A rare tumor of the skeletal muscle, usually found in the tongue
What is a fibrous histiocytoma?	A tumor consisting of a mixture of histiocytes and fibroblasts
Where are fibrous histiocytomas most commonly found?	The dermis
Are fibrous histiocytomas malignant?	No

MALIGNANT NEOPLASMS

What fraction of adult malignancies are soft tissue neoplasms?	$< 5\%$
How do malignant soft tissue neoplasms metastasize?	Hematogenously; often to the liver and lungs
How are malignant soft tissue neoplasms usually treated?	Surgical excision, followed by radiation. Chemotherapy is rarely useful.
What is a rhabdomyosarcoma?	A malignant tumor of skeletal muscle
Name 3 variants of rhabdomyosarcoma.	1. Pleomorphic 2. Embryonal 3. Alveolar

What is the most common soft tissue sarcoma of late middle and old age?

Malignant fibrous histiocytoma

Is malignant fibrous histiocytoma more common in males or females?

Males

What does malignant fibrous histiocytoma look like microscopically?

A mixture of extremely pleomorphic fibroblasts and histiocytes

What are the 2 types of liposarcoma?

Myxoid; nonmyxoid

What is another name for a neurofibrosarcoma?

Malignant schwannoma

What do the tumors of neurofibrosarcoma look like microscopically?

Many foci of necrosis. Mitoses are mixed with cellular spindle cells in a wavy pattern.

What is a synovial sarcoma?

A highly malignant soft tissue tumor of the synovial tissue

Where in the body is synovial sarcoma most commonly found?

The lower extremities

Where in relation to the joints is synovial sarcoma most often located?

In the tissue adjacent to the joint, not in the joint itself

What is special about the growth of synovial sarcoma tumors?

Their growth is biphasic.

What is an angiosarcoma?

A relatively rare tumor arising from the endothelial cells. It usually occurs in the skin.

Where are leiomyosarcomas most commonly found?

In the uterus

POWER REVIEW

What are the "soft tissues"?

Tissues between skeleton and skin, not including the viscera

What are the 4 most common types of pseudotumor?	1. Hematoma 2. Fat necrosis 3. Foreign-body granuloma 4. Xanthogranuloma
What is the difference between fat necrosis and a xanthogranuloma?	Xanthogranuloma contains "foam cells."
What are "foam cells"?	Lipid-filled histiocytes
What is the most common soft tissue tumor?	Lipoma
What are the 2 types of hemangioma?	Cavernous; capillary
What is the difference between the 2 types of hemangioma?	The size of the blood channels. Cavernous are bigger.
Who most commonly gets keloids?	African-Americans
Where are keloids classically found?	On the earlobe, after ear piercing
How is von Recklinghausen disease inherited?	Autosomal dominant
What tumor is associated with von Recklinghausen disease?	Neurofibroma
What is a uterine fibroid?	A leiomyoma
How do soft tissue tumors metastasize?	Through the blood
Where do soft tissue tumors metastasize?	The lungs (most common) and liver
Who is particularly at risk for developing a malignant schwannoma?	People with neurofibromatosis
Are synovial sarcomas usually found in the joints?	No, they are most often found in the tissue around the joints.

CONGENITAL DISORDERS

NEURAL TUBE DEFECTS (NTD)

What are they?

A group of disorders characterized by incomplete closure of the neural tube in early gestation which results in dorsal midline defects at birth

What structures can be involved?

Vertebrae, skull, brain, spinal cord, and meninges

NTDs are associated with an increase in what in the maternal serum?

α-fetoprotein

What are 3 possible reasons for NTDs?

1. Presence of pathologic state in utero at time of neural tube closure (metabolic, nutritive, toxic, or infective causes)
2. Faulty implantation of placenta
3. Genetic abnormalities

What is the most common NTD?

Spina bifida

What is the defect in spina bifida?

Failure of posterior vertebral arches to close

What is spina bifida occulta?

Same as spina bifida, but with no clinical abnormalities. Often there are only one or two vertebral arch defects.

What physical finding can be the only clue to spina bifida occulta?

Dorsal midline tuft of hair, overlying the site of defective vertebra

What malformation can be associated with lumbar spina bifida?

Arnold-Chiari malformation

What is a meningocele?

Herniation of meninges (arachnoid, dura) through a vertebral defect

What is meningomyelocele?

Herniation of meninges and spinal cord through a vertebral defect

What is the most severe NTD?

Anencephaly

Describe the clinical features of anencephaly.

Diminished or absent fetal brain tissue, usually associated with absence of overlying skull. Cerebral hemispheres, diencephalon, and midbrain can also be absent.

In anencephaly, what is exposed instead of fetal brain tissue?

A mass of undifferentiated vascular tissue

HYDROCEPHALUS

What is it?

Increased volume of cerebrospinal fluid within the cranial cavity

Name 4 types of hydrocephalus.

1. Internal hydrocephalus
2. External hydrocephalus
3. Communicating hydrocephalus
4. Noncommunicating hydrocephalus

What is the difference between internal and external hydrocephalus?

1. Internal: Increased CSF in the ventricles
2. External: Increased CSF in the subarachnoid space

What is the difference between communicating and noncommunicating hydrocephalus?

1. Communicating: CSF can freely flow between ventricles and spinal subarachnoid space
2. Noncommunicating: The flow of CSF is obstructed between the ventricles and spinal subarachnoid space, causing proximal dilation of the ventricular system

What can often be seen in infants with hydrocephalus?

Marked enlargement of the skull

Why does this enlargement occur?

Cranial sutures are not closed yet.

What are the causes of noncommunicating hydrocephalus?	Anything that can obstruct the CSF flow, including: 1. Congenital malformations 2. Inflammation 3. Tumors 4. Choroid plexus papilloma (rare; produces excess CSF)
What is hydrocephalus ex vacuo?	Apparent enlargement of ventricles because of decreased cerebral mass, not because of obstruction or increased CSF production.
Name 2 diseases characterized by decreased cerebral mass.	1. Ischemic brain atrophy 2. Alzheimer disease (advanced)

ARNOLD-CHIARI MALFORMATION

What is it?	Caudal (downward) displacement of medulla and cerebellum through foramen magnum into the cervical vertebral canal. It can be associated with lumbar spina bifida.
What defect is commonly associated with Arnold-Chiari malformation?	Thoracolumbar meningomyelocele
Name 2 consequences of Arnold-Chiari malformation.	1. Pressure atrophy of displaced brain tissue 2. Hydrocephalus, resulting from obstruction of CSF outflow tract

OTHER CONGENITAL DISORDERS OF THE NERVOUS SYSTEM

What is fetal alcohol syndrome?	A spectrum of characteristic dysmorphic features and developmental defects resulting from maternal alcohol intake during pregnancy
Name 6 features that can be found in fetal alcohol syndrome.	1. Microcephaly 2. Atrial septal defect 3. Mental retardation 4. Intrauterine growth retardation (IUGR) and subsequent growth failure 5. Short palpebral fissures 6. Micrognathia (small mandible)

What is Bourneville disease?	Another name for tuberous sclerosis syndrome
What is the pathogenesis of the tuberous sclerosis syndrome?	Disorder of migration and arrested maturation of neural ectoderm, resulting in hamartomas (tubers) of the brain, retina, and viscera
Name 4 features of tuberous sclerosis syndrome.	1. Multiple tubers in the cerebral cortex and periventricular areas 2. Adenoma sebaceum of the skin (primarily facial) 3. Angiomyolipoma of the kidney 4. Rhabdomyoma of the heart
What is the pathology of the "tuber"?	Proliferations of atypical multinucleated astrocytes, appearing macroscopically as small, white nodules
What is seen on the skin under an ultraviolet Wood lamp?	Discrete areas of hypopigmentation known as "ash-leaf spots"
What is the common clinical presentation of patients with tuberous sclerosis syndrome?	Infantile seizures and mental retardation
What is agenesis of the corpus callosum?	Complete or partial absence of the corpus callosum, wherein the only connection between the 2 cerebral hemispheres is at the brainstem. It is often asymptomatic.
What is von Recklinghausen disease?	An autosomal dominant disorder characterized by café au lait spots, multiple cutaneous neurofibromas, and Lisch nodules
What is another name for von Recklinghausen disease?	Neurofibromatosis
What are café au lait spots?	Small areas with irregular margins of increased pigmentation on the skin
What are Lisch nodules?	Pigmented nodules of the iris, consisting of melanocytes

Name the 2 types of neuro-fibromatosis, and the characteristics associated with each.	1. Peripheral (Type 1): Skin lesions, dermal and peripheral nerve tumors 2. Central (Type 2): Bilateral schwanno-mas of the acoustic nerve, and associated meningiomas, gliomas, and neurofibromas
Name 4 hereditary degenerative disorders of the nervous system and identify their pattern of inheritance.	1. Huntington disease (autosomal dominant) 2. Wilson disease (autosomal recessive) 3. Lipid storage diseases (e.g., Tay-Sachs disease and Niemann-Pick disease) 4. Friedrich ataxia (autosomal recessive)

CEREBROVASCULAR DISORDERS

What is the most common disorder of the central nervous system (CNS)?	Cerebrovascular disease; third most-common cause of death in the United States
Name 2 major categories of cerebrovascular disease.	1. Infarction (more common) 2. Hemorrhage
What are transient ischemic attacks (TIAs)?	Episodes of focal neurologic defects caused by temporary lack of cerebral blood flow, with complete resolution of deficits
How long do TIAs last?	Normally, a few minutes, but they can last up to 24 hours
What are some common neurologic defects seen in TIAs?	Amaurosis fugax, hemiplegia, and other cranial nerve defects
If TIAs are present, there is increased risk for what?	Increased risk of cerebral infarct (stroke)
What are 2 mechanisms of brain infarction?	Occlusion of the arterial blood supply to the brain from thrombosis, or embolism
What is the most common cause of vascular thrombosis?	Atherosclerotic plaques in blood vessels. They can rupture and initiate the coagulation cascade.
Name the 3 most common sites of cerebral thrombosis.	1. Bifurcation site of common carotid into internal carotid and external carotid arteries

2. Branching sites of circle of Willis, especially the middle cerebral artery (MCA)
3. Vertebral and basilar arteries, especially bifurcation sites

What clinical findings can be seen with arterial obstruction of MCA?

Findings depend on extent of collateral circulation, but may include:
1. Contralateral paralysis
2. Motor and sensory deficits
3. Aphasias

Name 5 causes of embolic occlusion.

1. Cardiac mural thrombi
2. Valvular vegetations, seen in infective endocarditis
3. Tumor cells
4. Air bubbles
5. Fat droplets

What is the most common site of embolic occlusion?

MCA

What are lacunae?

Small healed infarcts that appear grossly as "pits" in brain matter

What are some clinical manifestations of lacunar strokes if the obstruction of vessels occurs

In the internal capsule?

Pure motor deficits

In the thalamus?

Pure sensory deficits

Where are the 2 types of hemorrhagic disease?

1. Intracerebral hemorrhage (brain substance)
2. Subarachnoid hemorrhage (subarachnoid space)

What are 4 predisposing conditions that increase the risk of intracerebral hemorrhage?

1. Hypertension (most common)
2. Coagulation disorders, including thrombocytopenia
3. Hemorrhage within primary or metastatic cerebral neoplasms
4. Leukemia, in which neoplastic cells obstruct small vessels

Where are the 4 most common sites of intracerebral hemorrhage?	1. Basal ganglia 2. Pons 3. Cerebellum 4. Frontal lobe
What develops as a result of chronic hypertension?	Charcot-Bouchard aneurysms
Are these likely to rupture into brain parenchyma?	Yes
What type of aneurysm can rupture into the subarachnoid space?	Berry aneurysm, commonly found on the circle of Willis
What increases risk of rupture?	Hypertension
Name 3 other causes of subarachnoid hemorrhage (SAH).	1. Arteriovenous malformations 2. Trauma 3. Hemorrhagic diatheses
What is the most common cause of SAH?	Trauma

HEAD AND SPINE INJURIES

What is the #1 cause of most head and spine injuries?	Motor vehicle accidents (MVAs)

HEAD INJURIES

Name 4 types of injury to the brain in head trauma.	1. Intracranial hemorrhage (epidural, subdural, subarachnoid) 2. Concussion 3. Contusion 4. Laceration
What artery is injured in an epidural hemorrhage?	Middle meningeal artery (MMA)
How is the MMA injured?	Laceration from skull fracture
What is the clinical presentation of epidural hemorrhage?	First, loss of consciousness immediately after the injury. Then, a lucid interval, followed by acute signs of increased intracranial pressure (ICP).

What is causing the increased ICP?	Hematoma external to the dura mater presses inward, causing local brain compression
What is the treatment for epidural hemorrhage?	Immediate surgical decompression to prevent subtentorial herniation
What vessels are injured in a subdural hematoma?	Most commonly, the bridging veins from the cerebrum to venous sinuses in the dura mater
Name 2 causes of subdural hematoma.	1. Blow to the head, commonly in the frontal or occipital regions 2. Birth injury
What is the clinical presentation of subdural hematoma?	More insidious signs of decreasing mental status and enlargement of the hematoma can occur days to weeks after seemingly insignificant head injury.
Does the enlargement result from the bridging veins still hemorrhaging days to weeks after the injury?	No; the enlarging hematoma is thought to result from osmotic properties of water movement into the collection of blood.
Describe the course of a concussion?	It is usually associated with loss of consciousness, characterized by temporary widespread brain paralysis without obvious organic pathology, usually associated with complete recovery.
What is hypothesized to be the mechanism of injury of a concussion?	Rotational or shearing strains on the brain
What is a contusion brain injury?	Likened to a "bruise" on the brain, it results from torn capillaries from a blow to the calvarium.
What are 2 types of contusions?	1. Coup: Lesion is located directly beneath area of impact 2. Contrecoup: Lesion is opposite to the area of impact
What is the clinical presentation?	Loss of consciousness, possibly progressing to coma or death

What is the gross appearance of an acute contusion?	1. Swollen edematous gyri 2. Petechial hemorrhages
What is the gross appearance of an old contusion injury?	Sunken areas of brain, with small cysts
What is the microscopic appearance of an old contusion injury?	Gliosis
What is the microscopic appearance of an acute contusion injury?	Edematous cortex and subcortical white matter; fresh pericapillary hemorrhages
What are Duret hemorrhages?	The petechiae seen in acute contusions

SPINE INJURIES

What is a cord crush injury?	Compression and contusion of the spinal cord
What is the common mechanism of injury?	Dislocation of vertebra, most commonly in lower cervical area, following forcible flexion as in an MVA
What is herniated in a "slipped disc"?	Nucleus pulposus, the center of the intervertebral disc, through a defect in the annulus fibrosis, causing pressure on nerve roots
What is the most common area?	Lumbosacral; L4–5 or L5–S1 discs
What is the common clinical presentation?	Sciatica, or lower back pain after mild or moderate trauma

INFECTIONS OF THE NERVOUS SYSTEM

BACTERIAL INFECTIONS

What is the most common bacterial infection of the CNS?	Bacterial meningitis
In what population is bacterial meningitis most common?	Children

Name 5 causative micro-organisms of bacterial meningitis.

1. *Neisseria meningitidis* (meningo-coccus)
2. *Streptococcus pneumoniae* (pneumo-coccus)
3. *Haemophilus influenza type b* (now rare because of vaccine)
4. *Escherichia coli*
5. Group B Streptococcus
6. *Listeria monocytogenes*

Which of these causes of bacterial meningitis is most common in each of the following populations?

Newborns?

Now, Group B Strep. (Formerly, *E. coli*.)

Children?

S. Pneumoniae. H. influenzae is now rare because most children are immunized.

Adolescents and adults?

Meningococcus and pneumococcus

Elderly?

Listeria monocytogenes, pneumococcus

How does the pathogen obtain access to the meninges?

1. Direct invasion (from facial sinuses or middle ear)
2. Hematogenous seeding

What are the 3 classic clinical signs of bacterial meningitis?

1. Mental status changes
2. Fever
3. Nuchal rigidity (neck stiffness)

What are other associated symptoms?

Vomiting, headache, confusion, and seizures

What are the 3 findings in CSF diagnostic for bacterial meningitis?

1. Increased protein
2. Decreased glucose (<2/3 serum glucose)
3. Many polymorphonuclear neutrophils (PMNs)

What will be noted about the opening pressure on lumbar puncture (LP) for a patient with bacterial meningitis?

Increased pressure

What imaging test should be performed if papil-ledema or focal neurologic signs are present?

Head CT scan before LP, to rule out increased ICP from hydrocephalus or mass lesion

What can occur if a mass lesion is present?	Risk of brain herniation into spinal canal when pressure is released at the site of LP
What are the gross pathologic findings in the subarachnoid space?	Purulent exudate

CEREBRAL ABSCESS

What is the most common etiology of cerebral abscess?	Secondary infection from primary sources elsewhere in the body
Name 6 common primary sources of infection.	1. Otitis media 2. Frontal sinusitis 3. Mastoiditis 4. Lung abscess, empyema or other bronchopulmonary infection 5. Infective bacterial endocarditis
What are the clinical symptoms?	Increased ICP and source of primary infection
What are the CSF findings?	Increased opening pressure, slightly increased protein and lymphocytes, and no change in glucose
What organisms are seen in CSF?	None are usually seen, unless rupture of abscess has occurred.
What are the gross pathologic findings?	Cavitary lesion in the brain filled with thick exudate, walled off by edematous tissue
What can occur if infection spreads beyond abscess wall?	Encephalitis

MENINGEAL TUBERCULOSIS

What part of the nervous system is the most common site of tuberculous infection?	Meninges
How does the mycobacteria gain access to the meninges?	Miliary dissemination from another source elsewhere in the body

What are the clinical features of tuberculous infection of the meninges?	Gradual onset of anorexia, weight loss, and night sweats. Patient may also have mood changes, periods of drowsiness and delirium, and intermittent lucid intervals.

What are the CSF findings?

1. Increased lymphocytes
2. Significantly increased protein
3. Decreased glucose
4. Acid-fast bacilli in CSF

What are the gross pathologic findings in tubercular meningitis?

1. Gray-white thin exudate in meninges, pooling in the basilar cisterns and sylvian fissure
2. Tubercles (round white nodules) at the periphery

What is the microscopic pathology?

1. Granulomas composed of lymphocytes and large mononuclear cells
2. Tubercle bacilli

FUNGAL INFECTION

What are common pathogens of fungal infection in the CNS?

1. Cryptococcus neoformans
2. Coccidioides immitis
3. Aspergillus
4. Histoplasma

What predisposes an individual to fungal infection?

Impaired immunity

PARASITIC INFECTIONS

What is toxoplasmosis?

Parasitic infection in which the pathogen is *Toxoplasma gondii*

What is the source of toxoplasmosis in neonates?

Transmission transplacentally from infected mother

What are some other modes of infection?

1. Ingestion of foods contaminated by animal urine or feces
2. Contamination from household pets (i.e., cats)

What are 3 neurologic characteristics of congenital infection?

1. Hydrocephalus
2. Seizures
3. Microcephaly

What is the characteristic finding on radiologic studies?	Periventricular calcifications
Name the 3 areas of involvement in the brain.	1. Cerebral cortex 2. Basal ganglia 3. Retina
What is the most common site of toxological infection in adults?	Lymph nodes

VIRAL INFECTIONS

What is another name for viral meningitis?	Aseptic meningitis
How are the clinical findings different from bacterial meningitis?	None; they are the same: fever, headache, and nuchal rigidity
What are the CSF findings?	1. Increased lymphocytes 2. Moderate increase in protein 3. Normal glucose
What are the changes found in the brain substance occurring in meningo-encephalitis or encephalitis?	1. Perivascular cuffing (mononuclear cell infiltrate in the Virchow-Robin spaces around the vasculature) 2. Inclusion bodies in neuron or glial cells 3. Glial nodules (nonspecific proliferation of microglia)
Name 6 examples of CNS viral infection.	1. Arbovirus encephalitis (St. Louis, Eastern equine, Western equine) 2. Herpes simplex 3. Poliomyelitis 4. Rabies 5. Cytomegalovirus 6. HIV

Arbovirus Encephalitis

What does "arbo" in arbovirus indicate?	**AR**thropod **BO**rne
What is meant by "vector"?	Mode of transfer from reservoir to human
What is the vector for all 3 types of arbovirus?	Mosquito

**What are the clinical
characteristics of each of
the following:**

    A mild case of arbovirus?   Influenza-like illness

    **A severe case of
arbovirus?**   High fever, headache, meningeal signs
followed by coma and death

**What are 3 types of
arbovirus encephalitis?**

1. St. Louis
2. Eastern equine
3. Western equine

**What is the reservoir for
the St. Louis arbovirus?**   Horses and birds

    Eastern equine?   Horses and birds

**Which is more severe
clinically: Western or
Eastern equine arbovirus
infection?**   Eastern

**What area traditionally has
a lot of horses, birds, and
most importantly, mosqui-
tos, thus a higher incidence
of arbovirus infection?**   Maryland and Virginia Eastern shore
(especially areas of standing water)

Herpes Simplex Encephalitis

What causes it?   HSV type 1

**In what age group does
herpes simplex encephalitis
occur most often?**   Teenagers, young adults (severe)

**What part of the brain is
affected?**   Temporal lobe

What happens to the brain?   It becomes swollen, hemorrhagic, and
necrotic.

Poliomyelitis

**What deteriorates in
poliomyelitis?**   Anterior horn cells of spinal cord

**What are the early
symptoms?**   Fever, malaise, and headache

What are the late symptoms?	Meningitis and paralysis
What is the prognosis?	Mortality from respiratory failure is 5%–25%. Some muscles improve, while others remain permanently paralyzed.
Why is poliomyelitis rare today?	An effective vaccine exists.

RABIES

Name 6 animals that can carry the rabies virus in their saliva.	Dog, raccoon, fox, bat, squirrel, and skunk
What are the clinical manifestations of rabies?	Severe encephalitis with increased excitability of the CNS. Muscle contractions and convulsions can occur after minimal stimuli.
What are 3 histologic findings of rabies?	1. Neuronal degeneration 2. Perivascular cuffing in brainstem and spinal cord 3. Negri bodies (eosinophilic intracytoplasmic inclusion bodies)
Where are Negri bodies found?	Hippocampus and cerebellum (Purkinje cells)

CYTOMEGALOVIRUS (CMV) INFECTION

What organs can be affected in CMV infection?	Brain, spinal cord, kidneys, liver, GI tract, and salivary glands
What is the characteristic histology?	Giant cells with eosinophilic inclusions involving nucleus and cytoplasm
What type of persons are at increased risk?	Immunosuppressed individuals
What are the clinical signs of severe infantile infection?	Microcephaly, chorioretinitis, hepatosplenomegaly, and mental retardation
What can be seen on radiologic evaluation of the brain?	Periventricular calcifications

HIV INFECTION

Can neurologic dysfunction caused by HIV infection be seen before the onset of immunodeficiency?	Yes, it can be the presenting symptom.
What cells are thought to carry the virus into the nervous system?	Cells of monocyte-macrophage origin
What is the most common clinical presentation?	AIDS dementia complex
What are the common complaints of AIDS dementia complex?	Difficulty concentrating, memory impairment, slow thinking, depression, personality changes, lethargy, and coordination problems
What defines AIDS versus HIV infection?	Tuberculosis, cryptococcus, toxoplasmosis, cytomegalovirus, and other opportunistic infections are present in AIDS.
What 2 neoplasms are traditionally associated with HIV infection?	Lymphoma, Kaposi sarcoma

SLOW VIRUS INFECTION

Name 4 examples of suspected slow virus infection.	1. Kuru 2. Creutzfeldt-Jakob disease 3. Subacute sclerosing panencephalitis 4. Progressive multifocal leukoencephalopathy
What characterizes slow virus infections?	Long incubation period, little inflammatory response, and progressive deterioration
What is the histology?	Spongiosis, with numerous clusters of small cysts in the CNS gray matter
What 2 diseases do you suspect if dementia occurs acutely?	Creutzfeldt-Jakob disease; normal pressure hydrocephalus

Where was kuru first documented?	A cannibal tribe in New Guinea, which ritualized the practice of consuming the human brain
What findings are most prominent on presentation of kuru?	Cerebellar degeneration with marked tremor, ataxia, slurred speech, and progressive mental deficiency. Death will occur in a few months.
What is believed to be responsible for causing Creutzfeldt-Jakob disease?	Prion, a proteinaceous protein, once thought to be a self-replicating, non-nucleotide particle
What is subacute sclerosing panencephalitis?	Persistent infection with measles virus, usually infected in infancy but asymptomatic until late childhood or early adolescence. Prognosis is slowly progressive and usually fatal.
What is atypical about the measles virus?	Lack of M component of the virus, responsible for extracellular spread; perhaps responsible for slow infection
What is progressive multifocal leukoencephalopathy (PML)?	Rapidly progressive demyelination in multiple foci throughout the brain
What is the etiology of PML?	Most commonly, the Jakob-Creutzfeldt polyoma type of the papovavirus
What diseases can often be associated with PML?	Leukemia, lymphoma, or immuno-deficiency diseases

TUMORS

What percentage of all nervous systems disorders are neoplasms?	Approximately 10%
What is the incidence of neoplastic disease of the spinal cord?	Very rare
Are the majority of intra-cranial neoplasms above or below the tentorium	
In adults?	Supratentorial (above)

In children?

Infratentorial (below)

Are CNS tumors the most common malignancy in children?

No, but they are the 2nd most common after leukemia.

Where do most primary malignant CNS tumors metastasize?

They usually don't metastasize.

What can be some direct effects of intracranial tumors?

1. Neurologic dysfunction, with focal deficits depending on location of neoplasm
2. Electrically unstable neurons, with predisposition to epileptiform activity

Name 6 secondary effects of intracranial tumors.

1. Brain edema
2. Compression with resultant deficiency of vascular supply
3. Ischemia
4. Necrosis
5. Herniation of brain and/or cerebellar tonsils
6. Hydrocephalus

What can often be seen on funduscopic examination in a patient with intracranial tumors?

Papilledema (swelling caused by edema of optic nerve papillae)and retinal vein engorgement

Name the 4 most common intracranial tumors in adults (in order of frequency).

1. Glioblastoma multiforme
2. Metastatic tumors (from extracranial primary sites)
3. Meningioma
4. Acoustic neuroma

Name the 4 most common intracranial tumors in children (in order of frequency).

1. Astrocytoma
2. Medulloblastoma
3. Ependymoma
4. Craniopharyngioma

Name 3 other neoplasms of the CNS found in children.

1. Retinoblastoma
2. Neuroblastoma
3. Hemangioblastoma

How does a glial tumor grow differently from a non-glial tumor?

Glial tumors grow by infiltration, and thus cannot be completely removed. Non-glial tumors grow by expansion and are more likely to be totally resected.

ASTROCYTOMA

What is the function of a normal astrocyte?	In reaction to injury, astrocytes expand their cytoplasm and form glial fibrils.
What is the most common location of astrocytomas?	
In adults?	Central white matter of the cerebrum
In children?	Cerebellum in children
How are astrocytomas characterized?	Based on histology; Grade I–Grade IV
Compare the histologic characteristics of Grade I–Grade III astrocytomas.	1. Grade I: Least aggressive, cells resemble normal astrocytes 2. Grade II: Similar to grade I, but more pleomorphism and vascular changes 3. Grade III: Anaplastic; marked pleomorphism, prominent mitoses, hyperplastic vasculature, tissue necrosis
What is the treatment?	Surgical resection, with excellent prognosis if completely removed
What is another name for Grade IV astrocytoma?	Glioblastoma multiforme (GBM), the most common primary intracranial neoplasm
What is the peak age group for GBM?	Later middle age (i.e., 40s–50s)
Describe the histology of GBM.	Marked anaplasia and pleomorphism; vascular changes with endothelial hyperplasia; many mitoses
What pattern of tumor cells encompass areas of necrosis and hemorrhage?	Pseudo-palisade arrangement at the periphery
What is the prognosis of GBM?	Very poor, usually death within 1 year

OLIGODENDROGLIOMA

What is an oligodendrocyte?	A neuroglial cell, whose surface membrane coils around neuronal axons to form the myelin sheath in white matter

How fast does the oligodendroglioma proliferate?	Very slowly
What age group is most commonly affected?	Middle age
What is the most common site of origin?	Cerebral hemispheres
Describe the typical morphology.	Large round nuclei surrounded by a halo of clear cytoplasm, often called "fried egg appearance"
What is also seen as typical morphology?	Foci of calcification

EPENDYMOMA

Where is the most common location?	Fourth ventricle
What is the peak age group?	Children and adolescents, but any age group can be affected
What may result from tumor growth?	Hydrocephalus due to obstructed CSF flow
What is the pattern of the histology?	Rosettes with cells encircling vessels, or tubules with cells pointing toward a central lumen

MENINGIOMA

What is the proliferating cell type?	Arachnoid cell
Characterize these tumors.	Commonly benign and slow growing
What is the second most common primary intracranial neoplasm?	Meningioma
Why is surgery a feasible option with this type of tumor?	Meningioma is external to brain, and thus can be surgically removed.
Name the 2 most common locations.	1. Convexities of the cerebral hemispheres 2. The parasagittal region

Name several other common locations.	Falx cerebri, sphenoid ridge, olfactory area, suprasellar region
What is the gross appearance?	Firm, rubbery tumors, white or reddish colored, clearly distinguishable from brain parenchyma
What is the appearance under the microscope?	Whorled pattern spindle cells, ovoid nuclei, intranuclear vacuoles, and calcified psammoma bodies
What are psammoma bodies?	Microscopic concentric laminated mass of calcified material

MEDULLOBLASTOMA

What is the age group most commonly affected?	Young children under 14 years of age
Is medulloblastoma benign or malignant?	Highly malignant
What area of the brain is usually involved?	Cerebellum
What is the gross pathology?	Reddish gray, granular mass arising from roof of 4th ventricle
What is the histology?	Rosette-patterned sheets of closely packed cells with little cytoplasm and a pseudorosette pattern
What is meant by a pseudorosette?	Perivascular arrangement of tumor cells
What does PNET stand for?	Primitive neuroectodermal tumor. Medulloblastoma is one of the small cell tumors of the nervous system.
What is the prognosis of medulloblastoma?	Poor; survival of 1–2 years after onset of symptoms is typical.

RETINOBLASTOMA

What is the age group most commonly affected?	Young children
What percentage of cases results from sporadic mutation?	Approximately 60%

How are the rest of cases inherited?	Familial
What is the genetic defect?	Homozygous deletion of retinoblastoma (Rb) gene (chromosome 13)
Is an attenuated form of the disease present if only one deletion exists?	No; both deletions are required for tumor to develop (an example of the "two-hit" theory of carcinogenesis).

HEMANGIOBLASTOMA

What is it?	Tumor of blood vessel origin
What area of the brain is most frequently affected?	Cerebellum
What are common clinical complaints?	Difficulty with balance and walking
What disease is associated with hemangioblastoma?	von Hippel-Lindau disease, with similar lesions in retina and other organs
What are 2 neoplasms associated with von Hippel-Lindau disease?	1. Renal cell carcinoma 2. Pheochromocytoma (adrenal gland tumor)
What protein is sometimes produced by the neoplastic cells?	Erythropoietin
What can result from this?	Secondary polycythemia
What is the microscopic pathology?	Variable presentation, from purely vascular to highly cellular, with large polygonal cells full of lipids

SCHWANNOMA

What are 2 other names for schwannoma?	Neurilemoma, acoustic neuroma (if localized to CN VIII)
What is the cell of origin?	Schwann cell
Are schwannomas benign or malignant?	Benign
How fast does the tumor proliferate?	It is a slow-growing, encapsulated tumor

Where are schwannomas commonly located?	Posterior nerve roots and peripheral nerves
What 2 patterns of histology are seen?	1. Antoni type A neurilemoma: elongated cells with palisade nuclei, grouped in bundles 2. Antoni type B neurilemoma: less cellularity, similar pattern

NEUROFIBROMA

What disease is associated with multiple neuro-fibromas?	von Recklinghausen disease
From what cell are these neoplasms derived?	Schwann cell, involving peripheral nerves

METASTATIC TUMORS

What are the 6 most common primary sites of malignancy that metastasize to the brain?	1. Lung 2. Breast (usually to dura and skull) 3. Skin (malignant melanoma) 4. Kidney 5. GI tract 6. Thyroid
How do they metastasize?	Usually metastasis to the brain is hematogenous, but direct invasion is also possible.

CRANIOPHARYNGIOMA

From what tissues is the tumor derived?	The hypophyseal trunk or Rathke pouch
What is a Rathke pouch?	Diverticulum from the embryonic buccal cavity, from which the anterior lobe of the pituitary develops
What age group is most commonly affected by craniopharyngioma?	Children, averaging between 4–16 years of age
What clinical signs are evident?	Visual complaints, hypothalamic syndromes
What is the gross appearance?	Calcified, multiloculated mass of several centimeters, sometimes encapsulated by the surrounding brain, with cystic areas

What is seen on skull radio-graph that can suggest the diagnosis?	Plain films of the head will show characteristic calcifications.

LYMPHOMA

What conditions increase the risk of developing primary lymphoma of the brain?	Conditions that cause patients to be immunocompromised (e.g., AIDS, status post transplant)
What is the most common primary brain neoplasm of immunocompromised patients?	Lymphoma
In the absence of immune deficiency, in what age group do primary lympho-mas most commonly occur?	Patients in their 60s or 70s

What are 3 clinical features?

1. Headache
2. Seizures
3. Deficiency of higher neural function such as problems with memory

What is the gross pathology?	Usually multifocal, seen most often in the cerebrum, arising in the perivascular spaces
What is the microscopic appearance?	Similar to the classic forms of lymphoma

DEMYELINATING DISEASES

What are 2 characteristics of these diseases?

1. Destruction of myelin
2. Preservation of axons

Which is primarily affected, white or gray matter?	White matter
Which is the most common of the demyelinating diseases?	Multiple sclerosis

What are 2 other examples?

1. Acute disseminated encephalomyelitis
2. Guillain-Barré syndrome

MULTIPLE SCLEROSIS (MS)

What is the age group of peak incidence?	20–30 years of age
What is the etiology?	Unknown; immune or viral theory postulated but not proven. It is thought to be multifactorial.
Is the disease more common in men or women?	Slightly more common in women
What evidence supports the theory of an immune system etiology?	Increased incidence associated with human leukocyte antigen (HLA) haplotypes (A3, B7, DR2, DW2)
What is increased in the CSF in patients with MS and how is it detected?	Immunoglobulin, seen as multiple oligoclonal bands on electrophoresis
What is the relationship of incidence of MS to geographic location?	Incidence is directly proportional to distance from the equator
What are the morphologic changes of MS in the brain and spinal cord?	Multiple focal areas of demyelination known as plaques
What is the microscopic appearance of these areas of demyelination?	Localized edema, congestion, and microglial proliferation; progressive astrocytosis and infiltration; eventually, sclerotic plaque and reactive gliosis
What 3 sites are particularly affected in MS?	1. Optic nerve 2. Brainstem 3. Paraventricular areas
What cells infiltrate the plaques before reactive gliosis occurs?	1. Helper CD4+ cells 2. Cytotoxic CD8+ T lymphocytes 3. Macrophages
What are the early clinical findings of MS?	Motor deficits of the distal lower extremities, visual disturbances and retrobulbar pain, sensory deficits, and sometimes bladder incontinence
What is the classic Charcot triad of MS symptoms?	1. Nystagmus 2. Intention tremor 3. Scanning speech

| What is the characteristic pattern of the disease? | Periods of exacerbation alternate with long periods of asymptomatic remission, but there is eventual progression to invalidism and mental deterioration. |

ACUTE DISSEMINATED ENCEPHALOMYELITIS

What is another name for this condition?	Postinfectious encephalitis
In this case, what is meant by the term "postinfectious"?	The disease follows a viral illness
Name 4 viral illnesses that can cause this disease.	1. Measles 2. Mumps 3. Rubella 4. Chicken pox
What are the pathologic findings of acute disseminated encephalomyelitis?	Widespread demyelination
What is the most likely etiology?	Delayed hypersensitivity reaction to viral pathogens
What is the prognosis?	Variable; ranges from complete recovery to death

GUILLAIN-BARRÉ SYNDROME

What is it?	Acute inflammatory demyelinating disease; usually occurs following a viral infection, immunization, or allergic reaction; probably of autoimmune etiology
What is primarily involved?	Peripheral nerves
What age group has the peak incidence?	Young adults
What are the clinical features?	Ascending muscle weakness and paralysis, beginning in the distal lower extremities and progressing proximally
Can the disease be fatal?	Yes, rarely expiratory muscles can be paralyzed, causing respiratory failure and death.

What can be seen in the CSF?	Albumino-cytologic dissociation of CSF; can be an important diagnostic finding
What is albumino-cytologic dissociation?	Greatly increased protein, with only small increase of cell count

DEGENERATIVE DISEASE

What is meant by degenerative disease?	One that causes slowly progressive loss of neural function, can occur in CNS as well as peripheral nervous system (PNS)
List 4 causes of degenerative disease in the nervous system.	1. Dementia 2. Huntington disease 3. Parkinsonism 4. Amyotrophic lateral sclerosis (ALS)

DEMENTIA

What is dementia?	Organic disease of the CNS causing progressive loss of intellectual capabilities
What is the most common cause of dementia?	Alzheimer disease
What is the 2nd most common cause of dementia?	Multi-infarct dementia
What are other disorders that may cause dementia?	Chronic alcoholism, Binswanger disease, Pick disease

Alzheimer disease

What are the defining characteristics of Alzheimer dementia?	Multiple cognitive defects manifested as memory impairment and other possible disturbances in speech, language, recognition, and executive function. There is gradual onset and continuing cognitive disease. These symptoms must not be the result of another disease that could affect the nervous system in this way.
Approximately how many Americans are afflicted?	Over 2 million; the number is growing as the overall population ages
What are 2 clinical findings of Alzheimer dementia?	1. Slow, progressive loss of intellect 2. Deterioration of motor function, including contractures and paralysis

What can be the early sign of declining intellect?	Short-term memory loss
What can also develop?	Long-term memory loss, eventually leading to inability to read, count, or speak
What are 5 characteristic morphologic abnormalities?	1. Neurofibrillary tangles 2. Senile plaques 3. Granulovacuolar degeneration 4. Hirano bodies 5. Generalized cerebral atrophy
What are neurofibrillary tangles?	Intracytoplasmic bundles of filaments, derived from microtubules and neurofilaments
Where are the tangles found in the brain?	Within neurons, in the cerebral cortex
What are senile plaques?	Also known as neuritic plaques; swollen nerve processes forming spherical foci with a central amyloid protein core
Where are senile plaques commonly located?	1. Cerebral cortex 2. Amygdala 3. Hippocampus
What is granulovacuolar degeneration?	Intraneuronal cytoplasmic vacuoles containing granules
Where are they characteristically located?	Pyramidal cells of the hippocampus
What are Hirano bodies?	Intracytoplasmic eosinophilic inclusions seen in the proximal dendritic processes
Cerebral atrophy is seen most prominently in which areas of the brain?	Frontal and hippocampal areas
What is the gross appearance?	Sulci look widened because of loss of neurons and subsequent narrow gyri
What syndrome can exhibit similar findings to Alzheimer dementia?	Down syndrome in patients who survive to 40 years of age or older

In what other disease can neurofibrillary tangles also be seen?	Parkinson disease
What is the etiology of Alzheimer disease?	Unknown
What are 3 possible mechanisms that have been theorized?	1. Choline acetyltransferase deficiency 2. Alterations in nucleus basalis of Meynert 3. Abnormal amyloid gene expression
What is the tau protein?	Normally synthesized in gray matter, it has been shown to have hyperphosphorylation and it accumulates in the tangles and plaques of patients with Alzheimer disease.

Binswanger Disease

What is it?	Multiple lacunar infarcts and progressive demyelination of subcortical area. Also known as subcortical leukoencephalopathy.
What disease process is associated with Binswanger disease?	Hypertension
What area of the brain is characteristically spared?	Cortex

Pick Disease

What is the clinical presentation?	Similar to Alzheimer disease
What is the etiology?	Unknown
What are 3 characteristic pathologic features?	1. Marked cortical atrophy 2. Edematous neurons 3. Pick bodies (round intracytoplasmic inclusion bodies, composed of neurofilaments)
What two lobes of the brain are markedly atrophied in Pick disease?	Temporal and frontal lobes

HUNTINGTON DISEASE

What is it?	Progressive degeneration and atrophy of frontal cortex, caudate nucleus, and putamen, also referred to as Huntington chorea
What neurons are especially affected in these areas?	Cholinergic and GABA-ergic neurons
In the genome, what characterizes a worse prognosis?	Increased number of tri-nucleotide repeats
At what age will clinical abnormalities commonly start?	30–40 years of age; fatal prognosis usually by 55–60 years of age
What are the earliest seen clinical features?	Athetoid movements (characteristic involuntary, continuous, slow writhing movements, typically severe in the hands and arms)

PARKINSONISM

What is it and what are the associated clinical features?	A group of disorders characterized by 1. Resting pill-rolling tremor 2. Masked facies 3. Shuffling gait 4. Muscular rigidity 5. Slowed movements
What is the most common cause of parkinsonism?	Idiopathic Parkinson disease (also known as paralysis agitans)
What are other causes of parkinsonism?	Von Economo encephalitis, trauma, drugs and toxins, and Shy-Drager syndrome
What is von Economo encephalitis?	Infectious disease seen in 1915–1918, associated with the influenza pandemic; it causes postencephalitic parkinsonism in people 85 years of age or older who were affected by that pandemic
Participation in what sport can cause parkinsonism?	Boxing, because of repeated trauma to the head

What contaminant in illicit street drugs causes a similar clinical picture?	MPTP, methyl-phenyl-tetrahydro-pyridine, a dopamine antagonist
What is the Shy-Drager syndrome?	Autonomic dysfunction and associated orthostatic hypotension with parkinsonism

Parkinson Disease (Paralysis Agitans)

By what age will clinical symptoms be evident in Parkinson disease?	Usually after 50 years of age
What is the histology of Parkinson disease?	Gradual loss and depigmentation of cells in the substantia nigra and locus ceruleus
What do the damaged cells characteristically contain?	Lewy bodies, eosinophilic intracyto-plasmic inclusions
What neurotransmitter is depleted in the corpus striatum?	Dopamine, because damaged cells in the substantia nigra inhibit neuronal path-ways from the substantia nigra to the corpus striatum
What therapy can be effective?	L-dopa, a dopamine precursor

AMYOTROPHIC LATERAL SCLEROSIS (ALS)

What is the most common form of motor neuron disease?	Amyotrophic lateral sclerosis (ALS), also known as Lou Gehrig disease
Which motor neurons are degenerating in ALS?	Both upper and lower motor neurons of the lateral corticospinal tracts and anterior motor neurons of the cord
What happens to the muscles in ALS?	Muscles atrophy from denervation
What is the clinical presen-tation of ALS?	Both upper and lower motor neuron signs are present.
List the upper motor neuron signs that signify ALS.	Hyperreflexia Spasticity Pathologic reflexes (e.g., positive Babinski reflex)

List the lower motor neuron signs that signify ALS.	Atrophy of muscles Fasciculations
Which muscles are commonly involved at first presentation?	Intrinsic muscles of the hand, and muscles of the arm and shoulder
How quickly does the disease progress?	Rapidly, with death coming in 1–6 years

METABOLIC DISORDERS OF THE CNS

What is pernicious anemia?	Megaloblastic anemia and neurologic disorder, resulting from vitamin B_{12} deficiency
What is the neurologic disease of pernicious anemia?	Subacute combined degeneration of the spinal cord
What part of the spinal cord is involved?	The posterior and lateral columns
What is the gross pathologic appearance?	Gray discoloration of the dorsolateral columns
What is Wernicke syndrome?	Mental deficits characterized by memory loss, confabulation, and loss of location sense.
What is the predisposing factor for development of Wernicke syndrome?	Chronic alcoholism
What is the gross pathology of Wernicke syndrome?	Marked congestion of periventricular gray matter, with many petechial hemorrhages
What is the microscopic histology of Wernicke syndrome?	Prominent capillaries, from endothelial hypertrophy and hyperplasia, and acute ischemic necrosis of associated neurons
What is acute Wernicke encephalopathy and what causes it?	Rapid development of encephalopathy, characterized by severe ataxia, mental confusion, delirium, and restlessness. It results from thiamine deficiency.

| What can precipitate an acute Wernicke encephalopathy? | Administration of intravenous glucose load prior to administration of thiamine during inpatient treatment (i.e., must give thiamine before glucose) |

| What are the pathologic features of Wernicke encephalopathy? | Inflammatory hemorrhagic lesions in the hypothalamus, mamillary bodies, periaqueductal and periventricular regions |

AUTOIMMUNE DISORDERS AFFECTING THE NERVOUS SYSTEM

| What is myasthenia gravis? | A common disorder, affecting more women than men, usually caused by autoimmune processes |

| What is the diagnostic finding in most patients with myasthenia gravis? | Antibodies against the neuromuscular acetylcholine receptors |

| What is the clinical presentation of myasthenia gravis? | Muscles, such as extraocular muscles, are easily fatigued and demonstrably weak, with some relief if rested |

| What is the characteristic finding in the muscle in myasthenia gravis? | Lymphocytic infiltrates around the degenerating fibers |

| What do EMG (electromyographic) studies of patients with myasthenia gravis show? | Decremental responses to repeated nerve stimulation |

| What is the prognosis of myasthenia gravis? | Death, usually from respiratory infection, predisposed by weak muscles of respiration |

POWER REVIEW

List 7 common CNS tumors, giving the age group of their peak incidence, the most frequent sites, and their characteristics.

Table 30–1.
CNS Tumors

Type of CNS Tumor	Age Group	Frequent Sites	Characteristics
Astrocytoma, Grade IV (Glioblastoma Multiforme)	Older	Cerebral Hemispheres	Highly malignant; fast growing; most common primary intracranial neoplasm
Meningioma	Middle/older	Convexities of hemispheres, parasagittal, falx cerebri	Benign tumor; external to brain; second most common intracranial neoplasm
Medulloblastoma	Children	Cerebellum	Highly malignant; most common intracranial tumor in children
Neuroblastoma	Children	Cerebral hemispheres	Less common than peripheral neuroblastomas; N-myc amplification
Retinoblastoma	Young children	Retina; Bilateral and multifocal (familial); Unilateral and unifocal (sporadic)	Most common eye tumor of children; linked to Rb homozygous deletion
Neurilemmoma (Schwannoma)	Middle/later life	Cranial nerve VIII if intracranial	Commonly benign; usually resectable
Metastatic Tumors	Variable	From primary sites: lung, breast, skin, kidney, thyroid, GI	Similar incidence to GBM tumor

List the degenerative nervous system disorders, the age group most frequently associated with occurrence, their clinical findings, and the anatomic changes that they cause.

Table 30–2.
Degenerative Nervous System Disorders

Type of Degenerative Disorder	Age Group	Clinical Findings	Anatomic Changes
Alzheimer disease	Sporadic form: 60 years of age or older Familial: early as 40 years of age	Progressive dementia	Generalized cerebral atrophy; neurofibrillary tangles; senile plaques; Hirano bodies; decreased neurons in nucleus basalis of Meynert
Pick disease	Increased incidence in females	Progressive dementia	Cerebral atrophy, especially frontal and temporal lobes; Pick bodies, especially in Ammon's horn
Huntington disease	Autosomal dominant, delay of onset until 30–40 years of age	Chorea; athetosis; motor degeneration	Atrophy, neuron loss, and gliosis of lentiform nucleus and frontal cortex
Idiopathic Parkinson disease	Usually after 50 years of age	Parkinsonism	Neuronal loss and depigmentation of substantia nigra and locus ceruleus; Lewy bodies

Table 30–2.
Degenerative Nervous System Disorders

Type of Degenerative Disorder	Age Group	Clinical Findings	Anatomic Changes
Amyotrophic Lateral Sclerosis (ALS)	Middle-aged men	Rapidly progressive, upper and lower motor neuron loss	Degenerative loss of the lateral corticospinal tracts and anterior motor neurons of the spinal cord

What is myasthenia gravis?	A common disorder affecting more women than men, usually caused by an autoimmune formation of antibodies against the neuromuscular acetylcholine receptors
What is acute Wernicke encephalopathy?	Rapid development of encephalopathy, characterized by severe ataxia, mental confusion, delirium, and restlessness, precipitated by a glucose load before thiamine supplementation in alcohol withdrawal patients
What is pernicious anemia?	Vitamin B_{12} deficiency, causing subacute combined degeneration of the spinal cord, characterized by paresthesias, unsteady gait, position, and vibration sensation loss
What are the nerve tracts that are degenerating in pernicious anemia?	Posterior and lateral columns
What is ALS (amyotrophic lateral sclerosis)?	Degeneration of both upper and lower motor neurons, specifically lateral corticospinal tracts and anterior motor neurons of the cord
What is the pathology of Parkinson disease?	Gradual loss and depigmentation of cells in the substantia nigra and locus ceruleus, Lewy bodies (eosinophilic intracytoplasmic inclusions), and consequential

depletion of dopamine in the corpus striatum

Describe the clinical features of parkinsonism.

Resting pill-rolling tremor, masked facies, shuffling gait, muscular rigidity, and slowed movements

What are 3 characteristic pathologic features of Pick disease?

1. Marked cortical atrophy, especially of frontal and temporal lobes
2. Edematous neurons
3. Pick bodies, round intracytoplasmic inclusion bodies, made up of neurofilaments

What is Binswanger disease, also known as subcortical leukoencephalopathy?

Multiple lacunar infarcts and progressive demyelination of subcortical area, associated with hypertensive disease

What are the clinical findings of Alzheimer disease?

Slow, progressive loss of intellect, including memory loss
Deterioration of motor function, including contractures and paralysis

What are 5 characteristic morphologic abnormalities in Alzheimer disease?

1. Neurofibrillary tangles
2. Senile plaques
3. Granulovacuolar degeneration
4. Hirano bodies
5. Generalized cerebral atrophy

What is the most common neural tube defect (NTD)?

Spina bifida

What is the most severe NTD?

Anencephaly; is incompatible with life

What is hydrocephalus?

Increased volume of cerebrospinal fluid within cranial cavity

What is Arnold-Chiari malformation?

Caudal (downward) displacement of medulla and cerebellum through foramen magnum into the cervical vertebral canal

Name 5 features that can be found in fetal alcohol syndrome.

1. Microcephaly
2. Atrial septal defect
3. Mental retardation
4. Intrauterine growth retardation (IUGR) and subsequent growth failure
5. Short palpebral fissures

What is the pathology of the "tuber" in tuberous sclerosis?	Proliferations of atypical multinucleated astrocytes, appearing macroscopically as small, white nodules
What are Lisch nodules?	Pigmented nodules of the iris, consisting of melanocytes, seen in von Recklinghausen disease
What is the most common disorder of the CNS?	Cerebrovascular disease; the third most common major cause of death in the United States
What is the most common cause of vascular thrombosis?	Atherosclerotic plaques in blood vessels, which can rupture and initiate the coagulation cascade
Name the most common sites of cerebral thrombosis.	Bifurcation site of common carotid; branching sites of circle of Willis (especially middle cerebral artery); vertebral and basilar arteries' bifurcation sites
What is the most common cause of subarachnoid hemorrhage (SAH)?	Trauma
What is the most common site of embolic occlusion?	Middle cerebral artery (MCA)
What are Charcot-Bouchard aneurysms?	Outpouchings of the vasculature, developing as a result of chronic hypertension, likely to rupture into brain parenchyma
What type of aneurysm can rupture into the subarachnoid space?	Berry aneurysm, commonly found on the circle of Willis
What is the #1 cause of most head and spine injuries?	Motor vehicle accidents (MVAs)
Name 4 types of injury to the brain in head trauma.	1. Intracranial hemorrhage (epidural, subdural, subarachnoid) 2. Concussion 3. Contusion 4. Laceration

What artery is injured in an epidural hemorrhage?

Middle meningeal artery (MMA)

What vessels are injured in a subdural hematoma?

Most commonly, bridging veins from the cerebrum to venous sinuses in the dura mater

What is the difference between coup and contrecoup injury?

1. Coup: Lesion is located directly beneath area of impact
2. Contrecoup: Lesion is opposite to the area of impact

What is the most common area of a herniated inter- vertebral disc?

Lumbosacral; L4–5 or L5-S1 discs

What is the most common bacterial infection of the CNS and who gets it?

Bacterial meningitis; most common in children

What are 3 classic clinical signs of bacterial menin- gitis?

Mental status changes, fever, and nuchal rigidity (neck stiffness)

What are the diagnostic findings on LP of bacterial meningitis?

Increased protein, decreased glucose ($<2/3$ serum [glucose]), many PMNs

What is the most common etiology of cerebral abscess?

Secondary infection from primary sources elsewhere in the body

What are the CSF findings of tuberculous meningitis?

Increased lymphocytes, increased protein, decreased glucose, acid fast bacilli

What are the CSF findings in viral meningitis?

Increased lymphocytes, moderate increase in protein, normal glucose

What are Negri bodies?

Eosinophilic intracytoplasmic inclusion bodies found in the hippocampus, cerebellum (Purkinje cells), in rabies infection

Where are the majority of intracranial neoplasms in adults—above or below the tentorium?

Supratentorial in adults, infratentorial in children

What is the most common malignancy in children?

Leukemia

What is the second most common malignancy in children?	CNS tumors
Where do most primary malignant CNS tumors metastasize?	They usually don't metastasize.
What are psammoma bodies?	Microscopic concentric laminated mass of calcified material, seen in meningiomas
Name the 4 most common intracranial tumors in adults (in order of frequency).	1. Glioblastoma multiforme 2. Metastatic tumors (from extracranial primary sites) 3. Meningioma 4. Acoustic neuroma
Name the 4 most common intracranial tumors in children (in order of frequency).	1. Astrocytoma 2. Medulloblastoma 3. Ependymoma 4. Craniopharyngioma
What are the 6 most common primary sites of malignancy that metastasize to the brain?	1. Lung 2. Breast (usually to dura and skull) 3. Skin (malignant melanoma) 4. Kidney 5. GI tract 6. Thyroid
What is the most common primary brain neoplasm of immunocompromised patients?	Lymphoma
Which is the most common of the demyelinating diseases?	Multiple sclerosis
What is the classic Charcot triad of multiple sclerosis?	1. Nystagmus 2. Intention tremor 3. Scanning speech
What is the most common cause of dementia?	Alzheimer disease
What is the 2nd most common cause of dementia?	Multi-infarct dementia

31

Head and Neck

MOUTH

CONGENITAL ABNORMALITIES

What is a cleft lip?

Failure of the globular processes to unite within the maxilla during embryological development

Which lip is usually affected in cleft lip: the upper or lower lip?

Upper lip

A cleft palate is a premature closure of which two sutures during embryological development

Coronal and lambdoid sutures

Which of the palates may be involved?

Can involve the hard or soft palates or both

With what other congenital anomaly is cleft palate usually associated?

Cleft lip

What is Fordyce disease?

An asymptomatic condition characterized by the presence of painless yellow-to-white granules in mucosa of cheeks, lips, and gingivae

What are these granules?

Displaced ectopic sebaceous glands

Are they benign or malignant?

Benign

INFLAMMATORY DISORDERS

Name some common inflammatory disorders of the mouth and their causes.

1. Herpetic gingivostomatitis: herpes simplex virus (usually type 1)
2. Monilial (candidal) stomatitis: *Candida albicans*

3. Aphthous stomatitis: unknown etiology
4. Syphilis: *Treponema pallidum*

Define stomatitis.

Inflammation of the oral mucosa

Define gingivostomatitis.

Inflammation of the gums

Name 2 reasons people get stomatitis and gingivostomatitis.

1. Ill-fitting dentures
2. Poor dental hygiene

Characterize herpetic gingivostomatitis.

Development of vesicular lesions that fuse and rupture, forming small ulcers

In what population is it most commonly seen?

Infants and children

What systemic symptoms are often present in herpetic gingivostomatitis?

Malaise and fever

What is the prognosis?

Resolves in 7 to 10 days

Characterize monilial stomatitis.

White patches scattered over mucosa, tongue, palate, and pharynx

In what population is it most commonly seen?

In children with neglected oral hygiene or immunosuppressed patients

Describe the presentation and course of aphthous stomatitis.

Yellow-to-white ulcers of different sizes. Epithelium is preserved but with fibrous exudate. Usually lasts from 7 to 10 days.

Name and describe the 3 stages of oral syphilis and their symptoms.

1. Primary stage: chancre
2. Secondary stage: patches in oral mucosa and macules on tongue
3. Tertiary stage: gummas in hard or soft palate and glossitis

What is the characteristic histology of oral syphilis?

Marked lymphoplasmacytic infiltration mostly on small and medium-sized vessels

BENIGN TUMORS AND TUMOR-LIKE CONDITIONS OF THE MOUTH

What is gingival hyperplasia?

The gingiva appears as a pink, lobulated mass due to collagenous tissue proliferation and development of new blood vessels.

Can the tongue be involved in gingival hyperplasia?	Yes
Gingival hyperplasia is a common side effect of what drug?	Phenytoin
What is a ranula?	A unilateral cyst on the floor of the mouth near the frenulum
What causes a ranula?	It is believed to be a retention cyst of the sublingual glands or a remnant of a branchial cleft cyst.
What is a mucocele?	A cyst, usually on the lips, characterized by pools of mucus and inflammatory cells within the minor salivary glands
An epulis is a tumor-like mass. At what location in the mouth is it most common?	The gingiva. The mandibular gingiva is involved more often than the maxillary.
What is the gross appearance of an epulis?	A sessile or pedunculated, rubbery, red-blue or pink mass
Describe the histology of an epulis.	A fibrous stroma with numerous multinucleate giant cells and chronic inflammatory cells
What is a fibroma?	An exophytic soft tissue proliferation, usually occurring on the inner surface of the cheek and lips, covered by squamous mucosa
What is a granular cell tumor?	A benign tumor of the tongue consisting of hyperplasia of the squamous mucosa

LEUKOPLAKIA

What is it?	A lesion of the mucous membranes; may be due to chronic irritation and trauma
What does leukoplakia look like?	One or several white patches not less than 5 mm in diameter with raised, ill-defined borders

In what population does it occur more frequently?	Men

CARCINOMA OF THE MOUTH

What percentage of all malignant tumors are cancer of the mouth?	5% to 10%
What is the most common malignant lesion of the oral mucosa?	Squamous cell carcinoma
Name 5 risk factors for squamous cell carcinoma of the mouth.	1. Smoking 2. Tobacco chewers 3. Pipe smokers 4. Chronic exposure to sunlight 5. ETOH
List the clinical features of squamous cell carcinoma of the mouth.	It begins as a small indurated plaque, nodule, or ulcer, which increases in size. It can project into the oral cavity and interfere with speech and chewing.
Define carcinoma in situ.	The precursor lesion to invasive cancer. It is characterized by immaturity and disorganization of the squamous epithelium with pleomorphism, cellular atypia, and mitoses.
What limits a carcinoma in situ lesion?	An intact basement membrane
Define infiltrating carcinoma.	A well-differentiated cancer with abundant keratin formation and invasion into adjacent tissues
What is the prognosis of squamous cell cancer of the mouth?	It depends on degree of differentiation, size of primary tumor, depth of invasion, and metastasis. If it is multifocal, the prognosis is poor.
Where and how do these tumors metastasize?	To neck lymph nodes by lymphatic drainage

NASOPHARYNX

Define the tonsillar ring of Waldeyer.	Aggregations of lymphoid tissue that encircle the pharynx

What cells cover this normal lymphoid tissue?	Pseudostratified columnar epithelium or stratified squamous epithelium

INFLAMMATORY DISORDERS OF THE NASOPHARYNX

What is tonsillitis?	Bacterial infection that makes tonsillar bed enlarged and red
What is the histology of tonsillitis?	Crypts of squamous epithelium containing numerous neutrophils and desquamated epithelial cells
What are the organisms that most commonly infect the tonsils?	β-hemolytic streptococci (strep pyogenes) and pneumococci
What is pharyngitis?	Intense infiltration of the pharynx by inflammatory cells, edema, and hyperplasia of tissue in response to bacteria or viruses
What are the organisms that most commonly infect the pharynx?	Streptococci and staphylococci

BENIGN TUMORS

Name 2 benign tumors of the nasopharynx.	1. Nasal polyp 2. Angiofibroma
What is a nasal polyp?	A nonspecific proliferation of edematous stroma and nasal mucosa
Nasal polyps are commonly associated with which patients?	Those with a clinical history of allergies
Define angiofibroma.	A firm, rubbery, gray or purple tumor, usually with a broad attachment to the nasopharyngeal wall
What are 3 clinical presenting symptoms of an angiofibroma?	1. Nasal obstruction 2. Epistaxis 3. Nasal discharge
What is the microscopic appearance of an angiofibroma?	Vascular fibrous connective tissue intermingled with spindle shaped cells and chronic inflammatory cells, such as lymphocytes and plasma cells

What vessels are most frequently affected?	Medium-sized vessels
What may angiofibromas be confused with and why?	Because of their intense vascularity, angiofibromas may be confused with hemangiomas.

NASOPHARYNGEAL CARCINOMA

What is the most common malignancy of the naso-pharynx?	A lymphoepithelioma
Describe a nasopharyngeal lymphoepithelioma.	It has lymphoid elements mixed with malignant epithelial cells identical to those of a poorly differentiated squamous cell carcinoma.
Where is it most frequently found?	In the lateral wall of the eustachian tube
What is the clinical presentation of a nasopharyngeal lymphoepithelioma?	Nasal obstruction, bleeding, middle ear discomfort, cranial nerve palsies or enlarged lymph nodes in the neck
What populations are most commonly affected?	Young adults, often of Asian origin
What is the prognosis?	Poor, because these lesions tend to grow rapidly and metastasize early

LARYNX

What is the most common symptom of laryngeal disease?	Hoarseness
Define laryngitis.	An inflammatory process in the respiratory tract causing edema in the larynx
Why is laryngitis worrisome in children?	Edema can cause laryngeal obstruction and difficulty breathing.
Name 2 benign laryngeal tumors.	1. Laryngeal polyps 2. Papillomatosis
Describe laryngeal polyps.	Sessile or pedunculated nodules of proliferative stroma covered by benign epithelium

Where do they most frequently occur?	On the vocal cords
What is papillomatosis?	Friable nodules composed of a central core of fibrous tissue covered by hyperplastic squamous epithelium.
What virus is it thought to be associated with?	Human papilloma virus (HPV)
Why is papillomatosis worrisome?	It is believed to predispose the patient to carcinoma.

LARYNGEAL CARCINOMA

What is the most common epithelial tumor of the larynx?	Squamous cell carcinoma
Other than squamous cell carcinoma, what other type of cancer is found in the larynx?	Verrucous carcinoma
Describe verrucous carcinoma.	A large, fungating papillary growth. It is a very well-differentiated squamous cell tumor.

JAW

What infection can follow dental or periodontal infection?	Osteomyelitis of the jaw

CYSTS OF THE JAW

How are cysts of the maxilla and mandible classified?	Odontogenic cysts arise from a defect in tooth development, while nonodontogenic cysts arise secondary to inflammation of the dental pulp.
Name 5 types of odontogenic cysts.	1. Radicular (periapical) cyst 2. Follicular (dentigerous) 3. Eruption cyst 4. Primordial cyst 5. Odontogenic keratocyst
What is the most common cyst of the jaw?	Radicular cyst

Describe a radicular (periapical) cyst.

It arises in an epithelial dental granuloma as a result of inflammation and necrosis of the dental pulp. It is attached to the roots of the tooth and can be quite large.

What usually lines the radicular cyst?

Squamous epithelium

What is the derivation of follicular (dentigerous) cyst?

Misplaced epithelial buds

What usually lines the follicular cyst?

Stratified squamous epithelium

What is contained within the cyst?

Serous or mucoid material

What is an eruption cyst?

A small dentigerous cyst occurring on teeth already erupted

What is the most common clinical presentation of an eruption cyst?

Inflamed gingiva

What usually lines an eruption cyst?

Stratified squamous epithelium

What is within a primordial cyst?

The lumen is filled with keratocytes.

Where do primordial cysts usually form?

In the area of a missing tooth

What does an odontogenic keratocyst look like radiologically?

A radiolucency of the jaw

What usually lines the odontogenic keratocyst?

Keratinizing squamous epithelium

Which cyst has a tendency to recur and how often?

Odontogenic keratocyst recurs in up to 60% of cases.

Name 3 types of non-odontogenic cysts.

1. Nasopalatine cyst
2. Globulomaxillary cyst
3. Nasolabial cyst

Where is a nasopalatine cyst found?	In the midline of maxilla behind central incisors superior to the incisive papilla
What does the nasopalatine cyst contain?	Numerous mucus glands, nerves, and vessels
What lines a nasopalatine cyst?	Squamous, transitional, or cylindrical epithelium
Where is a globulomaxillary cyst found?	Beneath the maxillary lateral incisor and cuspid
What lines a globulomaxillary cyst?	Stratified squamous cuboidal epithelium
Where does a nasolabial cyst develop?	From epithelial remnants at the site of fusion of the facial processes
Where is a nasolabial cyst usually situated?	On the alveolar process near the base of the nostril

TUMORS OF THE JAW

Name the 3 types of tumors specific to the jaw.	1. Adamantinoma (ameloblastoma) 2. Odontoma 3. Cementum
Name some other conditions that may involve tumors of the jaw.	Osteoid osteomas, giant cell tumors, fibrous dysplasia, Paget disease, ossifying fibromas and osteosarcomas.

Adamantinoma

Describe an adamantinoma.	A neoplasm resembling the morphology of a developing tooth
What is the most common site of an adamantinoma?	The mandible
Describe the clinical features.	Presents as painless swelling, which may ulcerate and cause limitation
In what population is adamantinoma most common?	It has a slight predilection for women from 30–50 years of age.
How does it appear radiologically?	A unilocular or multilocular radiolucency with well-defined margins is seen. An embedded tooth may be present.

What is the histology?	Epithelial strands that vary in size and resemble the enamel of a tooth. The peripheral layer has centrally placed nuclei with pink cytoplasm surrounding the stroma. In the center, the cells undergo hydropic degeneration and thus form a cyst.
What is the prognosis?	Locally aggressive; destroys bone and adjacent structures; tumor is radio-resistant; usual treatment is curettage or resection.

Odontoma

Define odontoma.	A hamartoma arising from tissues involved in tooth formation
Describe the clinical features of odontoma.	It is diagnosed in people in their 20s; more commonly found in women than men; asymptomatic mass in the premolar or molar area of mandible
What is the pathology?	Lesion consists of varying proportions of dentin, enamel, cementum and pulp tissue. If in random arrangement, it is referred to as **complex odontoma.** If in normal formation patterns, then it is referred to as **compound odontoma.**
What is the prognosis?	Prognosis is good with simple curettage; recurrences are rare.

Cementoma

Describe a cementoma.	A tumor in which soft tissues have been partly or entirely replaced by cementum-like structures, cementicles
Which is affected more commonly—the mandible or the maxilla?	The mandible
Describe the clinical features of a cementoma.	Occurrence is predominantly in women; tumor usually appears around the root of a premolar or molar and can be fused to a tooth; can be single or multiple.
What is the radiological appearance?	A central radiopaque mass is present surrounded by a uniform shell.

What is the pathology?	Irregular osteoid formation and large hyperchromatic osteoblast with a background of proliferative fibrovascular tissue
What is the prognosis for cementoma?	Low malignant potential; possess capacity to recur and invade locally; rare metastasis to lungs has been reported.

SALIVARY GLANDS

Describe and identify the major salivary glands.	Large, bilateral glands including the parotid glands, submaxillary glands and sublingual glands
Describe and identify the minor salivary glands.	Small glands present in the oral cavity, pharynx, nasopharynx, nose, paranasal sinuses, and larynx
Which of the salivary glands contain	
Serous glands?	Parotid glands
Mucous glands?	Sublingual glands
Both serous and mucous glands?	Submaxillary and minor salivary glands

SIALADENOSIS

What is it?	Asymptomatic enlargement of the salivary glands unrelated to inflammation, salivary stones, or tumors
Sialadenosis is also referred to as what?	"Chipmunk facies"
What is the etiology of sialadenosis?	1. Nutritional deficiencies, malnutrition (alcoholism) 2. Ingestion of certain substances (iodides, lead, or mercury) 3. Hormonal imbalances (e.g., hypothyroidism, diabetes mellitus, and pregnancy)

SIALOLITHIASIS

What is it?	Stones in the salivary duct

Which glands are most commonly affected?	Submandibular (80%), parotid (less than 20%) and sublingual (1%–2%)
What is the etiology?	Unknown. Possible causes include: Abnormalities of salivary secretion Dehydration or electrolyte imbalances leading to precipitation of insoluble calcium salts
What are the clinical features of sialolithiasis?	Acute pain, gland swelling, and palpable mass at affected site
What is the treatment?	Manual removal of stones under local anesthesia. Sometimes, surgical excision is necessary.

PAROTITIS

In what populations is acute suppurative parotitis most often seen?	The very young or the elderly
What is the most common organism implicated in acute suppurative parotitis?	*Staphylococcus aureus*
In what condition does acute parotid inflammation and swelling occur?	Mumps
What are some predisposing factors for mumps?	1. Debilitation and dehydration 2. Systemic infection 3. Malignancies and chemotherapy treatment
What is the treatment for mumps?	Antibiotics and possibly surgical drainage

SJÖGREN SYNDROME

What is it?	A benign systemic disease with inflammatory and neoplastic characteristics.
Ratio of women: men	9:1
What is the clinical triad of symptoms in Sjögren syndrome?	1. Xerostomia (dry mouth) 2. Xerophthalmia (dry eyes) 3. Arthritis

What malignancy is associated with Sjögren syndrome?	Malignant lymphoma
What is sicca syndrome?	The combination of xerostomia and xerophthalmia due to a marked decrease in the secretion of the salivary and lacrimal duct
What is found in the serum of patients with Sjögren syndrome?	Autoantibodies to normal salivary duct epithelium
How are these antibodies visualized?	Immunofluorescent techniques
How do these antibodies appear histologically?	Atrophy of acinar tissue is seen, with fibrosis of interlobular and intralobular tissue and lymphoplasmacytic infiltration.
What do you call it if these findings are limited to one salivary gland presenting as a mass?	Lymphoepithelial lesion of Godwin
How is the diagnosis of Sjögren syndrome confirmed?	By presence of epimyoepithelial islands on needle biopsy. These result from altered or metaplastic ducts that become suspended in lymphoid tissue.

BENIGN TUMORS OF THE SALIVARY GLAND

True or false: Almost all salivary tumors are believed to be epithelial in origin (either acinar or ductal)?	True
What is the most common site of a salivary gland tumor?	Parotid gland (80%)
What are the clinical features of a benign salivary gland tumor?	A painless lump that gradually increases in size
What is the treatment for benign tumors?	Lobectomy or total excision

Define Mikulicz syndrome.	Bilateral swelling of the lacrimal, sub-mandibular and parotid glands due to known causes such as sarcoidosis or tuberculosis
Name 2 benign salivary gland tumors.	1. Benign mixed tumors (BMTs; pleomorphic adenomas) 2. Papillary cystadenoma lymphomatosum (Warthin tumor)

Benign mixed tumors

What is the most common benign salivary tumor and its incidence?	Benign mixed tumors
Where is a benign mixed tumor usually found?	Superficial lobe of the parotid gland; occasionally on or near the seventh cranial nerve
What are the clinical features of a benign mixed tumor?	Asymptomatic, slow-growing enlarging mass; does not invade facial nerve or infiltrate the skin; can be enormous
How does it appear on gross examination?	Well-circumscribed and sometimes encapsulated; small outpouching or satellite nodules are present
How does it appear on microscopic examination?	Mucins (cartilaginous material) of epithelial origin
What is the prognosis?	It can recur secondary to satellite lesion or incomplete excision.
Where is papillary cysta-denoma lymphomatosum tumor found?	Exclusively in the parotid gland
How is papillary cysta-denoma lymphomatosis diagnosed?	It concentrates technetium 99m, so it can be identified preoperatively.
What is the pathology?	Soft, fluctuant, brown, and cystic in some areas
What is the histology?	Tall eosinophilic cells in lymphoid stroma

Ratio of women to men that develop benign mixed tumors

1:8–10

What is the prognosis for benign mixed tumors?

Often multicentric in origin; tend to recur after local excision; very rarely, malignant lymphoma or undifferentiated carcinoma will arise in this tumor bed.

MALIGNANT TUMORS OF THE SALIVARY GLANDS

Describe the clinical features of malignant tumors of the salivary gland.

Pain, functional disturbance (dysphagia), ulceration, cranial nerve palsies, and local extension

What is the treatment for malignant tumors of the salivary gland?

Treatment is determined by grade, type, and extent. Radical excision or radical neck dissection may be performed. Radiotherapy can be a helpful adjunct.

What is the serious morbidity associated with malignant salivary gland tumors?

Extension into base of brain or exsanguination from invasion of the jugular vein or carotid artery

Name the 4 types of malignant tumors specific to the salivary glands.

1. Adenoid cystic carcinomas (cylindromas)
2. Mucoepidermoid carcinomas
3. Malignant mixed tumors (MMTs)
4. Acinic cell carcinomas

What other tumors are seen in the salivary glands?

1. Squamous cell carcinomas
2. Malignant lymphomas
3. Metastatic tumors of the intraparotid nodes
4. Polymorphous low-grade adenocarcinoma

What is the most common malignant tumor of the salivary gland?

Mucoepidermoid carcinoma (one third of all malignant salivary gland tumors)

What salivary gland is most often affected by mucoepidermoid tumor?

Parotid gland (60%–70%)

What is the pathology of mucoepidermoid tumor?

Circumscribed but nonencapsulated tumor containing mucus secreting and epidermoid cells as well as an inter-mediate type of basal or non–mucus-secreting cell; low, intermediate, and high grade cancers are seen.

What is the prognosis?	Depends directly on grade of tumor; 5-year survival rate is almost 90%. In 10% of patients, tumor is highly malignant—two thirds of these patients develop regional node metastasis and one third have distant metastasis over a 5-year course.

Malignant mixed tumors

What percent of malignant salivary tumors are malignant mixed tumors (MMTs)?	10%–15%
Are MMTs more frequent in women or men?	Two times more frequent in women than men
What are some clinical features of MMTs?	The typical clinical history is of untreated salivary tumor of many years with recent rapid enlargement. Pain and paralysis are often seen.
What is the pathology?	A single cell type such as epidermoid, adeno- and spindle cell carcinomas that appear to have developed and become malignant in a benign tumor; there is no pleomorphic spectrum.
What is the prognosis?	Poor prognosis if tumor is extensive or has been previously treated; local recurrence, nodal metastasis, and wide-spread bone and visceral metastasis are common.

Adenoid cystic carcinoma

Adenoid cystic carcinoma (cylindromas) is most common in which gland?	Submaxillary and minor salivary glands (It is the most frequent tumor in the minor salivary glands and accounts for roughly 20% of all tumors of these glands and 50% of the malignant tumors of these glands.)
What are some clinical features?	Local pain and facial paralysis

What is the pathology?

Epithelial islands with enclosed mucin or hyaline cylinders; not encapsulated; the small, darkly stained cells appear as anastomosing cords lying in mucoid or hyaline stroma.

What is the special characteristic of cylindroma?

Affinity for nerves with growth into and within the perineural spaces; thus, the surgeon must carefully examine the cylindroma by frozen section to detect perineural invasion at the margins.

What is the prognosis?

Poor; slow growing but relentless; recurrence is common; 5-year survival is 75% but drops to 15%–20% at 10–20 years.

What are the most common sites of metastasis?

Lungs, bones, and viscera

Acinic cell carcinoma

Where does acinic cell carcinoma usually arise?

Parotid glands

Is acinic cell carcinoma more common in men or women?

Women (70% of cases)

What are the clinical features?

Same as a benign mixed tumor

What is the pathology?

Grossly circumscribed but microscopically invasive; tumor resembles cellular lining of acini; cyst formation is common.

What is the prognosis?

5-year survival is 90% but decreases after that; recurs locally; infrequent regional node involvement; rarely metastasizes.

Metastatic tumors of the intraparotid nodes

Metastatic tumors of the intraparotid nodes usually arise from what 2 sources?

1. Melanomas of the head or eye
2. Squamous cell carcinomas from the head and neck

POWER REVIEW

A cleft palate is a premature closure of which 2 sutures?

Coronal and lambdoid sutures

What is Fordyce disease?

A benign, asymptomatic condition characterized by the presence of painless yellow-to-white granules (displaced ectopic sebaceous glands) in mucosa of cheeks, lips and gingivae.

Define stomatitis.

Inflammation of the oral mucosa.

Characterize herpetic gingivostomatitis.

Vesicular lesions that fuse and rupture, forming small ulcers

Characterize monilial stomatitis.

White patches scattered over mucosa, tongue, palate, and pharynx

Identify and describe the 3 stages of oral syphilis.

1. Primary stage: chancre
2. Second stage: patches in oral mucosa and macules on tongue
3. Third stage: gummas in hard or soft palate and glossitis.

Gingival hyperplasia is a common side effect of what drug?

Phenytoin

What is a mucocele?

A cyst, usually on the lips, characterized by pools of mucus and inflammatory cells within the minor salivary glands

Where is a granular cell tumor found?

The tongue

What is leukoplakia?

A lesion of the mucous membranes that may be due to chronic irritation and trauma

What is the most common malignant lesion of the oral mucosa?

Squamous cell carcinoma

What are 4 risk factors for squamous cell carcinoma of the oral mucosa?

1. Cigarette smoking
2. Tobacco chewing
3. Pipe smoking
4. Chronic exposure to sunlight
5. ETOH

Define the tonsillar ring or ring of Waldeyer.

Aggregations of lymphoid tissue that encircle the pharynx

What is the histology of tonsillitis?	Crypts of squamous epithelium that contain numerous neutrophils and desquamated epithelial cells
What is a nasal polyp?	A nonspecific proliferation of edematous stroma and nasal mucosa
What is the most common malignancy of the naso-pharynx?	A lymphoepithelioma
What is the most common symptom of laryngeal disease?	Hoarseness
Where do laryngeal polyps most frequently occur?	On the vocal cords
What is an eruption cyst?	A small dentigerous cyst occurring on teeth already erupted
How does odontogenic keratocyst appear radio-logically?	As a radiolucency of jaw
What is the most common cyst of the jaw?	Radicular cyst
Define odontoma.	A hamartoma arising from tissues involved in tooth formation

Which glands contain:

Serous glands	Parotid glands
Mucous glands	Sublingual glands
Both serous and mucous glands	Submaxillary and minor salivary glands
What is sialolithiasis?	Stones in the salivary duct
What is the most common organism implicated in acute suppurative parotitis?	*Staphylococcus aureus*
In what condition does acute parotid inflammation and swelling occur?	Mumps

What is the clinical triad of symptoms in Sjögren syndrome?

1. Xerostomia (dry mouth)
2. Xerophthalmia (dry eyes)
3. Arthritis

What is the most common benign salivary tumor and its incidence?

Benign mixed tumors (80%–85%)

What is the most common malignant tumor of the salivary gland?

Mucoepidermoid carcinoma (one third of all malignant salivary gland tumors)

What is the pathology of mucoepidermoid carcinoma?

Circumscribed but nonencapsulated tumor containing mucus-secreting and epidermoid cells as well as an intermediate type of basal or non-mucus-secreting cell

Where do acinic cell carcinomas usually arise?

Parotid glands

Define Mikulicz syndrome.

Bilateral swelling of the lacrimal, submandibular and parotid glands due to known causes such as sarcoidosis or tuberculosis

32

The Eye

LENS

CATARACTS

What is a cataract?

An opacification of the lens

Name 6 substances that are known to cause cataracts.

1. Corticosteroids
2. Phenothiazines
3. Ergot
4. Naphthalene
5. 2,4-dinitrophenol
6. Phospholine iodide (topical)

What 4 physical agents may cause cataracts?

1. Ultraviolet light
2. Trauma
3. Intraocular surgery
4. Ultrasound

Name 9 systemic diseases associated with cataracts.

1. Congenital rubella virus
2. Diabetes mellitus
3. Down syndrome
4. Atopic dermatitis
5. Scleroderma
6. Alport syndrome
7. Cretinism
8. Fabry disease
9. Galactosemia

What is the most common type of cataract in the United States?

Senile cataract

PRESBYOPIA

What is it?

Often referred to as "old age vision," it is a refractive condition associated with aging in which there is diminished power of accommodation resulting from loss of elasticity of the lens.

At what age does it usually occur?	Occurs in most persons after 40–45 years of age
What is the ultimate result of presbyopia?	People begin to have difficulty reading and require spectacles ("reading glasses") for near vision.

CORNEA

What is keratitis?	Inflammation of the cornea secondary to an infectious or mechanical etiology
Name 5 infectious agents frequently involved in keratitis.	1. *Staphylococcus* 2. *Streptococcus* 3. *Pseudomonas* 4. Herpes virus 5. *Chlamydia*
What predisposes the cornea to infection?	Exposure or trauma
What is the treatment for corneal opacities secondary to scarring?	Corneal transplant
What is the most common complaint of a patient suffering from a corneal abrasions?	Pain
What is used to diagnose a corneal abrasion?	Fluorescein test

BAND KERATOPATHY

What is it?	Calcium phosphate depositions in a horizontal band across the superficial central cornea
With what condition is it usually seen?	Hypercalcemia

WILSON DISEASE

What is the pathognomonic ocular finding in Wilson disease?	Kayser-Fleischer rings—golden rings of copper deposits in Descemet membrane of the cornea

What percent of untreated Wilson disease patients with neurologic symptoms have Kayser-Fleischer rings?	100%, eventually
What ophthalmologic procedure helps visualize Kayser-Fleischer rings?	A slit-lamp examination

RETINA

RETINAL DETACHMENT

What is it?	A separation of the neurosensory retina from the pigment epithelium and its supportive choroid, resulting in retinal infarction
What is the pathophysiology of retinal detachment?	Damage to the retina allows fluid to collect in the subretinal space.
Name 4 causes.	1. Age 2. Trauma 3. Ocular surgery 4. Diabetes
What are common complaints of a patient with a detached retina?	Floaters, blind spots, and flashing lights
What is the treatment of choice?	Surgery, either sclera buckling therapy or vitrectomy

RETINITIS PIGMENTOSA

What is it?	Hereditary, progressive retinal degeneration in both eyes
Name 3 symptoms of retinitis pigmentosa.	1. Night blindness (usually in childhood) 2. Loss of peripheral vision, progressing over many years to tunnel vision 3. Eventual blindness

RETINOBLASTOMA

What is it?	Hereditary, malignant intraocular tumor of retinal cells

What is the most common childhood ocular malignancy and what is its incidence?	Retinoblastoma, affecting 1:20,000 to 1:34,000 children

Name 5 presenting signs of retinoblastoma.

1. White pupil (leukocoria)
2. Squint (strabismus)
3. Poor vision
4. Spontaneous hyphema (blood in the anterior chamber of the eye)
5. Red, painful eye

DIABETIC RETINOPATHY

What is it?

A progressive microangiopathy of the blood vessels of the retina in diabetic patients

Name and describe the 2 types of diabetic retinopathy.

1. Non-proliferative (background): retinoscopic hemorrhages without neovascularization
2. Proliferative: advanced retinoscopic vascular changes with neovascularization

What is the most common complaint with diabetic retinopathy?

Decreased visual acuity

What are 2 modalities used for diagnosis?

1. Retinoscopy
2. Fluorescein angiogram

In severe cases, what is the treatment of choice?

Photocoagulation with argon laser to peripheral retina

HYPERTENSIVE RETINOPATHY

What is it?

Retinal changes caused by high blood pressure

Name 6 features of hypertensive retinopathy.

1. Arteriolar narrowing
2. Copper wiring: dull light reflections from blood vessel surfaces
3. Flame-shaped hemorrhages: hemorrhages in the retinal nerve fiber layer
4. Exudates: often radiating from the center of the macula (macular star)

5. Cotton-wool spots: fluffy white bodies (infarctions) in the superficial retina
6. Microaneurysms

CHERRY-RED SPOTS

What is a cherry-red spot?

An apparent color change in the retinal area of sharpest vision (fovea) that results from the opacification of the retinal layers around it

Name 2 conditions in which cherry-red spots are seen.

1. Central retinal artery occlusion
2. Tay-Sachs disease

INCREASED INTRAOCULAR PRESSURE

GLAUCOMA

What is it?

An ocular disease complex characterized by increased intraocular pressure

What are 3 classifications of glaucoma?

1. Chronic open angle glaucoma
2. Narrow angle glaucoma
3. Congenital glaucoma

Name the 3 types of chronic open angle glaucoma and identify the most common type.

1. Bilateral
2. Insidious
3. Slowly progressive. Slowly progressive is the most common type and accounts for 90% of the cases of chronic open angle glaucoma.

What is the pathophysiology of glaucoma?

Increased intraocular pressure (caused by either increased intraocular aqueous humor production or decreased outflow of aqueous humor) leads to optic nerve degeneration.

Glaucoma is diagnosed by what 3 modalities?

1. Increased intraocular pressure
2. Retinoscopy (optic disc cupping)
3. Peripheral vision field testing

How is glaucoma treated?

Intraocular pressure is decreased through topical eye drops, surgery, or both.

PAPILLEDEMA

What is it?

Optic nerve head swelling with engorged blood vessels

When is it seen?	With elevated pressure within the skull

PSEUDOTUMOR CEREBRI

What is it?	Intracranial inflammation that resembles a brain tumor
Name 4 symptoms associated with pseudotumor cerebri.	1. Optic nerve head swelling (papilledema) 2. Headaches 3. Protrusion of the eyeball (proptosis) 4. Transient loss or reduction in vision
Who gets it most frequently?	Obese women in their 30s

OTHER OPHTHALMALOGIC CONDITIONS

RED EYE

What are the 8 signs of serious ocular pathology in a red eye?	1. Visual loss 2. Pain 3. Opacities 4. Pupil irregularities 5. Perilimbal erythema 6. Increased pressure 7. History of eye disease 8. Refractory to treatment
Describe the clinical signs for each of the following conditions.	
Bacterial conjunctivitis	Conjunctival redness with purulent discharge
Viral conjunctivitis	Conjunctival redness with serous discharge
Allergic conjunctivitis	Conjunctival redness with clear discharge
Acute narrow angle glaucoma	Acute pain, cloudy cornea, perilimbal redness, blurred vision
Iritis	Perilimbal redness, irregular pupil, pain, decreased vision
Corneal ulcer	Epithelial defect with infiltrate, pain

Orbital cellulitis	Periocular swelling, erythematous ocular surface, decreased vision

STRABISMUS

What is it?	Misalignment of the eyes
Why is it important to correct strabismus?	To allow proper development of visual acuity and binocular vision
What condition develops if strabismus is not corrected?	Amblyopia
Define amblyopia.	Decreased vision in one or both eyes without detectable anatomic damage in the eye or visual pathways

OPTIC NEURITIS IN MULTIPLE SCLEROSIS

What is optic neuritis?	Inflammatory demyelination of the optic nerve. It is the most common ocular finding in multiple sclerosis.
Name 2 symptoms of optic neuritis.	1. Blurred vision 2. Pain on eye movement
Characterize the visual acuity in optic neuritis.	Reduced
Will refraction help acuity in optic neuritis?	No
What pupillary abnormality occurs in optic neuritis?	An afferent pupillary defect
What is an afferent pupillary defect?	Reduced pupilloconstriction on ipsilateral eye illumination with persistence on contralateral illumination
What visual field defect is common in optic neuritis?	A central scotoma
What is the name for optic neuritis behind the optic nerve head?	Retrobulbar neuritis
What is the appearance of the optic disc in optic neuritis?	Pink and swollen with indistinct margin if optic nerve head is involved. In retrobulbar neuritis, the disc is normal.

HORNER SYNDROME

What 3 things characterize Horner syndrome?

1. Ptosis of the upper eyelid
2. Miosis: constriction of the pupil
3. Anhidrosis: absence of sweating on the affected side

What causes a Horner syndrome?

A destructive lesion of the superior cervical ganglion

XANTHOMA (XANTHELASMA)

What is it?

Small yellowish lipid deposits on the eyelids

In what 3 conditions are they commonly seen?

1. Familial hypercholesterolemia
2. Primary biliary cirrhosis
3. High blood fat levels

In what population is it most common?

The elderly

AMAUROSIS FUGAX

What is it?

Sudden, transient decrease in vision in one eye, varying from visual field constriction to total blindness

What causes it?

Reduced cerebral circulation resulting in insufficient blood flow to the ophthalmic artery

KERATOCONJUNCTIVITIS SICCA

What is it?

Often called "dry eye syndrome," it is corneal and conjunctival dryness due to deficient tear secretion.

What condition is associated with keratoconjunctivitis sicca?

Sjögren syndrome

DEFINITIONS

Define the following terms.

Esotropia

Eyes turned inward

Exotropia

Eyes turned outward

Hypertropia	Eyes turned upward
Hypotropia	Eyes turned downward
Diplopia	Double vision
Blepharitis	Inflammation of the eyelids
Hordeolum	A suppurative inflammation of a gland of the eyelid
Sty	An external hordeolum of the oil glands of Zeis (in the follicles of eyelashes)
Chalazion	An internal hordeolum that causes an inflammatory lump in a meibomian gland resulting in a painless swelling in the eyelid
Pinguecula	Yellowish, benign conjunctival lump
Pterygium	A triangular fold of vascularized conjunctiva that grows horizontally onto the cornea in the shape of an insect wing
Arcus senilis	A white ring due to lipid deposition in the peripheral cornea that occurs with aging
Proptosis	Abnormal protrusion or bulging forward of eye
Sympathetic ophthalmia	Autoimmune destruction of the contralateral good eye after penetrating injury causes blindness to ipsilateral eye

POWER REVIEW

What is a cataract?	Opacification of the lens
Define glaucoma.	Increased intraocular pressure
Name the 2 types of diabetic retinopathy.	1. Background (non-proliferative) 2. Proliferative
What are the 4 characteristics of background diabetic retinopathy?	1. Venous engorgement 2. Dot and blot hemorrhages 3. Capillary microaneurysms 4. Exudates

What is the prominent feature of proliferative diabetic retinopathy?	Neovascularization
Name the 3 main types of conjunctivitis.	1. Bacterial 2. Viral 3. Allergic
What are 4 possible causes of retinal detachment?	1. Age 2. Trauma 3. Ocular surgery 4. Diabetes
What are the signs and symptoms of a retinal detachment?	Floaters, blind spots, and flashing lights
What is the most common ocular finding in multiple sclerosis?	Optic neuritis
What is optic neuritis?	Inflammatory demyelination of the optic nerve
What are 2 symptoms of optic neuritis?	1. Blurred vision 2. Pain on eye movement
What pupillary abnormality occurs in optic neuritis?	An afferent pupillary defect
What is blepharitis?	Inflammation of the eyelids
What is a sty?	An external hordeolum
What is a chalazion?	An internal hordeolum
What is a xanthoma?	Yellowish deposits on the eyelids
What is the leading cause of blindness in adults?	Diabetes mellitus
What infection is the most common cause of blindness in the world?	*Chlamydia trachomatis*

Section III

Pathology Atlas

33

Gross Pathology

Please identify the pathologic
condition depicted in each of the
photographs:

CELLULAR REACTION TO INJURY

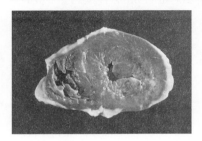

Left ventricular hypertrophy.
This condition occurs most
commonly as a physiologic response
to hypertension, and is an example
of the process of cellular
hypertrophy. In the specimen
depicted here, the cellular
hypertrophy is evident at the gross
level. In this particular heart there
are also several small foci of white
fibrous scar tissue in the
myocardium, which are indicative of
small remote infarctions.

VASCULAR SYSTEM

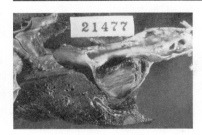

21477

Aneurysm. This large saccular
aneurysm, containing a laminated
thrombus, arises from the thoracic
aorta and impinges upon the lower
lobe of the left lung. The majority of
aortic aneurysms are related to
atherosclerosis and are located in
the abdominal aorta, often
immediately distal to the renal
arteries. Other causes of aortic
aneurysms include **syphilis** and
cystic medial degeneration.

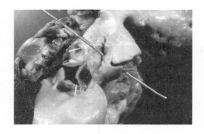

Aortic dissection occurs when blood gains entry into the wall of the aorta via a tear in the intima and dissects along the tissue planes of the media. Ultimately, the dissection may culminate in rupture with massive hemorrhage. Conditions predisposing to aortic dissection include hypertension and **Marfan syndrome.** The photo illustrates the aortic valve and proximal aorta, viewed from above. The silver probe passes through an oblique aortic intimal tear to pass into the pericardial cavity. The patient expired due to cardiac tamponade.

MEDIASTINUM

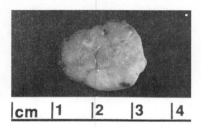

Nodular sclerosis Hodgkin disease. This enlarged mediastinal lymph node from a young adult female is notable for bands of white fibrous tissue which separate the pink-gray lymphoid tissue into numerous nodules. The appearance is distinctive, and, given the age and sex of the patient, essentially diagnostic of nodular sclerosis Hodgkin's disease.

THE HEART

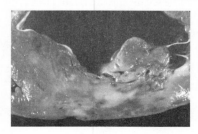

Acute myocardial infarction. The photo shows a portion of the wall of the left ventricle, which is notable for a mottled appearance consisting of alternating regions of tan-yellow pallor and pink-red hyperemia. This is the typical appearance of an acute myocardial infarction, probably several days in age. Had the patient survived, this area would be replaced over time by granulation tissue, followed by fibrous scar tissue.

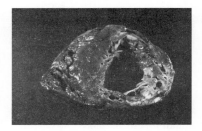

Myocardial infarction, remote. If the patient survives the initial insult of an acute myocardial infarction, the necrotic myocardium undergoes the stereotypical repair processes that result in the initial inflammatory response, followed by granulation tissue ingrowth and subsequent fibrosis. In this image, extreme thinning of the left ventricular free wall with visible dense white scar tissue is the end result of a past myocardial infarction.

THE RESPIRATORY SYSTEM

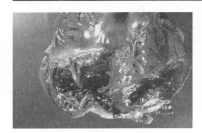

Pulmonary thromboembolus. This large thromboembolus was present at autopsy in the right ventricular outflow tract of an adult female who died suddenly and unexpectedly. Similar thromboemboli were present in both right and left pulmonary arteries. Pulmonary thromboemboli usually arise in the pelvic or deep leg veins; if the embolus lodges at the bifurcation of the right and left pulmonary arteries, the term **saddle embolus** is used.

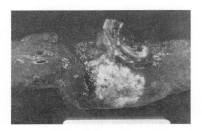

Primary lung carcinoma. This lung resection specimen contains a large tan-white tumor mass, with central discoloration suggesting hemorrhage, necrosis, or both. The tumor is an adenocarcinoma: note that the epicenter of the tumor is peripherally located. Adenocarcinomas are more often peripheral lesions, whereas squamous cell carcinomas tend to arise from larger, central bronchi. This represents a metastasis to a hilar lymph node.

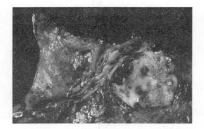

Metastatic tumor to the lung. The large tumor present near the hilum in this lung is grossly consistent with a primary lung tumor. However, additional smaller nodules were discovered upon thin sectioning of the specimen. Metastatic tumors are often multiple. Furthermore, the clinical history in this case, of a pulmonary nodule developing in a teenage male with history of high grade osteosarcoma of the femur, strongly suggests this is a metastasis. Metastases to the lung are more common than primary lung malignancies.

THE FEMALE REPRODUCTIVE SYSTEM

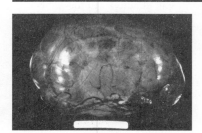

Serous cystadenoma. Benign ovarian tumors, such as this large serous cystadenoma, typically are cystic (often unilocular), with smooth external and internal surfaces and thin walls. There is usually little if any component of solid growth. In this instance, the cyst walls are so thin as to be translucent in areas. These tumors typically present in a younger patient population (women of reproductive age) than the corresponding malignant serous tumors (peri- and post-menopausal women).

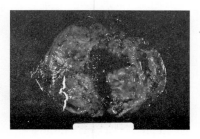

Ovarian carcinoma. This large ovarian mass in a 44-year-old woman has gross features suggesting a malignant process, including significant solid growth, and areas of hemorrhage and necrosis with cystic degeneration. The most likely diagnosis is serous cystadenocarcinoma.

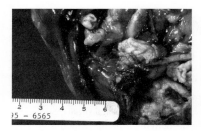

Mature cystic teratoma (ovarian dermoid cyst). Benign cystic teratomas are typically found in a younger patient population than those with ovarian carcinomas. Bilaterality is not unusual, and the tumors are generally cystic. The internal cyst lining is usually predominantly stratified squamous epithelium, resembling skin. Hair is commonly present (*adjacent to the ruler*), and tooth-like structures are sometimes seen. In most cases, tissues such as thyroid, cartilage, and respiratory epithelium (derived from the other germ layers) are also present.

KIDNEY AND URINARY TRACT

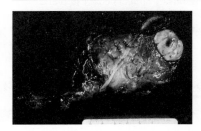

Renal cortical adenoma versus renal cell carcinoma. Small renal cortical lesions, such as this yellow, 3-cm nodule, may be difficult to precisely classify as malignant or benign. As a general rule and in the absence of specific worrisome histologic features, small lesions (less than or equal to 3 cm) have been considered benign (*adenomas*); lesions larger than 3 cm have been considered malignant (*carcinomas*).

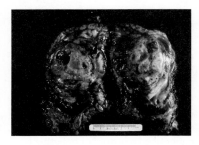

Renal cell carcinoma. The distinction between adenoma and carcinoma is moot in this case. This kidney has been bivalved, revealing a large (approximately 8 cm) tumor with extensive necrosis and hemorrhage replacing greater than one-half of the kidney. Residual normal renal parenchyma is present, and the specimen is surrounded by the perinephric fat, which appears to be invaded by the tumor, a renal cell carcinoma.

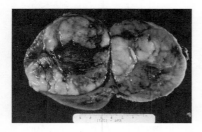

Wilms tumor (nephroblastoma) is the most common renal neoplasm of children. This example exhibits the classic gross features of this tumor: a fleshy, pink-gray lesion with hemorrhage and necrosis, which extensively replaces the kidney. Only a thin rim of residual renal parenchyma remains, which is grossly normal (*adjacent to the ruler*).

GASTROINTESTINAL SYSTEM

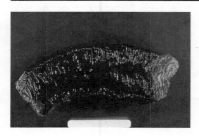

Segmental ischemia/infarction of the bowel. Ischemic bowel disease has multiple causes, including thrombosis, embolus, and severe hypotension (shock). In the early stages, as pictured here, the bowel typically appears congested and hemorrhagic, due to reperfusion of the ischemically damaged segment. Note the normal-appearing bowel at each resection margin.

LIVER, GALLBLADDER, AND EXOCRINE PANCREAS

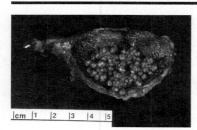

Cholelithiasis. Gallstones are common, with a propensity towards older adults and women. Obesity and hyperestrogenic states are risk factors. The brown-yellow stones pictured here are of the more common cholesterol type; **pigment stones** are dark brown to black and are composed chiefly of bilirubin salts. Pigment stones may be seen in persons with conditions predisposing to excessive hemolysis.

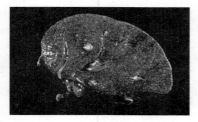

Cirrhosis. This section of liver is notable grossly for the presence of cirrhosis (nodules, fatty liver). The patient had a history of hepatitis B infection. Although cirrhosis may be separated into micronodular and macronodular types, this distinction is nonspecific for the various entities leading to cirrhosis. Note that there are two more dominant nodules in the section, which are more yellow in color. These nodules represent the foci of hepatocellular carcinoma, which patients with cirrhosis are predisposed to develop.

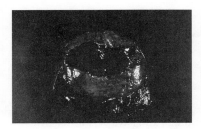

Hepatic adenoma. These benign proliferations of hepatocytes are almost always seen in women, and appear to grow in response to estrogenic influences. Although benign, they can undergo spontaneous hemorrhage (as in this case) sometimes with catastrophic results if the hemorrhage breaches the hepatic capsule, producing hemoperitoneum.

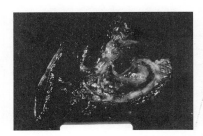

Pancreatic pseudocyst. The photo illustrates a large unilocular cyst, arising in the tail of the pancreas, and extending into the splenic hilum. At the side opposite the spleen, a small portion of normal pancreas is visible. Note the thick fibrous walls that are typical of a pseudocyst. Histologic examination of these cysts reveals absence of any epithelial lining; the cyst is instead composed of a wall of fibrous tissue with inner layer of necrosis and organizing hemorrhage.

SOFT TISSUES

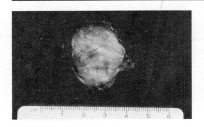

Lipoma is the most common soft tissue neoplasm, and these tumors usually resemble ordinary adipose tissue, both in their gross and histological appearance. Grossly, a lipoma is recognized because it forms a discrete, usually ovoid mass, and often is thinly encapsulated.

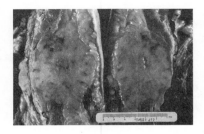

Sarcoma. This bisected specimen displays a tumor arising in the deep soft tissues of the back, in an adult man. The anatomic site and the gross features—a soft, fleshy neoplasm with hemorrhage and necrosis, which is clearly invading and destroying adjacent tissue structures—suggest a sarcoma.

HEAD AND NECK

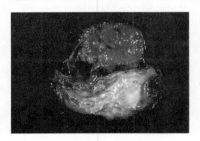

Warthin tumor is a distinctive benign tumor that almost always arises in the parotid gland and is commonly cystic. The gross appearance here is typical; the tumor also has a very distinctive histologic appearance consisting of epithelial as well as lymphoid components.

TRANSPLANT

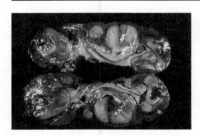

Post-transplant lymphoproliferative disorder. This nephrectomy specimen represents a renal transplant which was subsequently removed (explanted) due to the development of a post-transplant lymphoproliferative disorder (PTLD) in the patient. Note the numerous pink-white nodules of tumor. PTLDs are proliferations of B lymphocytes, which are allowed to proliferate unchecked due to a suppressed immune system. A causal relationship with Epstein-Barr virus is postulated. They may be polyclonal or monoclonal and run the histologic spectrum from benign lymphoid hyperplasias to aggressive malignant lymphomas.

THE ENDOCRINE SYSTEM

Multinodular goiter. This enormous specimen represents a thyroid affected by multinodular goiter. This is a benign, poorly understood condition typified by hyperplasia of the thyroid follicles, with cyst formation, scarring, and focal hemorrhage. The multicystic nature of the specimen can be appreciated grossly, and the color is characteristic of thyroid in general.

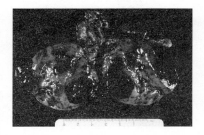

Pheochromocytoma. This tumor was present in the adrenal gland of a 40-year-old man with paroxysmal hypertension. The focal hemorrhages are typical. The tumor has been bisected.

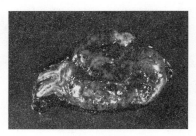

Adrenal cortical adenoma. These are relatively common lesions, and the variegated appearance of this specimen is typical. Note the short tail of normal adrenal gland present at one side of the tumor.

DEVELOPMENTAL AND GENETIC DISORDERS

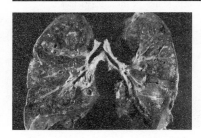

Cystic fibrosis, lungs. These lungs, from a patient with cystic fibrosis, show numerous small parenchymal nodules of bronchopneumonia as well as numerous enlarged and dilated airways (**bronchiectasis**). Several grey, enlarged hilar lymph nodes are also visible, a reaction to the chronic inflammatory process.

34 Histopathology

Please identify the pathologic condition depicted in each of the photographs:

INFLAMMATION

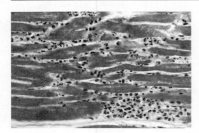

Acute inflammation. Neutrophils (polymorphonuclear leukocytes) are the earliest cellular component of the acute inflammatory response. In this image, neutrophils can be seen infiltrating among necrotic myocytes in an area of acute infarction of the myocardium. The appearance of the myocytes, with loss of nuclei but retention of basic cellular structure, exemplifies coagulative necrosis.

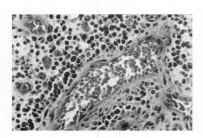

Chronic inflammation. The classic cellular constituent of chronic inflammation is the lymphocyte. In this image, numerous **plasma cells** surround a small vessel, and are recognizable by their eccentrically placed basophilic cytoplasm with small area of perinuclear clearing (termed the **hof**). Plasma cells are terminally differentiated B-lymphocytes. Also present in the image are hemosiderin-laden macrophages and occasional small lymphocytes and neutrophils.

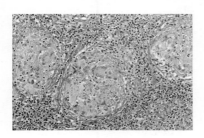

Granulomatous inflammation in sarcoidosis. This mediastinal lymph node contains several **non-caseating granulomas.** Note the numerous eosinophilic histiocytes with surrounding cuffs of lymphocytes. Multinucleated giant cells are present focally.

Mycobacterial and fungal infections, as well as sarcoidosis, classically elicit granulomatous inflammation.

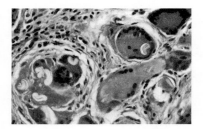

Foreign body giant cell reaction. Numerous multinucleated giant cells are present in this image. They were formed in reaction to numerous small cellulose fibers introduced into the patient's peritoneal cavity during a prior surgical procedure. The cellulose fibers are visible as small curved or doughnut-shaped objects within the cytoplasm of giant cells. This reaction represents the body's stereotypical response to foreign material.

CELLULAR REACTIONS

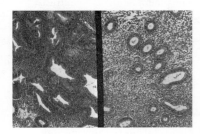

Hyperplasia refers to an increase in the total number of cells. As illustrated in the photomicrograph, note the tight crowding of hyperplastic endometrial glands (right side) as compared to the normal proliferative phase endometrium (left side). Endometrial hyperplasia is commonly attributed to increased estrogenic stimulation.

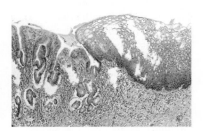

Metaplasia refers to replacement of one tissue type (generally epithelial) by another, often in response to some recurring stimulus. A classic example is Barrett esophagus, pictured here, in which the normal esophageal squamous epithelium is replaced by columnar epithelium. Barrett esophagus is significant because these patients are at increased risk for the development of esophageal carcinomas.

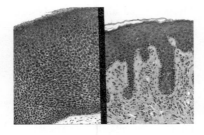

Dysplasia refers to alterations of epithelial cell size and shape, or alterations in the organization (or architecture) of cells, or both. The term has significance, as often the presence of dysplasia within epithelia is considered a pre-malignant condition. The image demonstrates severe dysplasia of the uterine cervix; note the poor maturation of the dysplastic cells as they ascend through the epithelium, nuclear hyperchromasia, and the presence of frequent mitotic figures which are not restricted to the basal layers.

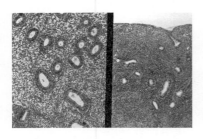

Atrophy refers to diminished cellular size, generally due to decreased stimulation or utilization. The photomicrograph contrasts atrophic endometrium (right) of a post-menopausal female with normal proliferative phase endometrium (left).

REPAIR AND FIBROSIS

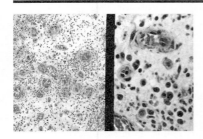

Granulation tissue represents an early response in the process of wound healing, and consists of a highly vascularized loose connective tissue with edema and variable acute and chronic inflammatory cells. In the low-power image of granulation tissue (left), note numerous small capillaries and a loose stroma. In the high-power image (right), numerous plasma cells, lymphocytes, neutrophils, and macrophages are identifiable, as well as a few spindle-shaped fibroblasts.

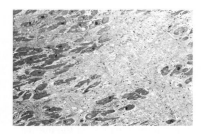

Fibrosis. For many forms of cellular or tissue injury, the end result is the formation of fibrous tissue (scar tissue). The photomicrograph illustrates myocardial fibrosis in the heart of a patient with severe coronary artery disease. This fibrosis is representative of the end-stage tissue response to a myocardial infarction. This lesion would be recognizable grossly as an area of firm white fibrous tissue in the myocardium.

NEOPLASIA

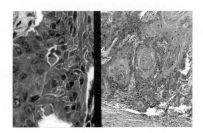

Squamous cell carcinomas may arise in a multitude of anatomic sites, but generally share key histopathologic features. These include the presence of **keratin pearls,** intercellular bridges, and a neoplastic cell population characterized by relatively large cells with abundant eosinophilic cytoplasm and well-defined cell borders. Poorly differentiated squamous cell carcinomas may lack some or all of these light microscopic features.

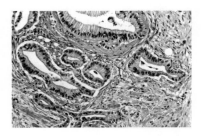

Adenocarcinoma. Adenocarcinomas, by definition, show evidence of differentiation towards glandular epithelium. The classic histologic feature indicative of adenocarcinoma is the presence of **discrete glandular lumina** within the tumor. Other features to look for include a columnar cell shape, as well as the presence of mucin secretion (often identified by positive mucicarmine staining). This image shows a ductal adenocarcinoma of the pancreas.

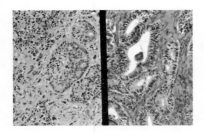

Differentiation. This term refers to the relative resemblance of a neoplastic process to the parent tissue from which it presumably has arisen. For example, a well-differentiated adenocarcinoma of the colon (right) contains well-defined glandular structures, lined by columnar cells which resemble those of the normal colonic epithelium. By contrast, the poorly differentiated adenocarcinoma (left), also of colonic origin, bears little resemblance to the normal colonic epithelium, and only very rare, poorly formed glandular lumina identify the process definitively as adenocarcinoma. Generally, the degree of differentiation is important in assessing the prognosis of a malignant tumor.

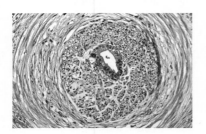

Local invasion. In addition to the loss of regulatory control over growth, malignant tumors, as well as some benign processes, are characterized by a variable capacity to invade local tissues. This feature can be responsible for many important clinical features of these tumors (e.g., perforation of the colon by a colonic adenocarcinoma) and may dictate certain therapeutic strategies (e.g., wide-excision). The photomicrograph demonstrates invasion of a peripheral nerve (cut in cross-section) by a focus of mucinous adenocarcinoma of the pancreas (forming a single glandular lumen in the center of the nerve).

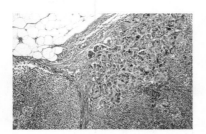

Metastasis. In addition to the capacity for local invasion described above, malignant neoplasms are characterized by the capacity for spread to distant anatomic sites, generally via hematogenous or lymphatic dissemination. As a general rule, **carcinomas** metastasize via lymphatic routes, whereas **sarcomas** metastasize via hematogenous routes. The image shows an axillary lymph nodal metastasis of high-grade ductal carcinoma of the breast, with tumor visible within lymphatic spaces of the nodal capsule.

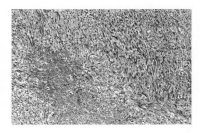

Sarcoma. Malignant tumors arising from and differentiating towards connective tissues (e.g., fibrous tissue, muscle, bone, adipose) are termed **sarcomas.** In addition, a prefix is given indicating the specific type of connective tissue the tumor is differentiated towards (e.g., **liposarcoma** for tumors showing adipose differentiation). In general, sarcomas are often grossly soft, **fleshy** tumors and frequently show evidence of necrosis and hemorrhage. Sarcomas often display a spindle cell pattern.

ANEMIA

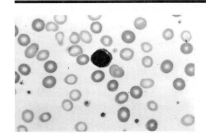

Hypochromic microcytic anemias are common. They display **hypochromia** (pale staining and increased central pallor) of the red blood cells and are also **microcytic** [(small and having a decreased mean corpuscular volume (MCV)]. Iron deficiency is by far the most common cause of hypochromic, microcytic anemia in the United States population. Other less common causes include **thalassemia syndromes** and lead poisoning. Note numerous hypochromic red blood cells as well as normochromic cells; the latter in this case indicate the patient has been transfused.

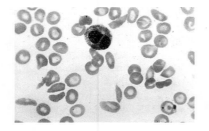

Sickle cell anemia represents the classic example of an anemia due to a genetically determined abnormality of hemoglobin structure or synthesis. A multitude of less common hemoglobinopathies have been described, with wide variation in clinical significance. The hemoglobin S found in sickle cell disease undergoes polymerization under conditions of low oxygen tension, producing the abnormally shaped sickle cells seen in the photomicrograph. A single eosinophil is present.

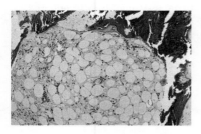

Aplastic anemia is a diagnosis of exclusion, made after other causes of anemia have been ruled out, and as such the diagnosis requires bone marrow biopsy as well as an extensive clinical work-up. Bone marrow biopsy in such a case shows extreme hypocellularity of the marrow space, with the majority of the marrow space occupied by fat. Small scattered foci of residual hematopoiesis may be present.

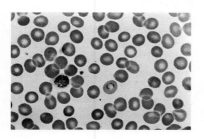

Malaria. The protozoal infection malaria remains a major cause of morbidity and mortality worldwide. Classically producing a paroxysmal febrile illness, latent chronic infection is also common in endemic areas. A portion of the *Plasmodia* life cycle is intra-erythrocytic, and the diagnosis is usually made by examination of a peripheral smear. Shown here is a ring-form trophozoite and a mature trophozoite, containing hemozoin pigment.

HEMATOLYMPHOID

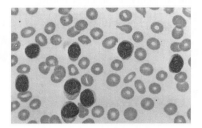

Chronic lymphocytic lymphoma (CLL), is a relatively common form of low-grade lymphoid neoplasm, usually of B-lymphocyte differentiation. The diagnosis is often suggested on peripheral smear, by noting the presence of a lymphocytosis composed predominantly of small, mature lymphocytes.

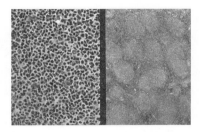

Follicular lymphoma. Also referred to as **follicle center cell lymphoma,** follicular lymphoma is a common form of non-Hodgkin's lymphoma, and is a neoplasm derived from B-lymphocytes. Note in the low-power image that the node is effaced by a process containing numerous closely-approximated lymphoid follicles. The high power image demonstrates a predominance of small-cleaved cells, identifiable by their nuclear folds and irregularities.

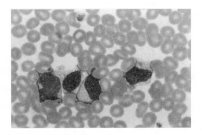

Infectious mononucleosis. Many infections can produce a peripheral blood lymphocytosis, or **mononucleosis syndrome.** Commonly, these are viral illnesses; the classic example is infection with Epstein-Barr virus (EBV), which produces the illness known to the layperson as "mono." In this image, from a case of EBV-related mononucleosis, three atypical, reactive lymphocytes are noted, with cytoplasmic granules. A single monocyte is also present.

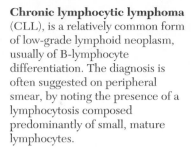

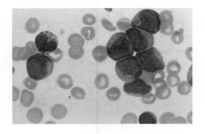

Acute myeloid leukemia. The image demonstrates circulating blasts typical of those seen in acute myeloid leukemia. Note the extremely fine, even chromatin pattern, prominent nucleoli, and sparse cytoplasm. A single cell contains a prominent *Auer rod,* which if seen in a leukemic process is specific for myeloid (as opposed to lymphoid) leukemia. The cell at the right (with prominent granules) is a basophil.

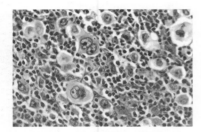

Hodgkin's disease. Although they may be extremely scarce, the *Reed-Sternberg cell* is essential for the diagnosis of Hodgkin's disease. It is characterized by binucleation with prominent eosinophilic inclusion-like nucleoli. The two nuclei often appear as mirror images of one another. Reed-Sternberg cells are present in the image, with a background of small lymphocytes. Eosinophils and plasma cells are also frequently present in Hodgkin's disease.

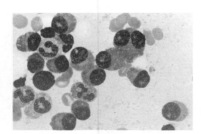

Myeloma. Numerous plasma cells, one of which is binucleate, are present in this image of a bone marrow aspirate specimen from a patient with multiple myeloma. Also seen are several neutrophils and band forms, as well as a single mast cell. The presence of increased plasma cells in the bone marrow is essential for the diagnosis of myeloma. Plasma cells are recognized by their eccentrically placed cytoplasm, cytoplasmic basophilia with perinuclear clearing (the **hof**), and a clock-face chromatin pattern (although **neoplastic** plasma cells may have nucleoli).

VASCULAR

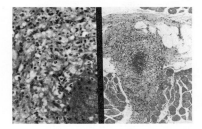

Vasculitis. The vessel in this muscle biopsy shows full-thickness (**transmural**) inflammation of its wall, diagnostic of vasculitis. The inflammatory infiltrate in the vessel wall is predominantly acute (neutrophils), and the vascular lumen is thrombosed. A variety of disorders may be associated with the histologic finding of vasculitis, including polyarteritis nodosa, Wegener granulomatosis, connective tissue diseases [e.g., systemic lupus erythematosus (SLE)], and infection.

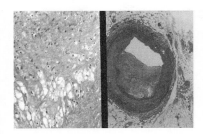

Atherosclerosis. Shown at low and high power is a typical lesion of atherosclerosis, involving a coronary artery. Note the eccentrically placed atheromatous plaque, which narrows the vascular lumen. The plaque is composed of an acellular core surrounded by fibrous tissue and foam cells, and lies between the medial and intimal layers of the vessel wall. High power illustrates foam cells.

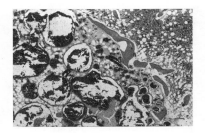

Hemangioma. Both benign (**hemangiomas**) and (**angiosarcomas; Kaposi sarcoma**) tumors showing vascular differentiation exist. The image demonstrates a hemangioma of the vertebral body. Note the large, thin-walled vascular spaces of the hemangioma, which contain numerous red blood cells, and adjacent bone marrow and reactive bone.

HEMORRHAGIC DISORDERS

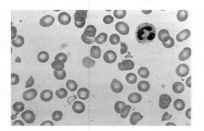

Microangiopathic hemolytic anemia. Several diseases and clinical syndromes show features on peripheral smear of hemolysis due to obstructions (usually thrombotic) in the microvasculature. These diseases/syndromes include disseminated intravascular coagulation (DIC), thrombotic thrombocytopenic purpura (TTP) and hemolytic-uremic syndrome (HUS). Note the numerous red cell fragments (**schistocytes**) as well as the near absence of platelets.

THE HEART

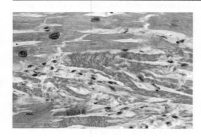

Contraction band necrosis. Contraction band necrosis is one of the earliest morphologically detectable alterations of acutely infarcted myocardium. Contraction bands are represented by thin, intensely eosinophilic transverse bands within infarcted myocytes. Contraction bands typically appear in areas of infarct that have undergone early reperfusion.

THE RESPIRATORY SYSTEM

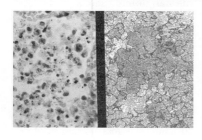

Bacterial lobar pneumonia. The low power photomicrograph in this case of lobar pneumonia illustrates filling of the alveolar spaces by acute inflammatory cells. At high power, numerous neutrophils and alveolar macrophages are seen, as well as abundant gram-positive bacterial organisms in pairs and short chains (**Brown-Hopps stain—similar to Gram stain**). The pre-mortem sputum cultures grew *Streptococcus pneumoniae*.

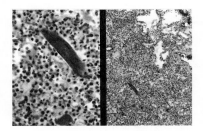

Bronchopneumonia due to aspiration. Bronchopneumonia produces similar histologic alterations as lobar pneumonia, but with a patchy, focal distribution predominantly centered around the bronchi/bronchioles. In this case, low power examination reveals an inflammatory infiltrate, as well as a large rectangular eosinophilic object which, on high power examination, exhibits cross-striations typical of skeletal muscle. Skeletal muscle, not normally found in the lung, represents aspirated food in this case.

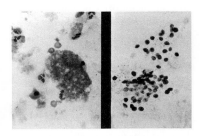

Pneumocystis pneumonia. *Pneumocystis carinii* is a ubiquitous organism which tends to cause disease only in the immunosuppressed populations. Histologically, pneumocystis pneumonia shows filling of the alveolar spaces by amorphous, frothy, acellular eosinophilic material on H & E staining (left); the encysted organisms are easily identified on silver stain (right) (bronchoalveolar lavage specimen).

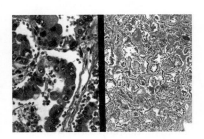

Bronchioloalveolar carcinoma (BAC) is a distinctive form of pulmonary adenocarcinoma which shows a tendency for growth along pre-existing alveolar septa. At low power, the alveolar growth pattern can be appreciated; high power reveals significant cytologic atypia and mitotic activity indicative of a malignant process.

MALE REPRODUCTIVE SYSTEM

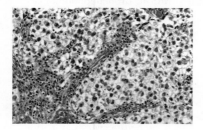

Seminoma. Testicular tumors represent the most common malignancies of young adult males, and of these tumors the *seminoma* is the most common. This photo-micrograph demonstrates the classical histologic features of seminoma, including pleomorphic polygonal cells with clear cytoplasm and prominent nucleoli, as well as fibrous septations with a prominent infiltrate of lymphocytes and plasma cells.

BREAST

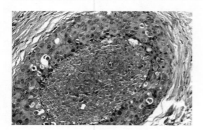

Ductal carcinoma-in-situ (DCIS) is a preinvasive form of mammary ductal carcinoma; the neoplastic cells remain confined to the ducts and have not yet breached the ductular basement membrane. The image shows a high-grade DCIS with central **comedonecrosis.** Note the smooth contour of the ductular basement membrane, indicating that the basement membrane remains intact. There is significant cytologic atypia.

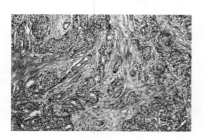

Ductal carcinoma. Ductal carcinoma-in-situ, when untreated, may progress to invasive ductal carcinoma. This occurs when the tumors gains the capacity to breach the ductular basement membrane, and invade the fibro-adipose stroma of the breast. Invasive ductal carcinoma usually elicits a prominent fibrous (or **desmoplastic**) stromal response, and in earlier years the tumors were known as **scirrhous carcinomas** in recognition of this fibrous response. Note the cords and islands of tumor, with occasional lumen formation, and the marked desmoplasia.

KIDNEY AND URINARY TRACT

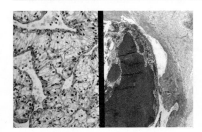

Clear-cell carcinoma of the kidney. While a host of tumors from different anatomic sites may contain cells with clear cytoplasm, renal cell carcinoma (RCC) remains the classic example and is commonly referred to as **clear cell carcinoma.** RCC also has a propensity to invade the renal vein, and may extend into the inferior vena cava and even to the right atrium of the heart. In these images, a low power view of a portion of the renal vein shows what appears to be blood and thrombus, however high-power examination reveals renal cell carcinoma.

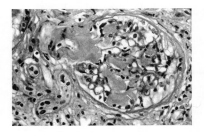

Renal amyloidosis. Amyloidosis is an example of a systemic disease which may present with renal manifestations (other examples include diabetes and lupus), and the diagnosis is often established by renal biopsy. The classic H&E histologic features of amyloid are seen here, in the glomerular mesangium—extensive deposits of amorphous, acellular eosinophilic material. The amyloid nature of the material is confirmed by positive staining with the Congo red stain, with **apple-green** birefringence when polarized (not shown).

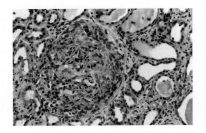

Rapidly progressive (crescentic) glomerulonephritis. Crescentic glomerulonephritis is typified by the presence of cellular **crescents** within Bowman space, with compression of the glomerular tuft, as seen in this image. Crescents are composed predominantly of epithelial cells of Bowman capsule, with macrophages and other inflammatory cells in variable numbers. Crescentic glomerulonephritis is not a specific entity; the features may be seen in several diseases.

GASTROINTESTINAL SYSTEM

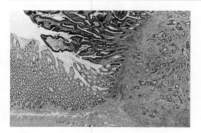

Colon, adenoma-carcinoma sequence. This low power photomicrograph of a large colonic polyp illustrates the concept of the adenoma-carcinoma sequence in colorectal carcinomas. At the left, lightly staining small regular glands of normal colonic mucosa can be seen. Adjacent to this, at the top of the photo, darkly stained glands of a colonic **adenoma** are easily seen. At the right side, irregular glands set in a desmoplastic stroma can be appreciated, representing a moderately differentiated adenocarcinoma that has arisen in the adenomatous polyp.

SKIN

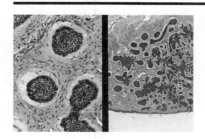

Basal cell carcinoma is an extremely common primary malignancy of the skin, which typically presents clinically on sun-exposed skin as a **pearly papule**. The neoplasm is histologically composed of nests, cords, or small nodules of **basaloid** cells characterized by small cell size, cytoplasmic basophilia, nuclear hyperchromasia, and **peripheral palisading** (lining-up of cells at the periphery of nests) that is well-illustrated here.

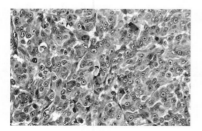

Melanoma is clinically a much more serious diagnosis than either basal cell or squamous cell carcinoma of the skin, and fortunately is much less common than either of those entities. Nonetheless, upwards of 7,000 persons will die of melanoma each year in the United States. In this image, typical histologic features of melanoma are present, including large pleomorphic atypical cells with abundant eosinophilic cytoplasm, prominent nucleoli, and occasional cells containing finely granular melanin pigmentation. Note mitotic figure.

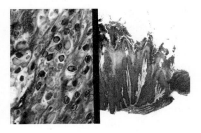

Verruca vulgaris. Commonly known as a wart, verruca vulgaris typically has a low-power architecture of papillomatous epithelial hyperplasia. At high power, eosinophilic intranuclear inclusions can occasionally be seen. The lesions are a result of local infection with human papilloma virus (HPV).

IMMUNOPATHOLOGY

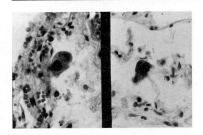

Immunohistochemistry, utilizing labeled antibodies which are highly specific for certain selected cellular antigens, has revolutionized the practice of surgical pathology. In this split field image, a pulmonary cell displaying histologic features of cytomegaloviral cytopathic effect is seen on H&E stain (left), and a similar cell shows strong labeling after application of an immunohistochemical stain specific for cytomegaloviral antigens.

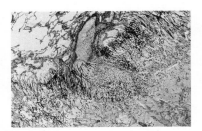

Disseminated fungal infection. This photomicrograph demonstrates invasive pulmonary aspergillosis in the lung of a patient undergoing chemotherapy for a hematologic malignancy. The fungal hyphae are stained black (silver stain). Note fungal hyphae invading the wall of a large vessel (center). Immunosuppression brings with it a host of potential opportunistic infections as well as certain neoplastic disorders that are infrequent in the immunocompetent patient population.

TRANSPLANT

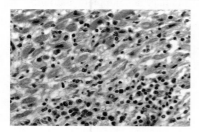

Acute cellular rejection, cardiac transplant. The photomicrograph demonstrates numerous lymphocytes, plasma cells and eosinophils infiltrating the myocardium of a patient who had undergone a heart transplant for congenital heart disease. Rejection and infection are major causes of morbidity and mortality in the transplant patient population, and illustrate the fine balance required of immunosuppressive therapies.

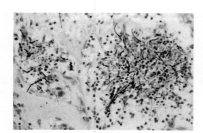

Disseminated candidiasis, cardiac transplant. This section of cardiac atrium, stained with the Brown-Hopps stain (similar to a Gram stain), shows a focus of fungal elements with associated inflammatory cells. Present in the section individual fungal yeast forms, chains of yeast forms (**pseudohyphae**), as well as hyphal forms. These features suggest the organism is a *Candida* species.

ENVIRONMENTAL

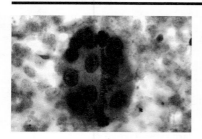

Asbestosis. This multinucleated giant cell has phagocytosed a **ferruginous body**. At the core of this structure is likely an asbestos fiber; however, since other inorganic particles can produce similar-appearing structures, the less specific term "ferruginous body" is preferable to the alternative "asbestos body". They have a golden-brown color derived from deposited iron (hence, "ferruginous"). Asbestos is implicated in the pathogenesis of some cases of pulmonary interstitial fibrosis, as well as benign and malignant mesothelial proliferations, and bronchogenic carcinomas.

Index

References in *italics* indicate figures; those followed by "t" denote tables